Student Learning Guide to accompany

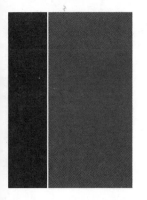

Fundamental Skills and Concepts for Nursing

Second Edition

Susan C. deWit, MSN, RN, CNS, PHN
Formerly, Instructor of Nursing
El Centro College
Dallas, Texas

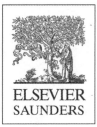

ELSEVIER
SAUNDERS

ELSEVIER
SAUNDERS
11830 Westline Industrial Drive
St. Louis, Missouri 63146

Student Learning Guide to Accompany
Fundamental Concepts and Skills for Nursing, 2nd edition

Executive Publisher: Barbara Nelson Cullen
Senior Developmental Editor: Robin Levin Richman
Developmental Editor: Catherine Ott
Publishing Services Manager: Catherine Jackson
Production Editor: Mary Stueck

ISBN-13: 978-0-7216-0310-0
ISBN-10: 0-7216-0310-6

Printed in the United States of America

Last digit is the print number: 9 8 7 6 5 4 3

To the Student

This study guide was created to assist you in achieving the objectives of each chapter in *Fundamental Concepts and Skills for Nursing*, 2nd edition, and establishing a solid base of knowledge in the fundamentals of nursing. Completing the exercises in each chapter in this guide will help to reinforce the material studied in the textbook and learned in class. Such reinforcement also helps students to be successful on the NCLEX-PN® examination.

STUDY HINTS FOR ALL STUDENTS

Ask Questions!
There are no stupid questions. If you do not know something or are not sure, you need to find out. Other people may be wondering the same thing but may be too shy to ask. The answer could mean life or death to your patient. That is certainly more important than feeling embarrassed about asking a question.

Chapter Objectives
At the beginning of each chapter in the textbook are objectives that you should have mastered when you finish studying that chapter. Write these objectives in your notebook, leaving a blank space after each. Fill in the answers as you find them while reading the chapter. Review to make sure your answers are correct and complete. Use these answers when you study for tests. This should also be done for separate course objectives that your instructor has listed in your class syllabus.

Student CD-ROM
The student CD-ROM packaged in the back of your *Fundamental Concepts and Skills for Nursing*, 2nd edition textbook contains the following sections: Audio Pronunciations from *Dorland's Medical Dictionary*; Film clips and audio clips from Jarvis' *Physical Examination and Health Assessment*, 4th edition text; Open book quizzes; and the Concept Maps featured in your *Fundamentals* textbook. Using these resources as you study can help you master the material.

Key Terms
At the beginning of each chapter in the textbook are key terms that you will encounter as you read the chapter. Text page number references are provided for easy reference and review, and the key terms are in color the first time they appear in the chapter. Phonetic pronunciations are provided for terms that you might find difficult to pronounce. The terms that were assigned simple phonetic pronunciations were selected because they are either (1) difficult medical, nursing, or scientific terms or (2) other words that may be difficult to pronounce. The goal is to help the student reader with limited proficiency in English to develop a greater command of the pronunciation of scientific and nonscientific English terminology. It is hoped that a more general competency in the understanding and use of medical and scientific language may result.

Key Points
Use the Key Points at the end of each chapter in the textbook to help with review for exams.

Reading Hints
When reading each chapter in the textbook, look at the subject headings to learn what each section is about. Read first for the general meaning. Then reread parts you did not understand. It may help to read those parts aloud. Carefully read the information given in each table and study each figure and its caption.

Concepts
While studying, put difficult concepts into your own words to see if you understand them. Check this understanding with another student or the instructor. Write these in your notebook.

Class Notes

When taking lecture notes in class, leave a large margin on the left side of each notebook page and write only on right-hand pages, leaving all left-hand pages blank. Look over your lecture notes soon after each class, while your memory is fresh. Fill in missing words, complete sentences and ideas, and underline key phrases, definitions, and concepts. At the top of each page, write the topic of that page. In the left margin, write the key word for that part of your notes. On the opposite left-hand page, write a summary or outline that combines material from both the textbook and the lecture. These can be your study notes for review.

Study Groups

Form a study group with other students so you can help each other. Practice speaking and reading aloud. Ask questions about material you are not sure about. Work together to find answers.

References for Improving Study Skills

Good study skills are essential for achieving your goals in nursing. Time management, efficient use of study time, and a consistent approach to studying are all beneficial. There are various study methods for reading a textbook and for taking class notes. Some methods that have proven helpful can be found in *Saunders Student Nurse Planner: A Guide to Success in Nursing School*. This book contains helpful information on test-taking and preparing for clinical experiences. It includes an example of a "time map" for planning study time and a blank form that you can use to formulate a personal time map.

ADDITIONAL STUDY HINTS FOR ENGLISH AS SECOND-LANGUAGE (ESL) STUDENTS

Vocabulary

If you find a nontechnical word you do not know (e.g., *drowsy*), try to guess its meaning from the sentence (e.g., *With electrolyte imbalance, the patient may feel fatigued and drowsy.*). If you are not sure of the meaning, or if it seems particularly important, look it up in the dictionary.

Vocabulary Notebook

Keep a small alphabetized notebook or address book in your pocket or purse. Write down new nontechnical words you read or hear along with their meanings and pronunciations. Write each word under its initial letter so you can find it easily, as in a dictionary. For words you do not know or for words that have a different meaning in nursing, write down how they sound and are used. Look up their meanings in a dictionary or ask your instructor or first-language buddy. Then write the different meanings or usages that you have found in your book, including the nursing meaning. Continue to add new words as you discover them. For example:

primary
- of most importance; main: *the primary problem or disease*
- the first one; elementary: *primary school*

secondary
- of less importance; resulting from another problem or disease: *a secondary symptom*
- the second one: *secondary school (in the United States, high school)*

First Language Buddy

ESL students should find a first-language buddy—another student who is a native speaker of English and is willing to answer questions about word meanings, pronunciations, and culture. Maybe your buddy would like to learn about your language and culture as well. This could help in his or her nursing experience as well.

To the Instructor

The *Student Learning Guide for Fundamental Concepts and Skills for Nursing* is designed to provide reinforcement for the terms and concepts presented in the text. It will assist students to set priorities, apply the nursing process, practice critical thinking, make good judgments and decisions, increase ability to communicate therapeutically, practice critical thinking, and meet chapter objectives.

ORGANIZATION OF THE TEXT

Included are a wide variety of exercises, questions, and activities. Most chapters include Terminology, Short Answer, NCLEX-PN® Exam Review, Critical Thinking Activities, Meeting Clinical Objectives, and a special section called Steps Toward Better Communication written by a specialist in English as a second language. Other sections that appear where appropriate are Completion, Sequencing, Identification, Review of Structure and Function, Setting Priorities, and Application of the Nursing Process.

Description of Exercises

The exercises are as follows:

- **Terminology**—matching or fill-in-the-blank questions to reinforce correct use of words from the chapter terms list.
- **Short Answer**—list of brief answers to reinforce knowledge and assist students to meet the chapter objectives.
- **NCLEX-PN® Exam Review**—questions in NCLEX format (both multiple choice and the new alternate item formats), based on real-life situations and requiring knowledge, synthesis, analysis, evaluation, and application.
- **Critical Thinking Activities**—brief scenarios and questions to foster problem-solving skills in nursing care which may be practiced individually or in study groups.
- **Meeting Clinical Objectives**—suggestions for practicing learned skills and obtaining experience in the clinical area. These exercises help students meet the clinical practice objectives and encourage focusing on the school's clinical objectives.
- **Completion**—this exercise reinforces the chapter content with fill-in-the-blank questions.
- **Sequencing**—the student practices decision making and problem solving by ordering the best way to carry out a task within the nursing process.
- **Identification**—the student names appropriate steps in a process or procedure or verifies normal or abnormal laboratory values.
- **Review of Structure and Function**—this is a reexamination of the anatomy and physiology of the body system pertinent to the text chapter.
- **Setting Priorities**—students analyze information and make decisions to set priorities within tasks or clinical situations.
- **Application of the Nursing Process**—critical thinking skills are used and the steps of the nursing process are applied to real-life patient care.

All answers to the exercises are included on the *Instructor's Resource* (CD-ROM) *for Fundamental Concepts and Skills for Nursing,* 2nd edition, and also in the Instructor's Resources section of the textbook's companion Evolve website. The answers can be printed out and put on reserve in the library or posted so that students can check them should the instructor choose not to use the *Student Learning Guide* for class credit activities.

STUDENTS WITH LIMITED ENGLISH PROFICIENCY

Because so many students who are natives of other countries are entering nursing programs in the United States and Canada, we have enlisted the aid of a specialist in English as a Second Language who has worked with many health care occupation students. She helped construct the exercises in the "Steps Toward Better Communication" within each chapter. Her letter to you follows. I hope you find this section helpful to your students with limited English proficiency.

Susan C. deWit, MSN, RN, CNS, PHN

STEPS TOWARD BETTER COMMUNICATION

Imagine yourself back in nursing school—trying to read the texts and understand the lectures in Spanish or German. Students studying in a language that is not their native tongue face not only the challenge of learning the medical and physiological lessons that are required of all nursing students, but they must also decipher and use a language whose nuances and grammar are unfamiliar to them. In order to ease some of that burden, we attempted to simplify and regularize the language of *Fundamental Concepts and Skills for Nursing,* 2nd edition and the student learning guide, and to explain some of the colloquial uses of English that occur.

A major part of the nursing process could be described as "knowing your patient inside and out," and one key to that knowledge is being able to accurately and sensitively communicate with the patient and colleagues. To this end, after the regular exercises, we added a section for the ESL student entitled "Steps Toward Better Communication," which offers help in pronunciation, vocabulary building, and use of grammatical issues such as verb tense, and encourages asking for help and clarification. In addition, one section on understanding cultural nuances and mannerisms will help the student face real-life situations and clarify feelings; another offers facility in appropriately asking questions and carrying on conversations.

A note about pronunciation: we assume that the important medical terms will be used and modeled correctly by the instructor. In terms of conversation, intelligibility rather than native-like accuracy should be the goal. Correct stress is the major determining factor in how easily a person can be understood. Therefore we chose to indicate stressed syllables in words and phrases rather than giving phonetic pronunciations which students often find difficult to understand.

Description of Exercises

The following exercises appear in the Steps Toward Better Communication as appropriate:

- **Vocabulary Building Glossary** explains and defines idiomatic or unusual uses of nonmedical terms used in the chapter and indicates the stressed syllables by capitalizing them.

- **Completion** sentences offer opportunities to use the words presented in the Glossary, often in different contexts than they are used in the text, thereby offering yet another way to increase vocabulary.

- **Vocabulary Exercises** use words from the chapter in various ways to increase ease of understanding.

- **Word Attack Skills** deal with word segments, suffixes, prefixes, and types of words to help the student learn to decode new words and their usage.

- **Pronunciation Skills** offer practice in pronouncing difficult terms as well as phrases and sentences, with emphasis on stress and intonation.

- **Grammar Points** are made occasionally, especially when there is a recurring point raised by the chapter, such as the use of the past tense in taking case histories.

- **Communication Exercises** encourage communicative interchange, and writing and use of dialogues that might actually be used by a practicing nurse. The value of this section is enhanced if students can be paired in first- and second-language speaker combinations, giving each the opportunity to experience the other's accent and offering the possibility for cross-cultural exchange. Answers to the Communication Exercise dialogue questions are found in the *Instructor's Resource*, and may be printed out for student use.

- **Cultural Points** present explanations and questions about issues and customs that may differ across the cultures represented in the class, and in the prospective patient community. They can explain the normative culture in which the individual will be working, while at the same time acknowledge and validate an individual's cultural difference.

In preparing these materials, I have drawn on my experience in teaching practicing and aspiring health care personnel. I have found them to be dedicated and eager to improve their own lives while helping others. I have learned much from them about hard work, perseverance, humor, and what they need in order to do a better job. My colleagues in teaching English and nurses with whom I have worked have been helpful with ideas for teaching projects, indicating language areas needing to be addressed, and offering suggestions and solutions for problems. However, any omissions and errors are my own.

I have been impressed with the similarity between learning language skills and nursing skills. Both require access to academic knowledge, but mastery occurs with hands-on practice and experience. The exercises are geared to provide this opportunity. Encourage your students to interact as often as possible. Look at each lesson with the question, "How can I structure this lesson so the students will have to generate their own language to complete the exercise?" Offer real-life challenges and tasks for speaking and communicative interaction with other students, colleagues, and patients whenever possible. An encouraging, open, and interactive classroom is the best setting for language learning and improvement. I wish you well in working with this special group of people.

Gail G. Boehme
English Language Instructor/Consultant
Santa Barbara City College
Continuing Education

Contents

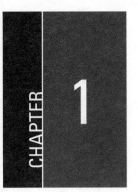

Nursing and the Health Care System

Answer Key: Textbook page references are provided as a guide for answering selected questions. A complete answer key was provided for your instructor.

TERMINOLOGY

Directions: Define and give an example of each of the following terms.

(2)   1.   Apprenticeship _____

_____

(4)   2.   Invasive procedure _____

_____

(6)   3.   Nursing process_____

_____

(4)   4.   Theory_____

_____

ACRONYMS

Directions: Write a brief answer for each question.

(8)   1.   Describe how DRGs (diagnosis-related groups) affect payment for health care.

_____

_____

(8)   2.   Describe an HMO (health maintenance organization).

_____

_____

(8)   3.   How does an HMO differ from a PPO (preferred provider organization)?

_____

_____

SHORT ANSWER

Directions: Write a brief answer for each question.

(1-2) 1. List four influences Florence Nightingale has had on nurses' training.

_____

_____

_____

(4) 2. List two major influences on nursing education in the United States.

_____

_____

(2) 3. Describe the early schools for practical nursing.

_____

_____

_____

(5) 4. Considering the functions of the practical nurse, describe four desirable attributes of the nurse.

a. _____

b. _____

c. _____

d. _____

(6-7) 5. Compare the education and training of LPN/LVNs and registered nurses.

LPN/LVN	**Registered Nurse**
_____	_____
_____	_____
_____	_____
_____	_____

(5-6) 6. The purpose of the nurse practice act is to _____

_____ .

Student Name_____

NCLEX-PN® EXAM REVIEW

*Directions: Choose the **best** answer(s) for each of the following questions.*

(2) 1. The first school of nursing was funded by
1. physician payments for services rendered.
2. contributions by Crimean war servicemen and their families.
3. the estate of Florence Nightingale.
4. charges to patients for nursing care.

(2) 2. The Civil War spurred the growth of nursing as many nurses were needed to care for the wounded. Nursing care during the Civil War was directed by _____ _____. (Fill in the blank)

(2) 3. In the United States in the early schools of nursing, education was achieved through
1. formal classes in anatomy and nursing.
2. a set curriculum covering medical and surgical nursing.
3. instruction by trained nurses in the hospital.
4. working directly on the hospital units.

(2) 4. There were several prominent nurses instrumental in the progression of nursing in the United States. Which nurse began community nursing? _____ _____ (Fill in the blank)

(4) 5. A nursing theory is
1. a group of facts about a particular topic that has been proven by scientific method.
2. a statement about relationships among concepts or facts that is not based on actual knowledge.
3. a proven hypothesis based on gathered facts.
4. a guess about what may happen in a particular situation.

(5-6) 6. The practice of nursing is governed by a nurse practice act and
1. standards of nursing care.
2. codes of ethics.
3. institutional rules and regulations.
4. licensure requirements.

(6) 7. Practical nursing arose to
1. provide a stepping stone to becoming a registered nurse.
2. provide more training than a nurse's aide receives.
3. fill a gap left by nurses who enlisted in the military.
4. provide less expensive employees to hospitals.

(8) 8. Under the DRG system, the hospital
1. receives a set amount of money for each patient hospitalized with a particular diagnosis.
2. must discharge patients within a set number of days.
3. decides what care for a particular diagnosis will cost.
4. is often overpaid for the care actually given a patient.

(8)   9. HMOs have become a prominent part of health care in the United States. HMOs (Select all that apply)
1. provide care at a lower price than independent doctors.
2. enroll patients for a set fee per month.
3. are very popular with physicians.
4. have a preferred list of providers for health care.

(8-9)   10. Managed care has brought several changes to the practice of medicine. Effects of managed care are (Select all that apply)
1. less continuity of care for the patient.
2. provision for the patient to stay with one physician long-term.
3. attention to delivery of cost-effective care.
4. greater job satisfaction of health care providers.

(9)   11. A complaint of many health care professionals about managed care is the increased amount of
1. documentation and paperwork necessary.
2. trained personnel to staff hospital units.
3. time required to care for each patient.
4. accountability patients have for their own care.

CRITICAL THINKING ACTIVITIES

1. Within a small group of your fellow students, discuss your definition of nursing. Compare differences among the definitions of the various group members.

2. Identify some ways in which the *Standards of Nursing Care* are applied in the clinical setting.

MEETING CLINICAL OBJECTIVES

Directions: The following suggested activities will help you meet the stated clinical practice objectives for the chapter. Review your school's clinical objectives for the week and outline a plan of activities that will help you meet them. If you are unsure how to meet them, consult with your instructor at the beginning of the clinical day.

1. Talk with an LPN/LVN and an RN on your clinical unit and ask them what they see as differences in the roles of these two types of nurses.

2. Check within your clinical facility and in the local classified ads to determine what opportunities for employment as an LPN/LVN exist in your community.

Student Name_____

STEPS TOWARD BETTER COMMUNICATION

VOCABULARY BUILDING GLOSSARY

Term	Pronunciation	Definition
active listening	AC tive LIS ten ing	to listen for the meaning of what a person is saying and repeat it back to him or her
attributes	AT tri butes	qualities, characteristics
ancillary	AN cil lar y	helping in a subordinate way
balanced ratio	BAL anced ratio	a correct proportion
charge out	CHARGE OUT	initiate a financial charge for something
collaborator	col LAB o ra tor	one who works together with others
contain (verb)	con TAIN	to limit
controversy	CON tro ver sy	disagreement
core curriculum	core cur RIC u lum	the basic set of what is taught
criteria	cri TER i a	rules or standards to judge by
Crusades	Cru SADES	religious wars made by European Christians against Muslims in the eastern Mediterranean in the 11th to 12th centuries
delegator	DEL e ga tor	one who tells others what to do
exacting	ex ACT ing	very careful with details
expertise	ex per TISE	a high level of experience
foster	FOS ter	encourage, promote
funded	FUN ded	provided with money for the support of something
funds	funds	money
gap	GAP	empty space in a line of things
implement	IM ple MENT	(verb) to do, to use
in other instances	in other IN stances	in other situations
inherent	in HER ent	naturally part of something, built into
lacking	LACK ing	absent
licensure	LI cens ure	giving licenses
midwife	MID wife	a woman who helps the birthing of a baby
nightmare	NIGHT mare	a very bad dream
phenomena	phe NOM e na	observable facts or events
pilgrims	PIL grims	people traveling on religious journeys
prior	PRI or	previous, coming before
regulatory body	REG u la tor y BOD y	a group that makes rules
scope	SCOPE	the range or limits of something
skyrocket	SKY rock et	to go up very quickly
sought (verb, past tense)	SOUGHT	desired, looked for (present = seek)
standards	STAN dards	the expected level against which other things are measured (e.g., above or below standard)
vigilant	VIG i lant	watchful, watching carefully

COMPLETION

Directions: Fill in the blanks with the correct term from the list to complete the sentence.

active listening	criteria	collaborator	gap
implement	prior	delegator	controversy
foster	skyrocket	sought	vigilant

1. The nurse gave instructions to the aides respectfully and is known as a good
   _____.

2. A calm, unhurried attitude and display of concern will _____ the
   formation of trust between nurse and patient.

3. The nurse went over every part of the patient's chart as he _____ to
   gather all the pertinent information.

4. The type of treatment appropriate for that particular form of cancer is a matter of
   _____.

5. After planning his work for the day, the nurse began to _____ the
   plan.

6. The nursing diagnosis of *Pain* was made based on the _____ listed
   for that diagnosis.

7. The patient had developed an allergy to penicillin during his _____
   respiratory infection.

8. The nurse must be _____ in observing for side effects of medication.

9. The use of the latest technology for diagnostic testing is one factor that has made the cost of medical care
   _____.

VOCABULARY EXERCISES

Directions: Underline the correct definition of these words used in the Standards of Care.

1. assessment: test   evaluation
2. diagnosis: finding, conclusion   drawing
3. outcome: removal   result
4. implementation: carrying out   making equipment
5. evaluation: measurement   analysis
6. collegiality: education   relationship with other workers

Student Name_____

WORD ATTACK SKILLS

Stress/meaning change: Some words that are spelled the same change meaning when the stress is placed on a different syllable. Often, this shows the difference between the word as a noun and as a verb.

AT tri bute (noun) = a characteristic

at TRIB ute (verb) = to credit, to be the cause for

IM ple ment (noun) = a tool

IM ple MENT (verb) = to put into action, use

1. Underline the stressed syllables in these words in the following sentences:
   a. He attributed his success to his attributes of hard work and honesty.
   b. The use of the surgical implements was implemented with a training session.

2. If *ethics* means "a system of moral or correct behavior," then which of the following would be an "ethical manner" of behavior for the nurse?
   a. The nurse took some of the patient's medication because her sister needed it.
   b. The nurse contributed information during collaboration with the dietitian about the patient's food likes.
   c. The nurse told the visitor he could not tell her about the patient's prognosis, that she would need to ask the patient about that.

COMMUNICATION EXERCISES

Directions: Find a partner and practice your communication skills by doing one of the following:

1. Explain the difference between a licensed practical nurse/licensed vocational nurse and a registered nurse.

2. Explain the important role Florence Nightingale played in nursing.

CULTURAL POINTS

1. This chapter talks about the historical overview that shaped the nursing tradition in Europe and North America, and the bases for the art and science of nursing as currently practiced there. It also talks about the ways nurses are educated and the health care systems that operate today.

2. If you are from another country, think about the differences in nursing there. How are nurses trained there? Is the job of a nurse different? In what way? What is the health care system in your country? In what ways do you think it is better or worse than the system in North America? What are the traditions and history that have shaped the health care and nursing systems in your country? Share your answers with your peers.

Review the chapter key points, answer the study questions, and complete the critical thinking activities at the end of the chapter in the textbook.

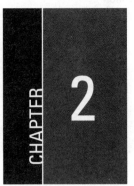

CHAPTER 2

Concepts of Health, Illness, and Health Promotion

Answer Key: Textbook page references are provided as a guide for answering selected questions. A complete answer key was provided for your instructor.

TERMINOLOGY

Directions: Match the terms in Column I with the definitions in Column II.

	Column I		Column II
(12)	1. _____ acute illness	a.	Disease of body or mind
(14)	2. _____ asymptomatic	b.	Illness for which there is no cure
(12)	3. _____ chronic illness	c.	Unknown etiology
(12)	4. _____ convalescence	d.	Without symptoms
(12)	5. _____ etiology	e.	Tendency to maintain stability of the internal biologic environment
(11)	6. _____ health		
(15)	7. _____ hierarchy	f.	Recovery from illness
(18)	8. _____ homeostasis	g.	Illness that develops suddenly
(12)	9. _____ idiopathic	h.	Illness that persists for a long time
(11)	10. _____ illness	i.	Arrangement of objects, elements, or values in order of importance
(12)	11. _____ terminal illness	j.	Cause of disease
		k.	Absence of disease and complete physical, mental, and social well-being

SHORT ANSWER

Directions: Write a brief answer for each of the following.

(12)   1. Illness behaviors include how people:

a. _____

b. _____

c. _____

d. _____

(13)   2. Rather than treating the illness itself, nursing is concerned with:

_____

_____

_____

(14)   3. List three examples of health behavior.

a. _____

b. _____

c. _____

(21)   4. A stressor can be helpful or harmful depending on the:

a. _____

b. _____

c. _____

d. _____

e. _____

COMPLETION

Directions: Fill in the blank(s) with the correct word(s) from the terms list in the chapter in the textbook to complete the sentence or idea.

(13)   1. The term _____ was first used by _____ to signify the ideal state of health in every dimension of a person's personality.

(13)   2. In Dunn's view, each person accepts responsibility for and takes _____ in improving and maintaining his or her own state of wellness.

(14)   3. With patients from so many different countries, _____ differences must be considered when planning nursing care.

(15)   4. Each patient must be dealt with as a(n) _____, whose concepts of health and illness and health care might be different from your own.

(15)   5. A holistic approach considers the _____, _____, _____, and _____ aspects of a person.

(15-17)   6. Maslow's hierarchy of needs consists of _____ needs, _____ needs, _____ needs, _____ needs, and _____ needs.

(18)   7. Adaptability to a(n) _____ is essential to stability and health.

Student Name_____

(18)   8.   When the equilibrium of the body is disturbed, _____ occurs.

(19)   9.   When the brain perceives a situation as threatening, the _____ stimulates the physiologic functions needed for _____.

(20)   10.   Hans Selye states that the body attempts to deal with stressors by the secretion of _____.

(22)   11.   Adjusting to or solving challenges is called _____.

(22)   12.   Strategies that protect us from increasing anxiety are called _____.

NCLEX-PN® EXAM REVIEW

*Directions: Choose the **best** answer(s) for each of the following questions.*

Situation: Your patient has had a flare-up of osteoarthritis in his knee. He is having difficulty walking.

(12)   1.   You know that in the transition stage of illness the person may (Select all that apply)
- .1. deny being ill.
- ·2. acknowledge that symptoms of illness are present.
- 3. begin recovering from illness.
- 4. withdraw from usual roles.

(15)   2.   In planning care for a patient you recall that Abraham Maslow states that
- ·1. people respond to needs as whole, integrated beings.
- 2. each person must take responsibility for improving his or her own state of wellness.
- 3. stress plays a role in every disease process because of faulty adaptation by the body.
- 4. humans are naturally inclined to be healthy.

(12)   3.   Osteoarthritis is a chronic illness. A chronic illness differs from an acute illness in that the acute illness
- 1. lasts a long time.
- 2. cannot be cured.
- 3. has no known cause.
- ·4. develops suddenly.

(15-17)   4.   According to Maslow's hierarchy, which of the following would be the priority need?
- 1. intimacy
- 2. independence
- 3. artistic expression
- 4. psychological comfort

(20)   5.   The general adaptation syndrome is said to occur in response to
- 1. initial stress.
- 2. short-term stress.
- 3. any perceived stress.
- 4. long-term stress.

(23)   6.   An example of the defense mechanism of rationalization would be
- 1. forgetting the name of someone you intensely dislike.
- 2.. blaming the teacher for a poor grade on a test when you did not study sufficiently.
- 3. kicking the dog when you are mad at your boss.
- 4. praising someone whom you intensely dislike.

(20)   7.   Disorders that are often stress-related are (Select all that apply)
- 1. hypertension.
- 2. appendicitis.
- 3. gastritis.
- 4. multiple sclerosis.

MATCHING

Directions: Indicate with a check mark which of the following are sympathetic nervous system actions and which are parasympathetic actions.

(20)

Result of Action	Sympathetic	Parasympathetic
1. Dry mouth	_____	_____
2. Increased heart rate	_____	_____
3. Bronchial constriction	_____	_____
4. Intestinal motility—diarrhea	_____	_____
5. Sweating	_____	_____
6. Pupil dilation	_____	_____

CRITICAL THINKING ACTIVITIES

1. Identify ways in which holistic care can be practiced in the clinical area.

2. Describe ways in which your body attempts to maintain homeostasis when you contract a cold virus.

3. Identify the common signs of stress that you experience when approaching a major examination.

4. List four ways in which you think you might be able to decrease stress and anxiety for patients.

MEETING CLINICAL OBJECTIVES

Directions: The following suggested activities will help you meet the stated clinical practice objectives for the chapter. Review your school's clinical objectives for the week and outline a plan of activities that will help you meet them. If you are unsure how to meet them, consult with your instructor at the beginning of the clinical day.

1. Look for signs of stress from staff or patients on the nursing unit to which you are assigned.

2. Attempt to decrease stress or anxiety for at least one patient.

STEPS TOWARD BETTER COMMUNICATION

VOCABULARY BUILDING GLOSSARY

Term	Pronunciation	Definition
adverse	AD verse	not favorable
alters	AL ters	changes
atrophy	A troph y	to shrink, grow useless
condone	con DONE	to pardon or overlook wrongdoing
convey	con VEY	to communicate an idea

Student Name _____

core	CORE	center
crucial	CRU cial	very important
deprivation	dep ri VA tion	a condition of want and need
detectable	de TECT able	something you can see or notice
deviation	de vi A tion	a difference, a move away from
dynamic	dy NAM ic	energetic, full of activity
emerge	e MERGE	appear, come out
esteem	es TEEM	respect
feedback	FEED back	information given in response
hierarchy	HI er ar chy	organization from high to low
hygiene	HY giene	health and cleanliness
integrated	in te GRA ted	combined
intervene	in ter VENE	to come between in order to change something
maladaptive	mal a DAP tive	giving the wrong reaction
merely	MERE ly	only
noncompliant	NON com PLI ant	not following the rules
perception	per CEP tion	seeing and understanding
prolong	pro LONG	to continue over a period of time
reimburse	RE im burse	pay back
resolves	re SOLVES	ends or concludes
reticular	re TIC u lar	like a net
susceptible	sus CEP ti ble	easily influenced or affected

COMPLETION

Directions: Fill in the blank(s) with the correct word(s) from the Vocabulary Building Glossary to complete the sentence.

1. The patient suffered a(n) _____ reaction from the drug; he broke out in a rash.

2. The patient did not have good _____ practices and his teeth were in very poor condition.

3. The patient did not stick to the diet and was _____ with the exercise program as well.

4. Her _____ of the situation after reviewing the data in the chart was that the patient was suffering from a serious infection.

5. Exposure to prolonged sunlight sometimes _____ certain drugs, making them noneffective.

6. When signs of complications occur, the nurse can quickly _____ to have the treatment changed.

7. It is hoped that the patient will _____ from the chemotherapy treatments with no further signs of cancer.

8. His type of abdominal pain is a(n) _____ from the classic signs and symptoms of appendicitis.

9. Crying all the time is a(n) _____ response to a crisis.

10. It is hoped that his pneumonia _____ without any permanent damage to the lungs.

VOCABULARY EXERCISES

This chapter discusses various aspects of a person and discusses assessing for factors within those various aspects. The various aspects are:

biologic	refers to	the body
psychologic	refers to	the mind and emotions
sociologic	refers to	culture, environment, life roles
spiritual	refers to	religion, soul

Directions: Match the word to a corresponding action or response, then give another example.

1. _____ biologic
   _____
   _____

2. _____ psychosocial
   _____
   _____

3. _____ spiritual
   _____
   _____

a. attending church
b. running a fever
c. joining a group
d. meditating each day
e. praying before meals
f. feeling sharp pains in the chest

WORD ATTACK SKILLS

Opposites

Directions: Give the opposite for these words from the textbook. Use words from the Vocabulary Building Glossary above when possible.

Term	Pronunciation	Definition	Opposite
1. optimum	OP ti mum	at the highest or best level	_____
2. monitor	MON i tor	watch over a period of time	_____
3. vague	VAGUE	not clear or specific	_____
4. passive	PAS sive	not active	_____
5. thrive	THRIVE	grow strong and healthy	_____

Student Name_____

6.	adversity	ad VER si ty	bad luck	_____
7.	underreact	UN der re ACT	not enough response	_____
8.	malaise	ma LAISE	general feeling of illness, unhappiness	_____

Meanings of Nouns and Verbs

Directions: Note how these words from the chapter change, depending on whether they are used as a verb or a noun.

Verb	Noun
intervene	intervention
motivate	motivation
ambulate	ambulation
validate	validation
deprive	deprivation
clarify	clarification
deviate	deviation
adapt	adaptation

COMMUNICATION EXERCISES

1. Considering Figure 2-2 in the textbook, consider the variables in health and illness. Give an example from your life (or that of a friend) for each of these variables:
   a. Culture
   b. Religion
   c. Standard of living
   d. Support system
   e. Genetic influence

2. Referring to Table 2-7 in the textbook, consider what health promotion measures should be used by the following age groups. Verbalize your thoughts to a peer.
   a. Teenagers
   b. Elders
   c. Pregnant women

3. Look at the list of stressful situations below. Numerically rank them according to which are most stressful to you, with the most stressful being #1, the next #2, and so forth. Then compare your list with the lists of some of your peers.
   _____ Not having enough time to study
   _____ Not having enough money
   _____ Concern over how you look
   _____ Lack of sleep
   _____ Worry about family
   _____ A dirty room
   _____ Feeling like you didn't do a good job
   _____ Worry over not enough quality time with loved ones

4. List things that are stressful to you, such as:
   unmade bed
   sink full of dirty dishes
   unmowed lawn

   _____

   _____

   _____

   _____

   _____

CULTURAL POINTS

1. What things about being with a group of people from a different culture do you find stressful? How do you cope with these stresses?

2. If you are from a different country, do you think there is a different level of stress in your native country than here? Is it higher or lower? Why?

3. What are some ways people in your culture deal with stress?

Review the chapter key points, answer the study questions, and complete the critical thinking activities at the end of the chapter in the textbook.

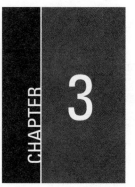
Student Name _____

Legal and Ethical Aspects of Nursing

Answer Key: Textbook page references are provided as a guide for answering selected questions. A complete answer key was provided for your instructor.

TERMINOLOGY

Directions: Define and give an example of each of the following terms:

(29)   1.   standards of care _____

(34)   2.   negligence _____

(34)   3.   malpractice _____

(32)   4.   confidential _____

(35)   5.   libel _____

(35)   6.   invasion of privacy _____

(35)   7.   slander _____

(35)   8.   assault and battery _____

(28)   9.   accountability _____

(34)   10.   prudent _____

SHORT ANSWER

Directions: Read the Code for Nurses and the Code of Ethics for the Licensed Practical Nurse in the chapter of the textbook. When you have completed your study of the two codes, fill in the following blanks.

(39)   1.   Ethics is a code of _____ that represents _____ conduct for a particular _____ .

(39)   2.   A violation of ethical behavior may result in discipline by _____ or loss of _____ .

(37) 3. Ways in which nurses can prevent patient lawsuits against themselves or the hospital include:

_____

_____

_____

(29) 4. The consequences of violating the nurse practice act could be:

_____

_____

_____

(29) 5. The purpose of the standards of nursing practice is to

_____

_____

_____

and to _____ .

NCLEX-PN® EXAM REVIEW

*Directions: Choose the **best** answer(s) for each of the following questions.*

(27) 1. Although both a statute and a tort are laws, a tort is a
   1. civil or criminal law.
   2. wrong against the public.
   3. violation of civil law.
   4. felony crime.

(28) 2. The scope of practice for nurses is set forth in the
   1. standards of practice.
   2. code of ethics.
   3. laws of the state.
   4. nurse practice act.

(28-29) 3. You decide to delegate frequent vital sign measurements on your postoperative patient to the nursing assistant. When delegating nursing tasks to others, you are responsible for (Select all that apply)
   1. knowing whether the task can be legally delegated.
   2. verifying the competency of the person delegated the task.
   3. observing the person performing the task.
   4. supervising the person's charting of the task performed.

(29) 4. Two of your colleagues ask you if you wish to join them at a seminar on current neurological care. Continuing education for nurses is important because
   1. self-esteem is dependent on continued learning.
   2. there are constant changes in health care practice.
   3. pay raises depend on continuing education activities.
   4. the up-to-date nurse is respected by colleagues.

(31) 5. One nurse says to another, "Well, did you make it with Dr. S. last night?" Making sexual comments on the nursing unit is considered sexual harassment, and is illegal when it
   1. is offensive to the people in the vicinity of the speaker.
   2. is concerned with some aspect of patient care.
   3. interferes with someone's job performance.
   4. is directed from supervisors to employees.

Student Name_____

(33-34) 6. A patient is brought to the emergency room unconscious after an automobile accident. She is seriously injured and needs immediate surgery. No next of kin can be quickly located. A signed informed consent is not necessary since the patient
   1. is unconscious and unable to communicate.
   2. is to undergo a lengthy exploratory surgical procedure.
   3. was admitted through the emergency room.
   4. has been very seriously injured.

(33) 7. Which consent form is used to show the patient has consented to have blood drawn for laboratory tests, treatments by the nurses such as dressing a wound or catheterization, and treatment by the physical or respiratory therapist?
   1. consent for surgery
   2. informed consent
   3. conditions of admission
   4. consent for special procedures

(37) 8. Which one of the following are considered an incident and need to be reported on an incident or occurrence form? (Select all that apply)
   1. a patient falling to the floor while getting out of bed
   2. a visitor slipping and falling on a wet hallway floor
   3. giving the patient the wrong medication
   4. a patient complaining about the care given by a nursing assistant

(32) 9. Which of the following are legal points in the Health Insurance Portability and Accountability Act (HIPAA)? (Select all that apply)
   1. The patient has a right to amend an error in his medical record.
   2. Information cannot be given to outside sources without the patient's permission.
   3. Patient information must not be exposed to public view.
   4. The patient cannot see information in the medical record.

(31) 10. Reportable events, by law, under the Child Abuse Prevention and Treatment Act, include (Select all that apply)
   1. a parent locking a 20-year-old drug-abusing son out of the house.
   2. a school child who continually comes to school unbathed and in dirty clothes.
   3. bruises on a child's legs after a fall down the front steps of the home.
   4. a child who has been brought to the ER for the fourth time in a year with a broken bone that a parent says must be from a fall that was unwitnessed.

ETHICAL SITUATIONS

Situation A

A young girl has been brought by ambulance to the emergency room. You are the admitting nurse and note that she has swallowed an overdose of sedatives and is now having her stomach emptied of its contents. Since this was an attempted suicide, the police reporters were in the hallway. When you go to lunch, your friends from other units want to know how old the girl is, and why she was brought in. You were the person who recorded the emergency room notes into her chart and so you have some information.

1. When asked if the girl took an overdose, you might answer:
   a. "Yes, but she's OK."
   b. "She must have had a desire to die."
   c. "That information is confidential."

2. In this situation, to discuss the patient not only violates her right to privacy, but could result in a(n) _____ and possibly _____ employment.

Situation B

The patient in the suite at the end of the hall orders his meals from the hospital's special gourmet menu. At noon on Sunday he did not touch any of the food, although the meal was excellent. The chef's salad and strawberry pie looked very good. You pick up his tray from his room.

3. Thinking that it is a shame to waste such food, you
   a. give it to the housekeeping staff.
   b. send it back to the kitchen.
   c. offer it to the entire unit staff.
   d. eat it yourself.

Situation C

A unit secretary is very tense about her new job on the cardiac telemetry unit. Her doctor has prescribed a mild tranquilizer for her. She knows that when clients go home, the medications are often left behind and returned to the pharmacy. She asks the nurses if they could give her the tranquilizers that are left upon a patient's discharge, saving her the expense of having the prescription filled.

4. This is a distinct breach of _____ on her part.

5. If the nurses grant her request, they are prescribing or dispensing medicine without a license and this is a(n) _____ offense.

Student Name_____

Situation D

You have been a patient's nurse for her entire stay in the hospital. She has come to rely on you and when she is ready to go home, she wants to give you a sum of money in appreciation for the "lovely things you have done for her."

6. In this situation you should
    a. explain to her that the service is part of her care.
    b. accept the money because although you receive a salary from the hospital, clients should pay for the service you render them individually.
    c. accept the gift of money and tell nobody so that no one else will feel hurt that she selected only you.
    d. suggest she give the money to the nursing assistant who needs it more than you do.

7. The patient insists that you take the money or you will hurt her feelings. Therefore you
    a. tell her of some specific need the hospital has to which she could make a contribution.
    b. suggest a fund in her name with suitable recognition.
    c. accept the gift so that there are no hurt feelings in the situation.
    d. tell her to give it to the nursing assistant since she needs the money more than you do.

CRITICAL THINKING ACTIVITIES

1. You overhear a nurse say to a patient, "If you won't stay in your bed, I will have to find a way to keep you there." Is this a breach of legal or ethical conduct? How would you handle the situation?

2. How would you tactfully explain the process of placing advance directives on file in the chart?

3. As a student, explain the rules that govern the care you give while in the clinical setting.

4. If you were caring for a child and discovered that the child seemed very fearful of his parent and also had some unexplained bruises, what would you do?

MEETING CLINICAL OBJECTIVES

Directions: The following suggested activities will help you meet the stated clinical practice objectives for the chapter. Review your school's clinical objectives for the week and outline a plan of activities that will help you meet them. If you are unsure how to meet them, consult with your instructor at the beginning of the clinical day.

1. Review the documentation in the nurse's notes for one of your assigned patients from the previous 24 hours. Determine if it meets the guidelines for legally sound charting. Look at legibility, judgmental statements, objectivity, thoroughness, and correction of any errors. Are there any problems noted for which interventions do not seem to have been done? Think about how you might have charted differently.

2. During a clinical day, observe for ways in which patient's rights are being protected. Were there any instances of when patient's rights were violated? Discuss these in your clinical group.

3. Properly obtain a signature on an informed consent form.

4. Look for areas in which HIPAA is being violated by leaving patient information exposed to other patients or visitors. Report what you saw to the clinical group. Discuss how the events could have been prevented.

STEPS TOWARD BETTER COMMUNICATION

VOCABULARY BUILDING GLOSSARY

Term	Pronunciation	Definition
access	AC cess	able to get to or see something
bound	BOUND	required
breach	BREACH	a break or neglect of a rule; a violation
contrary	CON trar y	opposite
disciplines	DIS ci plines	areas of interest or experience
emancipated minor	e MAN ci PA ted MI nor	a person who is normally under the legal age to take action for him- or herself, but has been declared by law to be able to make legal decisions for him- or herself
escalated	ES ca la ted	raised the level, increased
explicit	ex PLIC it	clear and definite
gravely	GRAVE ly	severely, seriously
harass	ha RASS	to trouble and annoy continually
inservice classes	IN service classes	classes offered at the place of employment
jeopardize	JEOP ar dize	to put in danger
likelihood	LIKE li hood	probability
means	MEANS	way, ability
pertinent	PER tin ent	directly related to what is being talked about
precedent	PREC e dent	an example that sets a standard for future action
prescribed (adj)	pre SCRIBed	as directed
proxy	PROX y	acting for someone else on his or her behalf either in person or by document
rapport	rap PORT (silent t)	a friendly, sympathetic relationship
resuscitated	re SUS ci ta ted	brought back to life or consciousness
scope	SCOPE	the extent or limits of something
seemingly	SEEM ing ly	appears true on the surface, but may not be
suggestive	sug GES tive	indicating an indecent or sexually improper meaning
surrogate	SUR ro gate	a substitute, a person who acts in place of another
whistle blowing	WHIS tle BLOW ing	telling about someone's wrong or illegal activity to the authorities
witnessed	WIT nessed	observed

Student Name_____

COMPLETION

Directions: Fill in the blank(s) with the correct word(s) to complete the sentence.

1. Use the correct verb in the following sentences (*jeopardize, witness, resuscitate, escalate*).
   a. That type of action can _____ a nurse's license.
   b. The argument was heated, and her remarks made the situation

      _____.
   c. The nurse was asked to _____ the signing of the consent form.
   d. When a patient's heart stops, it is mandatory to try to _____
      him.

2. Use the correct adjective in these sentences (*prescribed, suggestive, pertinent*).
   a. He took all of the _____ medication but was not well.
   b. The physician wanted only the _____ facts such as the vital
      signs and intake and output amounts.
   c. The abdominal pain and nausea were _____ signs of appendi-
      citis.

3. Use the correct noun in these sentences (*precedent, scope, access, proxy, means*).
   a. At the end of the first semester of nursing school, the nursing student's

      _____ of knowledge of nursing is very small.
   b. Since he was incapacitated, his _____ in the legal matter was
      his brother.
   c. The consulting physician needed _____ to the patient record in
      order to gather data needed for a diagnosis.
   d. The patient did not have the _____ with which to obtain his
      prescribed medications.
   e. Allowing a family member to visit after visiting hours were over set a(n)

      _____ in the unit.

4. Use the correct adverb in these sentences (*seemingly, gravely*).
   a. The patient was _____ more cheerful after his family visited.
   b. After reviewing the diagnostic tests, the doctor became _____
      concerned about his patient's condition.

VOCABULARY EXERCISE

Reasonable can be defined as being within the bounds of common sense. *Prudent* means careful in conduct
and exercising good judgment or common sense.

Write a definition of *ethics*:

_____

_____

_____

WORD ATTACK SKILLS

The verb *prescribe* means to:
1. advise the use of something (medicine).
2. set a rule to be followed.

The noun *prescription* means a:
1. doctor's written instruction for medicine.
2. rule or suggestion to follow.

Directions: Write sentences for the above words.

1. prescribe: _____

    _____

2. prescription: _____

    _____

PRONUNCIATION PRACTICE

Directions: Underline the accented syllable on the following words and practice pronouncing them with a partner or to yourself.

accountability	competent	consent	defamation	delegation
liable	libel	malpractice	negligence	reciprocity

COMMUNICATION EXERCISES

Directions: If there is some part of the chapter you do not understand, ask your teacher or another student to explain it to you. Clarify your understanding by repeating points, restating in your own words, and asking clarifying questions.

1. Read and practice the following dialogue.

    Mary and Jim prepare to move a patient up in bed. N.T. is Jim's patient. Mary goes to the far side of the bed.

    Jim: "We are going to move you up in bed, Ms. T."

    Mary : "Let me move your pillow to the top of the bed." Jim crouches down in preparation for moving Ms. T.

    Mary : "Jim, I find it easier to raise the bed up before trying to move my patients. Could we do that?"

    Jim: "The control is on your side; I'm sorry, I just got to thinking about Ms. T.'s dressing change and wasn't paying close attention."

    Mary : "That's OK, sometimes I forget too."

2. Read and practice the following dialogue.

    Ms. H.: "I'm feeling like I don't want this surgery now that I signed the consent."

    Nurse: "You've changed your mind? Are you feeling better than you were?"

Student Name_____

Ms. H.:	"It just seems like such an inconvenient time right now with my husband having to leave town for 2 weeks on business."
Nurse:	"Oh, it isn't because the pain has suddenly disappeared?"
Ms. H.:	"Oh no, the pain is still there, but I seem to be more used to it now."
Nurse:	"Didn't you tell me that this was your third attack of severe pain from your gallbladder?"
Ms. H.:	"Yes, it is the third time it has happened, but it has been over a period of two years."
Nurse:	"I know it will be difficult recovering while your husband is out of town, but you have a very large gallstone according to your ultrasound report and that could cause a problem with bile flow that can affect your whole body. It really would be best to attend to the problem now."
Ms. H.:	"Oh, I know, I'm just not looking forward to being put to sleep."
Nurse:	"Does anesthesia scare you?"
Ms. H.:	"When I had it once before I was really terribly sick afterwards."
Nurse:	"How long ago was that?"
Ms. H.:	"About 22 years ago."
Nurse:	"There are newer types of anesthesia that don't tend to cause as much nausea. Talk to the anesthesiologist about that."
Ms. H.:	"OK, I'll do that."

3. Write a dialogue where a patient refuses to have a nasogastric tube inserted even though she is vomiting. Share your dialogue with a peer by reading it to him or her.

CULTURAL POINTS

1. Many industries in the United States are heavily regulated by state and federal laws. The medical and health professions are regulated by laws and by professional guidelines and licensing. This is done for the protection of the patients and the health care professionals. Is this done in your country? To what extent? Do you think it is a good idea or not? Why? Discuss this with your classmates from other countries.

2. What are the ethical standards for nurses in your country?

Review the chapter key points, answer the study questions, and complete the critical thinking activities at the end of the chapter in the textbook.

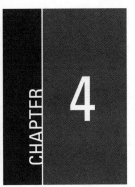

CHAPTER **4**

Overview of the Nursing Process and Critical Thinking

Answer Key: Textbook page references are provided as a guide for answering selected questions. A complete answer key was provided for your instructor.

TERMINOLOGY

Directions: Match the terms in Column I with the definitions in Column II.

Column I	Column II
(44) 1. _____ critical thinking	a. Step-by-step process used by scientists to solve problems.
(44) 2. _____ decision making	b. Directed, purposeful mental activity by which ideas are created and evaluated, plans are constructed, and desired outcomes are decided.
(47) 3. _____ priority	c. Something taking precedence over other things at a particular time because of greater importance.
(43) 4. _____ nursing process	d. Way of thinking and acting based on the scientific method.
(43) 5. _____ scientific method	e. Choosing actions to meet a desired goal.

SHORT ANSWER

Directions: Write a brief answer for each question.

(43) 1. List the components of the nursing process in order.

a. _____

b. _____

c. _____

d. _____

e. _____

(44)   2. In order to solve a problem, one should use the following steps:

     a. _____

     b. _____

     c. _____

     d. _____

     e. _____

(45)   3. Explain how critical thinking differs from ordinary thinking.

     _____

     _____

     _____

     _____

     _____

(45)   4. How could you have a peer help you learn to listen attentively?

     _____

     _____

     _____

     _____

     5. How might you improve your critical thinking skills?

     _____

     _____

     _____

     _____

(47)   6. How are patient problems usually prioritized?

     _____

     _____

(47)   7. When prioritizing nursing tasks, you should consider:

     _____

     _____

(47)   8. To maintain organization with a shift workload, you must be
_____ and _____
tasks as needed.

CONCEPT MAPPING

(46)   Make a concept map of your personal responsibilities. You might start by prioritizing your categories of responsibilities (home, family, community, work, school, etc.) Use a separate sheet of paper for this exercise.

Student Name_____

NCLEX-PN® EXAM REVIEW

*Directions: Choose the **best** answer(s) for each of the following questions.*

(43) 1. The nursing process
1. ensures high-quality nursing care.
2. is essential for the provision of nursing care.
3. provides a framework for planning, implementing, and evaluating nursing care.
4. guarantees expected outcomes will be met.

(48-49) 2. The development of clinical judgment requires (Select all that apply)
1. dedication to studying and learning.
2. critical thinking skills.
3. ability to delegate to others.
4. experience in the clinical setting.

(45) 3. Attentive listening requires (Select all that apply)
1. focusing on the topic of discussion.
2. a good bit of practice.
3. watching the speaker's face.
4. thinking of a response while listening.

(47) 4. When setting priorities for nursing care, problems that threaten health are considered
1. high priority.
2. not a priority.
3. low priority.
4. medium priority.

(47) 5. When all tasks have relatively high priority and it is not possible to accomplish them all, you must
1. postpone some of the tasks to the next shift.
2. rush through care for other patients to provide extra time.
3. delegate some tasks to others to complete.
4. apologize to the patient for what cannot be done.

CRITICAL THINKING ACTIVITY

Directions: Consider the following situation and determine what needs to be done. Then, using the problem-solving/decision-making process, prioritize what needs to be done.

You are a single mother and you have become a new nursing student. On the first day of classes you arrive at the college at 8:15 A.M. (0800). You must buy your books, find your classrooms, and buy a parking permit for the campus, as well as attend two classes at 9:00 A.M. (0900) and 11:00 A.M. (1100). Your daughter has had an earache and you need to call the doctor's office to obtain an afternoon appointment time for her. Your son needs some school supplies before tomorrow. You must grocery shop for food to fix dinner and the rest of the week's meals.

Priority Rating	What Needs to Be Done
_____	_____
_____	_____
_____	_____
_____	_____
_____	_____
_____	_____
_____	_____
_____	_____

MEETING CLINICAL OBJECTIVES

Directions: The following suggested activities will help you meet the stated clinical practice objectives for the chapter. Review your school's clinical objectives for the week and outline a plan of activities that will help you meet them. If you are unsure how to meet them, consult with your instructor at the beginning of the clinical day.

1. Ask several nurses in the clinical area how they organize their work for the shift.

2. Devise a personalized work organization form.

3. Practice attentive listening with different patients.

4. Think about the steps (components) of the nursing process as you carry out tasks on the unit. Decide what part of the process you are using for each task you perform.

STEPS TOWARD BETTER COMMUNICATION

VOCABULARY BUILDING GLOSSARY

Term	Pronunciation	Definition
attribute	AT tri bute	characteristic
coherent	co HER ent	fits together, connects logically
concisely	con CISE ly	briefly, in a few words
delegate	del e GATE (v)	to appoint another person to do something
dynamic	dy NAM ic	energetic, active
enhance	en HANCE	to make better, more complete
implement (v)	IM ple ment	use, put into action
input	IN put	information or advice from someone
overlapping	O' ver LAP ping	partly covering another thing or time
prognosis	prog NO sis	the expected outcome
unforeseen	UN fore seen	not expected

VOCABULARY SIMILARITIES EXERCISE

These words have different meanings depending on the pronunciation:

AT tri bute (n)—a characteristic; a TRI' bute (v)—to give credit to, or reason for

DEL e gate (n)—someone given responsibility; del e GATE (v)—to give responsibility to another

Directions: The following definitions for the individual words are all correct meanings. Check the ones that give the correct meaning for this phrase: "sound conclusions" (con CLU' sions).

sound: ___ correct   ___ noise   ___ healthy

conclusion: ___ an ending   ___ an opinion

The phrase "sound conclusions" means _____.

COMPLETION

Directions: Fill in the blank(s) with the correct word(s) from the Vocabulary Building Glossary to complete the sentence.

1. Performing a thorough patient assessment helps prevent _____ problems while giving care.

2. Once the nursing care plan is written, the nurse can _____ the individual actions.

3. Characteristics of effective writing are expressing thoughts coherently and _____.

4. The steps of assessment and evaluation of the nursing process are _____, in that assessment occurs during the evaluation phase to determine the effectiveness of actions.

5. Obtaining a complete patient history often requires _____ from the family.

6. Reading articles from the chapter bibliography will _____ learning.

7. The nursing care plan must be written in a(n) _____ manner so that all caregivers know exactly what the goals are and what actions to carry out.

8. Before explaining treatment plans to a patient, the physician should tell the patient the _____.

COMMUNICATION EXERCISES

1. You have prioritized care for your patients and attend to the man with chest pain before treating the boy with a cut arm. Your instructor asks, "Why did you decide to attend to the man with the chest pain first?"

   You respond: _____

   _____

   _____

   _____

   _____

2. Reread Critical Thinking Activity #2 in the chapter in the textbook. A nursing assistant has the only portable sphygmomanometer. What would you say to her to solve your problem?

   _____

   _____

   _____

   _____

ATTENTIVE LISTENING EXAMPLE

Directions: Practice the following dialogue with a partner.

You wish to delegate ambulating M.S. to the nursing assistant. You approach the aide to discuss this.

You: "I would like you to ambulate M.S. in room 232, bed 2, once this morning and again after lunch. She is recovering from pneumonia and is still quite weak. Please use a gait belt."

Aide: "I already have three baths to give and vital signs to take for eight patients. I don't know that I can fit ambulating her into my schedule."

You: "You have already been assigned to do eight sets of vital signs and three full baths?"

Aide: "Well, I'm to do the vital signs and set up the three patients for their baths, not give full bed baths."

You: "It seems like you will have time to do the ambulation. Let me check with you at 10:00 A.M. to see how things are going. If there is a problem, then I will have to find another way to ambulate her."

Review the chapter key points, answer the study questions, and complete the critical thinking activities at the end of the chapter in the textbook.

CHAPTER 5

Assessment, Nursing Diagnosis, and Planning

Answer Key: Textbook page references are provided as a guide for answering selected questions. A complete answer key was provided for your instructor.

TERMINOLOGY

Directions: Match the terms in Column I with the definitions in Column II.

Column I		Column II
(60)	1. _____ cues	a. Pieces of information on a specific topic.
(51)	2. _____ data	b. All the information gathered about a patient.
(63)	3. _____ goal	c. Conversation from which facts are obtained.
(60)	4. _____ signs	d. Conclusions made based on observed data.
(60)	5. _____ symptoms	e. Abnormalities objectively verifiable by objective means.
(52)	6. _____ interview	f. Data the patient says are occurring, but are not verifiable by objective means.
(51)	7. _____ database	g. Broad idea of what is to be achieved through nursing intervention.
(60)	8. _____ inferences	h. Pieces of information that influence decisions.

COMPLETION

Directions: Fill in the blank(s) with the correct word(s) to complete the sentence.

(51)   1. Assessment consists of gathering information about patients and their _____ using _____.

(52)   2. Assessment is a(n) _____ process.

(62)   3. Defining characteristics are the specific _____ and _____ attached to the nursing diagnosis that indicate the data from which the diagnosis was derived.

(60)   4. Etiologic factors are those factors that indicate the _____ of the patient's problem.

(60)   5.   A nursing diagnosis is a statement that indicates the patient's
_____ status or the risk of a(n)
_____, the causative or related factors, and the specific
_____.

        6.   In order to perform even the simplest nursing skill, you need to
_____ how to do it.

(65)   7.   Whenever nursing care is performed, it is essential to consider the
_____ needs of the patient.

(51)   8.   A nursing database is compiled by using the _____
process.

(60)   9.   The nursing problems present for a patient are determined by
_____ the assessment data.

(60)   10.   In many agencies, problems of the patient are stated as nursing
_____.

(62)   11.   Nursing care is delivered by considering the order of
_____ of the patient's needs or problems.

(63)   12.   Expected outcome statements should be written so that it is easy to
_____ whether they have been achieved.

(65)   13.   When formulating a nursing care plan, the nurse chooses interventions that are most likely
to achieve the _____.

(65-66)   14.   In order to function effectively, the nurse must use a method of
_____.

(52)   15.   Sources of data used for the formulation of a patient database are:

_____

_____

(52-59)   16.   Methods used to gather a patient database are:

      a.   _____

      b.   _____

      c.   _____

(64)   17.   List one piece of data or a patient need for each area of need indicated on the concept map in
Concept Map 5-3 for which you found a problem.

_____

_____

_____

_____

_____

_____

_____

Student Name_____

(63)   18. List three nursing diagnoses found in many long-term care residents that are problems of basic needs and are part of the reason the resident needed to be in a long-term care facility.

        a. _____

        b. _____

        c. _____

(52)   19. Under which of Gordon's 11 Functional Health Patterns would V.T.'s problem of left-sided weakness fit the best?

        _____

(52)   20. List the functional areas for each of the Gordon's functional health patterns that should be assessed when a problem is found related to that health pattern.

        _____

        _____

CORRELATION

Directions: For each of the following patient problems, choose the most appropriate nursing diagnosis from the NANDA list in your textbook.

(61)

1. B.A. is admitted with severe abdominal pain.

    _____

    _____

2. L.H. has fallen and fractured his hip.

    _____

    _____

3. J.T. is admitted with burns on his chest.

    _____

    _____

4. Although recovering, T.P. suffered a stroke that has paralyzed his right extremities. He is right-handed.

    _____

    _____

5. V.T. has emphysema and becomes very short of breath whenever she tries to perform a task.

    _____

    _____

NCLEX-PN® EXAM REVIEW

*Directions: Choose the **best** answer(s) for each of the following questions.*

(52) 1. Examples of objective data are (Select all that apply)
   1. blood pressure.
   2. pain.
   3. oxygen saturation level.
   4. itching.

(52) 2. History and physical examination provide both subjective data and objective data. Subjective data are data that _____ _____ _____. (Fill in the blank)

(60) 3. Analysis of the database is necessary for the formulation of
   1. expected outcomes/goals.
   2. nursing interventions.
   3. nursing diagnoses.
   4. evaluation statements.

(61) 4. Which of the following is a NANDA accepted nursing diagnosis?
   1. Gall stones
   2. Shortness of breath
   3. Impaired gas exchange
   4. Itching

(62) 5. The difference between a medical diagnosis and a nursing diagnosis is that a nursing diagnosis
   1. labels the illness.
   2. defines the patient's response to illness.
   3. indicates the priority of the problem.
   4. is made by the physician and nurse together.

(62) 6. When considering the order of priority of patient problems according to Maslow (Select all that apply)
   1. pain takes precedence over elimination needs.
   2. sleep is more important than food.
   3. inability to eat takes precedence over a risk of falling.
   4. oxygen needs take precedence over activity needs.

(63) 7. Short-term nursing goals are those that
   1. are accomplished before discharge from the hospital.
   2. take many weeks or months to accomplish.
   3. are achievable within 7–10 days.
   4. are achieved through medical intervention.

(63) 8. An expected outcome
   1. is a short-term goal.
   2. is data gathered after nursing intervention.
   3. is a broad, long-term goal statement.
   4. should contain measurable criteria.

(63) 9. The primary objective of choosing nursing interventions is to
   1. keep the patient safe and comfortable.
   2. help the patient meet the expected outcomes.
   3. carry out the physician's orders.
   4. organize the nurse's work for the shift.

(51, 65) 10. The LPN/LVN's role in nursing care planning is to (Select all that apply)
   1. assist with the writing of the nursing care plan.
   2. evaluate the plan written by the registered nurse.
   3. assist with the data collection process.
   4. write nursing diagnoses for the patient's problems.

Student Name_____

CRITICAL THINKING ACTIVITIES

1. Analyze the following assessment data obtained about a patient and determine the patient's needs. Then place the needs in order of priority.

   O.N., a 78-year-old female, is admitted with pain in the left hip after a fall. She is unable to move her left leg without severe pain. She is apprehensive and scared. There is a bruise on her left forearm. She cries out when she tries to move her left leg.

2. Choose appropriate nursing diagnoses from the NANDA list for the above patient's needs. Write expected outcomes for each nursing diagnosis chosen.

3. Determine which of the data from the above situation are objective and which are subjective. Write an "S" or "O" beside each one to indicate your choice.
   a. _____ Blood pressure is 132/84.
   b. _____ Cries out when leg is moved.
   c. _____ Has a bruise on left forearm.
   d. _____ Is apprehensive and scared.
   e. _____ Pulse is 92.
   f. _____ Winces when left leg is moved.
   g. _____ States that leg really hurts.
   h. _____ Respirations are 18.

MEETING CLINICAL OBJECTIVES

Directions: The following suggested activities will help you meet the stated clinical practice objectives for the chapter. Review your school's clinical objectives for the week and outline a plan of activities that will help you meet them. If you are unsure how to meet them, consult with your instructor at the beginning of the clinical day.

1. Before your first clinical patient assignment, perform an assessment on a classmate, friend, or family member.

2. Review the nursing assessment and history form on your assigned patient's chart. Note the types of information and the nursing comments it contains.

3. Find the physician's history and physical on your assigned patient's chart. Read it. Look up any unfamiliar terms.

4. Perform an assessment on your assigned patient. Now find the nursing care plan in the patient's chart. Determine if the nursing diagnoses designated for this patient are appropriate by determining if the data you collected support them. Are there other appropriate nursing diagnoses that seem to be missing?

STEPS TOWARD BETTER COMMUNICATION

VOCABULARY BUILDING GLOSSARY

Term	Pronunciation	Definition
affect	AFF ect	emotional feeling or expression
alleviate	al LEV i ate	to relieve, make less painful
concurrent conditions	con CUR rent con DI tions	conditions happening at the same time

correlate	corr e LATE	to show how one thing relates meaningfully to another
deviate	DE vi ATE	to be different, or move away from
differentiate	diff er EN tiate	to show differences among several things
elicit	e LI cit	to get, bring out (usually information)
formulate	FORM u late	to put together, organize
infer	in FER	to guess, or figure out from the information given
next of kin	NEXT of kin	closest relative
over-the-counter	O ver the COUN ter	medications available without prescription
pertinent	PER ti nent	directly relating to a situation
prosthesis	pros THE sis	an artificial limb (hand, arm, leg, etc.)
rapport	ra POR (t is silent)	a sympathetic relationship between people
scan	sCAN	to look over quickly
significant other	sig NIF i cant other	someone important to the patient, usually a spouse or close loved one—not a blood relative

COMPLETION

Directions: Fill in the blank(s) with the correct word(s) from the Vocabulary Building Glossary to complete the sentence.

1. Jan is Tom's _____ and has lived with him for 8 years.

2. It is not a good idea to _____ from the accepted procedure when administering medications.

3. Sometimes it is difficult to _____ between symptoms of a minor illness and a major illness in the beginning stages.

4. Ibuprofen is a commonly used _____ medication.

5. Whether a patient is experiencing side effects of medication is _____ information to have before giving another dose of the medication.

6. Heat is sometimes used to _____ pain.

7. Once all the assessment data are gathered, the nurse will _____ the nursing care plan.

8. When unexpectedly assigned a new patient, it is good to _____ the chart for the current diagnostic test results.

9. Nurses learn to _____ laboratory data with the signs and symptoms the patient has.

10. Diabetes is often a(n) _____ for a patient who is hospitalized for renal failure.

11. When the lower leg is amputated, the patient will be fitted with a(n) _____.

12. When the blank on the admission form for "religion" lists "none," one can _____ that the patient does not belong to an organized religious group.

Student Name _____

WORD ATTACK SKILLS

Directions: Pronounce these word pairs, and tell the difference in the definition of the noun and the verb or adjective.

1. rapport (n) _____

   report (n) _____

2. elicit (v)_____

   illicit (adj) _____

3. affect (v) _____

   effect (n) _____

Usage note: the verb "affect" means to have an influence or cause a change. The noun "affect" means the general feeling or emotion felt by a person. *Her diet affected her health. Her affect reflected how poorly she was feeling.*

COMMUNICATION EXERCISE

Directions: You need to assess Ms. N. for pain. Here is an example of such a communication interaction. Practice the dialog with a peer, taking turns being the nurse and the patient.

Nurse: "Are you having much pain this morning?"

Ms. N.: "Yes, I'm hurting quite a bit."

Nurse: "Can you show me where it seems to be hurting the most?"

Ms. N.: (Points to the area of her incision over the hip.) "It's mostly right here, but it does go down this leg muscle."

Nurse: "Can you describe the type of pain you are experiencing?"

Ms. N.: "It is a dull ache with throbbing in the incision area. When I move, I get a stabbing pain here in my thigh."

Nurse: "How would you rate it on a scale of 1–10 with 1 being the least pain and 10 being the most pain?"

Ms. N.: "I guess I would rate it at about 8."

Nurse: "OK, I think it is probably time for some more pain medication now. I'll check to see when you last had it."

Other terms that might be used to describe pain are: *sharp, dull, burning, knife-like, radiating, searing, needle-like.*

Review the chapter key points, answer the study questions, and complete the critical thinking activities at the end of the chapter in the textbook.

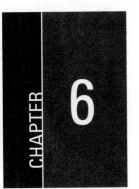

CHAPTER

6 Implementation and Evaluation

Answer Key: Textbook page references are provided as a guide for answering selected questions. A complete answer key was provided for your instructor.

TERMINOLOGY

Directions: Match the terms in Column I with the definitions in Column II.

Column I

(70)   1. _____ implementation
(70)   2. _____ interventions
(73)   3. _____ documentation
(71)   4. _____ evaluation
(71)   5. _____ clinical pathway
(75)   6. _____ outcome-based quality improvement
(75)   7. _____ nursing audit
(71)   8. _____ independent nursing action
(71)   9. _____ dependent nursing action
(71)   10. _____ interdependent action
(70)   11. _____ time-flexible
(70)   12. _____ time-fixed

Column II

a. Can be done at any time
b. Step-by-step approach to total care of the patient
c. Manage the quality of performance
d. Carry out nursing interventions
e. Must be done at a set time
f. Nursing action based on nursing judgment that does not require an order
g. Action requiring a health care provider's order
h. Examination of patient records to see if care meets accepted standards
i. Assessment of effectiveness of nursing actions in meeting expected outcomes
j. Actions that come from collaborative care planning
k. Recording of pertinent data on the clinical record
l. Actions involving more than one health care professional

SHORT ANSWER

A.   *Directions: Recalling information from Chapters 4 and 5, complete the following exercise. For each nursing action on the left, give the name of the step of the nursing process in which the action occurs (assessment, nursing diagnosis, planning, implementation, evaluation).*

1. Interviewing the patient to obtain a history.   _____

2. Setting a goal for improved mobility.   _____

3. Assisting the patient to turn, cough, and deep-breathe after surgery.   _____

4. Auscultating for bowel sounds. _____

5. Checking a lab report to see if there are abnormalities in the patient's urine. _____

6. Teaching a patient to take his or her own blood pressure. _____

7. Reaching the conclusion that the patient has a fluid volume deficit. _____

8. Gathering data to determine if expected outcomes have been met. _____

9. Writing *Activity Intolerance related to decreased oxygenation* on the nursing care plan. _____

10. Checking the intake and output record to see if the patient is taking in 1500 mL of fluid a day as planned. _____

11. Writing "Pain will be controlled by analgesia within 8 hours" on the nursing care plan. _____

12. Writing on the nursing care plan "Encourage family to bring in ethnic foods allowed on therapeutic diet." _____

B. *Directions: Write a short answer or fill in the blanks for each of the following questions.*

(70) 1. The first step in organizing actions for implementation is to set _____.

(70) 2. Clues for imminent deadlines for certain tasks can be found in the _____.

(70) 3. When planning time for uninterrupted care, consider:

    a. _____

    b. _____

    c. _____

    d. _____

(70) 4. Before carrying out a planned nursing action, in addition to knowing the reason for the intervention, the expected outcome, and the usual standard of care, it is necessary to consider _____.

(71) 5. The clinical pathway is a(n) _____ approach to patient care and is an outgrowth of _____ care.

(71) 6. The designated standard of care for performing a procedure can be found in the _____.

(74) 7. After implementing patient care, _____ must be done.

Student Name _____

(74) 8. You will know goals have been met when _____ have been reached.

(74) 9. Evaluation is a(n) _____ process.

(74) 10. Nursing care plans are usually revised every _____.

(72) 11. Interventions may be performed by _____ in the home health setting.

(71) 12. A(n) _____ or _____ procedure may not be delegated to a nursing assistant in the long-term care setting.

(71) 13. It is necessary for the nurse to _____ documentation of the nursing assistants, as ultimate responsibility for documentation lies with the nurse.

SETTING PRIORITIES

Directions: Considering the Standard Steps used when performing a nursing procedure, prioritize the following with #1 being highest priority and #7 being lowest.

1. _____ Clean and dispose of used supplies.
2. _____ Document.
3. _____ Prepare the patient.
4. _____ Explain the procedure.
5. _____ Wash your hands.
6. _____ Perform the procedure.
7. _____ Restore the unit and make the patient comfortable.

NCLEX-PN® EXAM REVIEW

*Directions: These questions require use of prior knowledge from preceding chapters. Choose the **best** answer(s) for each of the following questions.*

1. A part of the assessment step of the nursing process is
   1. setting goals to be accomplished.
   2. gathering data about the patient's condition.
   3. choosing nursing interventions to solve problems.
   4. carrying out nursing interventions to meet the goals.

2. Nursing diagnosis is a way of
   1. stating patient problems.
   2. labeling the patient's medical problem.
   3. devising a nursing care plan.
   4. analyzing assessment data.

3. Which one of the following is a correctly written expected outcome for the nursing diagnosis *Pain related to abdominal incision*?
   1. Pain will be relieved by giving analgesia.
   2. Analgesia will be given for pain relief.
   3. Pain will be relieved before discharge.
   4. Pain will be controlled by analgesia for at least 3 hours.

4. When implementing nursing orders on the care plan, it is *most* important to consider
   1. the safety of the patient.
   2. convenience for the patient.
   3. the degree of importance of the task.
   4. whether a procedure will be interrupted.

5. When evaluating whether the expected outcome "Wound infection will subside within 7 days" has been met, you would gather which of the following data? (Select all that apply)
   1. evidence that the antibiotic doses were given
   2. appearance and characteristics of the wound
   3. evidence that the patient is taking decreasing amounts of pain medication
   4. downward trend in the patient's temperature chart

(71) 6. Which one of the following would be an independent nursing action?
   1. giving a medication
   2. applying a heating pad
   3. assisting a patient with speech therapy practice
   4. teaching about the side effects of a medication

(71) 7. Which of the following is true regarding a care path?
   1. It is devised by the physician and the nurse.
   2. All disciplines involved in the patient's care provide input.
   3. It addresses only the critical problems of the patient.
   4. It is a standardized plan of care used for each patient.

(71) 8. Efficiently implementing patient care requires
   1. following the procedure manual's standards of care.
   2. following a work organization plan exactly.
   3. prioritizing and combining tasks.
   4. enlisting the help of a nurse's aide.

(74) 9. Evaluation as a step of the nursing process is a method of determining
   1. whether actions are effective in helping the patient reach expected outcomes.
   2. how expected outcomes should be written on the nursing care plan.
   3. which patient problems need to be addressed first.
   4. whether the nursing diagnosis was chosen correctly.

(75) 10. The goal of a outcome-based quality improvement program is to
   1. make nurses evaluate the care they give.
   2. identify care that is not up to the standard.
   3. determine if nurses are documenting care accurately.
   4. improve nursing practice within an agency.

(71) 11. There are independent and dependent nursing actions. Dependent actions require a health care provider's order. Your male patient has had a hip replacement. When you go to check on him, he is grimacing and says he needs pain medication. When asked, he states that his pain is at a 7 on a scale of 1–10. You check the orders and give him his narcotic analgesic. This action is a(n) _____ nursing action. (Fill in the blank)

Student Name _____

12. An expected outcome for the above patient's nursing diagnosis of *Pain related to surgical procedure* is "Pain will be relieved for at least 3 hours with medication." An important part of writing an expected outcome is that it must be
    1. subjective.
    2. relevant.
    3. measurable.
    4. patient-oriented.

(74) 13. The evaluation step of the nursing process determines
    1. if all the actions on the plan were implemented.
    2. whether the expected outcomes are measurable.
    3. the patient's response to medical treatment.
    4. if actions have helped the patient meet the expected outcomes.

(75) 14. When evaluation shows that the expected outcomes are not being met, you would
    1. consider different actions to assist the patient to meet the outcomes.
    2. revise the nursing diagnosis.
    3. rewrite the expected outcomes.
    4. reassess the patient's status and rewrite the entire nursing care plan.

15. The difference between a goal and an expected outcome is that a goal is
    1. more specific.
    2. patient-oriented.
    3. broader.
    4. long-term.

CRITICAL THINKING ACTIVITIES

1. What factors will you consider when planning your work for a shift?

2. Identify the positive aspects of a quality management program for nursing.

3. L.R. was injured in an automobile accident. You are assigned to care for him. Consider the following information and then construct a nursing care plan for this patient.

   L.R. had surgery 2 days ago for removal of a ruptured spleen. He has an abdominal incision that is oozing slightly onto the dressing. He has a badly swollen right knee and bruises on the right extremities. He cannot walk without pain. He states that he is very sore and that his incisional area is hurting. He states that the pain is a 6 on a scale of 1–10. His orders read "Daily dressing change; Vicodin q4h prn pain; right leg elevated; BRP with assistance."

   How would you evaluate the success of your care plan?

4. Can you make a concept map of the nursing diagnoses and interventions for this patient?

MEETING CLINICAL OBJECTIVES

Directions: The following suggested activities will help you meet the stated clinical practice objectives for the chapter. Review your school's clinical objectives for the week and outline a plan of activities that will help you meet them. If you are unsure how to meet them, consult with your instructor at the beginning of the clinical day.

1. Devise your own work organization form/tool.

2. Study how unit nurses perform procedures. Are they carrying out the Standard Steps?

3. Construct a nursing care plan for an assigned patient.

4. Revise the above-constructed nursing care plan at the end of the shift.

STEPS TOWARD BETTER COMMUNICATION

VOCABULARY BUILDING GLOSSARY

Term	Pronunciation	Definition
accreditation	a ccred i TA tion	approval to a set of standards
adept	a DEPT	skillful; clever
agency-wide	A gen cy wide	through all departments or people in an agency
blame	blAMe	to accuse; say someone is responsible for something bad
buckling	BUCK ling	fastening with a buckle
clue	CLUE	information that helps provide an answer
collaborative	col LAB bo ra tive	working together with others
deadline	DEAD line	the time or date when something must be completed
imminent	IM mi nent	immediate, ready to happen soon
impairment	im PAIR ment	weakness or damage
incorporated into	in COR por a ted into	made a part of; included in
intervening	in ter VEN ing	coming between
latter	LA tter	the last of two things mentioned
process evaluation	PRO cess e val u A tion	looking at how well a process is working
rationale	ra tion ALE	the reasons behind a decision
refresh your memory	re FRESH your MEM o ry	to go back and think about something again
sequence	SE quence	a connected series of acts; an order
strive	strIve	to try hard

COMPLETION

Directions: Fill in the blank(s) with the correct word(s) from the Vocabulary Building Glossary to complete the sentence.

1. The _____ for the assignment to be turned in was Friday.

2. It is important to master skills quickly as the first clinical day is
    _____.

3. Nursing care planning is a(n) _____ process among nurses and other health professionals.

4. Each student should _____ to be well-prepared for each clinical day.

Student Name _____

5. The stroke left the patient with left-sided _____.

6. That nurse is _____ at eliciting information quickly from patients.

7. The patient fell in the hall, but did not _____ the nurse for his fall.

8. Having clinical days on Tuesday and Thursday is difficult because of the _____ lecture day.

9. The fine rash provided a(n) _____ about what might be wrong with the patient.

10. Nurse's notes must be written in the _____ in which events occur.

11. Patient teaching is often _____ into providing patient care.

12. An instructor will often ask for the _____ of a step of a nursing procedure.

WORD ATTACK SKILLS

Some words and phrases have equal meaning (synonyms):

write = note = jot down

clinical pathway = care path = care map

Equivalent words may have different meanings and pronunciations depending upon how they are used.

Verbs	Nouns	Nouns
note	note	no TA tion
im ple MENT	IM ple ment	im ple men TA tion
doc u MENT	DOC u ment	doc u men TA tion
in ter VENE	in ter VEN tion	
pri OR i tize	pri OR i TY	pri or i ti ZA tion

The suffix "-ation/tion" means an action or a process, or something connected with an action or a process: *Intervention is the act, or result, of intervening.*

ABBREVIATIONS

Directions: Give the meaning for each abbreviation.

1. ST _____

2. LT _____

3. q _____

4. 4h _____

5. ROM _____

6. PT _____

7. CVA_____

8. r/t _____

9. UA_____

10. OBQI _____

COMMUNICATION EXERCISES

1. Make a list of questions you would like to ask a unit nurse about performing a patient assessment. Make brief notes of the answers you receive and later rewrite them into complete sentences.

2. Make a list of points to consider when you are making a work organization plan for giving patient care. Remember to include visiting time, diagnostic tests, doctors' rounds, and so forth.

CULTURAL POINTS

1. Some questions and procedures may seem very personal and even objectionable to some people of different ages and cultures. For example, an older woman of any culture may feel uncomfortable having a male nurse doing peri-care, or a man may feel uncomfortable being catheterized by a female nurse. In some cultures where the women dress very modestly and may not even have much social contact with men outside the family (as in some Muslim groups), having a male nurse or even a male doctor examine them and observe or touch their unclothed bodies could make them uncomfortable or be considered sinful.

2. Southeast Asian immigrants may believe that the spirit might leave the body on risky occasions, so they tie a string around the wrist of the patient to bind the spirit to the body. Nurses may be tempted to remove these strings before transporting the patient to the operating room, but this is very traumatic for the patient, and there is an emotional value in leaving on the strings. If the nurse is from such a culture or of an older generation, he or she may find it difficult or uncomfortable to perform some of these required procedures.

3. Remember that what is required is done for the good of the patient and is necessary for the success of the diagnosis and treatment. Such questions and procedures must be handled in a matter-of-fact and straightforward manner.

4. Nursing care plans need to take into account the needs and beliefs of patients of different ethnic backgrounds, and those of their families. Food preferences should be accommodated as much as possible within the prescribed diet and capabilities of the dietary department.

Review the chapter key points, answer the study questions, and complete the critical thinking activities at the end of the chapter in the textbook.

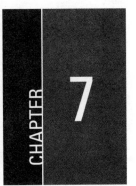

Student Name _____

CHAPTER **7**

Documentation of Nursing Care

Answer Key: Textbook page references are provided as a guide for answering selected questions. A complete answer key was provided for your instructor.

TERMINOLOGY

Directions: Match the charting acronym in Column I with the correct meaning in Column II.

Column I		Column II
(83) 1. _____ POMR		a. Data, action, response
(82) 2. _____ MAR		b. Subjective data, objective data, assessment, plan
(87) 3. _____ PIE		c. Medication administration record
(86) 4. _____ SOAP		d. Problem-oriented medical record
(86) 5. _____ SOAPIE		e. Plan, implementation, evaluation
(87) 6. _____ DAR		f. Subjective data, objective data, assessment, plan, implementation, evaluation

VOCABULARY

Directions: Using the textbook glossary or your dictionary, match the term in Column I that is useful in documentation with its meaning in Column II.

Column I		Column II
1. _____ radiates		a. Difficulty breathing
2. _____ productive cough		b. Large amount
3. _____ copious		c. Coughing up material
4. _____ serosanguineous		d. Spreads to other areas
5. _____ spasm		e. Situated close together
6. _____ dyspnea		f. Empty the bladder
7. _____ paresthesia		g. Containing an excess of fluid
8. _____ paroxysmal		h. Mixed blood and serum
9. _____ distended		i. Sudden attacks
10. _____ void		j. Localized muscle contraction
11. _____ edematous		k. Enlarged; stretched out
12. _____ exudate		l. Itching
13. _____ approximated		m. Numbness and tingling
14. _____ intact		n. Undisturbed, uninjured
15. _____ pruritus		o. Fluid with cellular debris

SHORT ANSWER

Directions: Write a brief answer for each question.

(81)   1.   Three purposes of documentation are:

   a. _____

   b. _____

   c. _____

(95)   2.   The medical record is a legal document and for that reason nurses must adhere to the following rules:

   a. _____

   b. _____

   c. _____

   d. _____

   e. _____

   f. _____

   g. _____

   h. _____

   i. _____

(83)   3.   Briefly correlate the nursing process to the process of charting.

   _____

   _____

   _____

   _____

   _____

(83)   4.   The six main methods of charting are:

   a. _____

   b. _____

   c. _____

   d. _____

   e. _____

   f. _____

COMPLETION

Directions: Fill in the blank(s) with the correct word(s) to correctly complete the sentence.

(81)   1.   Insurance companies rely on documentation to _____
reimbursement of expenses for care given.

Student Name _____

(81)   2.   Documentation is used to track the application of the
_____.

(81)   3.   Documentation should show progress toward _____
listed on the nursing care plan.

(83)   4.   Only health care professionals _____ for
the patient, or those involved in legitimate research or teaching, should have
_____ to the chart.

(83)   5.   The chart is the property of the _____.

(84)   6.   Narrative charting requires the documentation of care in
_____ order.

(84)   7.   An advantage of source-oriented—or narrative—charting is that it indicates the patient's
_____ for each shift.

(85)   8.   POMR methods of charting are said to improve continuity of care and communication by
keeping _____ related to a problem all in one place.

(87)   9.   Focus charting is directed at a nursing diagnosis, a patient
_____, a concern, a sign, a symptom, or a(n)
_____.

(88)   10.   An advantage of the FOCUS charting method is that it shortens charting time by using many
_____ and _____.

(88)   11.   Charting by exception is based on the assumption that all standards of practice are carried out and result in a normal or expected response unless
_____.

(88)   12.   The heart of the charting by exception method is unit-specific
_____ and standards of nursing care.

(89)   13.   An advantage of the charting by exception method of documentation is
that it highlights _____ and patient
_____.

(91)   14.   An advantage of some computer-assisted charting is that documentation is done as
_____ are performed.

(91)   15.   To protect patient confidentiality when using computer-assisted charting, each nurse must
have a(n) _____ in order to access the computerized chart.

(91)   16.   A major advantage of computer documentation is that notes are always
_____.

(91)   17.   When a case management system is used, documentation of
_____ is placed on the back of the care path sheets.

(91)   18.   When documenting, the patient's needs, problems, and activities should be presented in
terms of _____.

(96)   19.   A Kardex is a quick reference for current information about the patient and
_____.

(92)   20.   Home care charting must particularly note _____ in
place and the need for _____.

ABBREVIATIONS

Directions: Consult Appendix 6 and list the abbreviation for each of the following terms that are often used when charting.

(Appendix 6)

1. activities of daily living _____
2. as desired _____
3. estrogen replacement therapy _____
4. bathroom privileges _____
5. genitourinary _____
6. dyspnea on exertion _____
7. coronary artery disease _____
8. chief complaint _____
9. hypertension _____
10. upper respiratory infection _____
11. within normal limits _____
12. last menstrual period _____
13. transient ischemic attack _____
14. potassium _____
15. treatment _____
16. congestive heart failure _____
17. right lower quadrant _____
18. discontinue _____
19. date of birth _____
20. electrocardiogram _____
21. short of breath _____
22. fetal heart rate _____
23. health maintenance organization _____
24. left lower lobe _____
25. magnetic resonance imaging _____
26. immediately _____
27. nothing by mouth _____
28. physical therapy _____
29. range of motion _____
30. urinalysis _____

Student Name_____

NCLEX-PN® EXAM REVIEW

*Directions: Choose the **best** answer(s) for each of the following questions.*

(82) 1. The patient's occupation and religious preference may be found on the
   1. physician's history and physical sheets.
   2. nursing admission assessment sheets.
   3. face sheet of the chart.
   4. admission and treatment consent form.

(84) 2. A specific advantage of source-oriented or narrative charting is that it
   1. is lengthy and thorough.
   2. provides subjective information about the patient.
   3. reflects the patient's conditions in chronological order.
   4. is concise and often read by physicians.

(86) 3. A disadvantage of POMR documentation is that it
   1. provides for control of quality of care.
   2. reduces duplication of information and recording.
   3. speaks only to abnormalities in the patient's condition.
   4. fragments data due to much recording on flow sheets.

(87) 4. A FOCUS charting note contains
   1. description of the patient's present condition.
   2. data, action, and response.
   3. subjective information, objective information, assessment, and plan.
   4. statement of problem, action, and result.

(88) 5. Charting by exception's goal is to
   1. provide a comprehensive database.
   2. decrease lengthy narrative entries.
   3. utilize flow sheets only.
   4. make charting flow more smoothly.

(82) 6. There are many different flow sheets used in charting. The total amount of oral fluids consumed for the shift is recorded on the

   _____

   flow sheet. (Fill in the blank)

(82) 7. A notation of a physician's visit to the patient should be made by the nurse on the
   1. nurse's notes or activity flow sheet.
   2. consultation record.
   3. Kardex or computer care plan.
   4. physician's order sheet.

(82) 8. The type of IV catheter in use would be found charted on the
   1. physician's order sheet.
   2. daily activity flow sheet.
   3. medication administration record.
   4. intravenous flow sheet.

(95) 9. A legally acceptable way to correct a charting error is to
   1. use "white-out" to keep the chart neat.
   2. line through the word and write "mistaken entry" above it.
   3. use ink to obliterate the word and write a word above it.
   4. tear out the page the error is on and begin charting for that shift again.

(94)   10. Which of the following are considered essential information to be included in documentation? (Select all that apply)
1. number of friends who visited
2. change in a sign or symptom
3. changes in behavior
4. physician's visit

(App 6)   11. The patient has redness of the left eye. "Left eye" is abbreviated as
1. OD.
2. OS.
3. OU.
4. LE.

(95)   12. Rules to follow when documenting are to (Select all that apply)
1. use complete sentences.
2. use only accepted abbreviations.
3. spell all words correctly.
4. include your opinion.

(95)   13. If another nurse asks you to chart on a patient for him or her and gives you a list of the data, you should
1. chart chronologically according to the list.
2. refuse to chart what you have not done yourself.
3. ask what else you can do to help as you cannot chart for the other nurse.
4. chart on the activity flow sheets, but not in the nurse's notes.

(81)   14. A very important part of charting from the hospital's point of view is
1. noting the physician's visits.
2. noting the discharge time on the chart.
3. documenting when visitors come.
4. documenting equipment being used.

(95)   15. When documenting that a patient has refused a treatment, you should include
1. consequences of refusing the treatment.
2. why the treatment was refused.
3. attempts to change the patient's mind.
4. why the treatment is important to recovery.

CRITICAL THINKING ACTIVITIES

1. Compare the six different forms of charting and choose the one that seems to you to be the most logical and easy to use.

2. From the following scenario, list the assessment data, define the main problem in the form of a nursing diagnosis, and write an expected outcome.

   J.T., age 22, was involved in an automobile accident. She arrives via ambulance at the emergency room. She is able to answer questions and can follow commands, although she is strapped to a backboard to prevent spinal movement. Her pupils are equal and reactive to light. X-rays show a fracture of her right femur and she is unable to move her right leg without excruciating pain. There is a laceration on her right wrist. She complains of pain in the right wrist.

Student Name_____

Assessment data:

Nursing diagnosis:

Expected outcome:

MEETING CLINICAL OBJECTIVES

Directions: The following suggested activities will help you meet the stated clinical practice objectives for the chapter. Review your school's clinical objectives for the week and outline a plan of activities that will help you meet them. If you are unsure how to meet them, consult with your instructor at the beginning of the clinical day.

1. After obtaining permission, read nurse's notes that staff nurses have written and identify four characteristics of good documentation.

2. Review each of the flow sheet chart forms for the types of information to be recorded.

3. Write out nurse's notes daily on each assigned patient, trying to create a "picture" of the patient for someone else reading the notes. Edit your notes to make them more concise and objective.

4. Review the hospital charting/documentation manual for specific requirements of the assigned facility that may vary from what you learned in lecture or from textbooks.

5. Ask a staff nurse to show you how the computer is used in the facility to chart, update care plans, order supplies, discontinue charges, and so forth.

STEPS TOWARD BETTER COMMUNICATION

VOCABULARY BUILDING GLOSSARY

Term	Pronunciation	Definition
acronym	AC ro nym	a word formed from the first letters or parts of other words
adage	AD age	a saying
adhere to	ad HERE to	follow rules, pay attention to
ambiguous	am BIG u ous	not clear, not specific
audit	AU dit	an official examination of records
brevity	BREV i ty	not using a lot of words, shortness
compiled	com PILEd	to put together item by item
duration	du RA tion	the length of time
jot	JOT	make a quick written note
noteworthy	NOTE wor thy	important
offshoot	OFF shoot	a new development or direction
reimbursement	re im BURSE ment	to pay back someone for money that has been paid out
rule of thumb	RULE of thumb	a guideline
time frame	TIME frame	limits of a period of time

VOCABULARY EXERCISES

Directions: Substitute words from the glossary for the underlined words.

1. The <u>saying</u> was <u>not clear.</u>

   The _____ was _____.

2. The <u>examination of records</u> showed a need to <u>pay back</u> the patient's money.

   The _____ showed a need to
   _____ the patient's money.

3. The <u>guideline</u> is that <u>the length of time</u> of the office visit should <u>follow</u> the rules.

   The _____ is that the _____
   of the office visit should _____ the rules.

4. The student should <u>make a quick note of</u> the <u>letters standing for words</u> that she feels are <u>important</u> and <u>put together</u> a list.

   The student should _____ down the
   _____ that she feels are _____
   and _____ a list.

5. The <u>limited time</u> required the doctor use <u>only a few words</u> in talking about the <u>new development</u> in the problem.

   The _____ required that the doctor use _____ in talking about the
   _____ in the problem.

PRONUNCIATION AND INTONATION SKILLS

A statement ends with a falling voice pitch or intonation. For example: She has completed the documentation.

A question may end with either a rising or a falling intonation of the voice.

Questions that can be answered "yes" or "no" end with a rising pitch: (N=nurse; S=student)

1. N: Did you complete the charting?

   S: Yes, I did.

2. N: Is the patient ready for surgery?

   S: Yes, he is.

3. N: Are there any donuts left in the coffee room?

   S: No, sorry. They are all gone!

Questions that ask for information with a question word ("who," "what," "when," "where," etc.) end with a falling pitch.

1. N: When did you give the meds?

   S: Fifteen minutes ago.

2. N: Who is working the second shift?

   S: M.A.

Student Name _____

3. N: Why is the computer terminal still on?

    S: Oops, sorry. I forgot to turn it off.

Directions: Look at the following sentences and mark whether the pitch is rising (up) or falling (down). Practice asking and answering the questions with a partner.

1. Where is the doctor?   up   down

2. Have you finished taking the vital signs?   up   down

3. Can I bring you some fresh water?   up   down

4. What was K.J.'s temperature?   up   down

5. Did you initial the error in the chart? up   down

6. Who ate all the donuts?   up   down

COMMUNICATION EXERCISE

Look at the method of charting you chose in Critical Thinking Activity #1 in the textbook chapter. Explain to a partner why you chose that method of charting. Listen to your partner explain his or her choice.

Review the chapter key points, answer the study questions, and complete the critical thinking activities at the end of the chapter in the textbook.

CHAPTER 8

Communication and the Nurse-Patient Relationship

Answer Key: Textbook page references are provided as a guide for answering selected questions. A complete answer key was provided for your instructor.

TERMINOLOGY

A. Matching

Directions: Match the terms in Column I with the definitions in Column II.

		Column I		Column II
(107)	1.	_____ aphasic	a.	Communication in words
(99)	2.	_____ congruent	b.	Return of information and how it was interpreted
(106)	3.	_____ empathy		
(100)	4.	_____ feedback	c.	Relationship of mutual trust or affinity
(110)	5.	_____ input	d.	Communication without words
(99)	6.	_____ nonverbal	e.	Ability to understand by seeing the situation from another's perspective
(105)	7.	_____ rapport		
(99)	8.	_____ verbal	f.	In agreement
			g.	Difficulty expressing or understanding language
			h.	Information given or put in

B. Completion

Directions: Fill in the blank(s) with the correct word(s) to complete the sentence.

active listening   confidentiality
body language   shift report
communication   therapeutic

(109)   1.   The essential communication regarding patients that takes place between nurses going off a shift and those coming on the next shift is termed ___shift report___.

(99)   2.   A patient may express pain by using ___body language___ rather than explicitly telling a nurse.

(99)   3.   ___Communication___ of messages is a continuous, circular process occurring both verbally and nonverbally.

(8)   4.   ___therapeutic___ communication promotes understanding between the sender and the receiver.

(101)   5.   Concentration and focusing on what is being said by the other person is essential for
_____active listening_____.

(106)   6.   _____Confidentiality_____ must be kept for all communication between the patient and the nurse.

SHORT ANSWER

Directions: Write a brief answer for each question.

(99)   1.   Necessary components of the communication process are:

_____

_____

_____

(100)   2.   Factors that influence communication are:

a.   _____

b.   _____

c.   _____

d.   _____

(103)   3.   When conducting an admission interview, both closed-ended questions and open-ended questions are used. List three types of information for which you would want to ask a closed-ended question:

a.   _____

b.   _____

c.   _____

(106)   4.   An example of an open-ended question that might be asked during an admission interview would be:

_____

(110)   5.   Identify four ways to delegate effectively:

a.   _____

b.   _____

c.   _____

d.   _____

(106)   6.   Three key factors in the nurse-patient relationship are that this relationship:

a.   _____

b.   _____

c.   _____

(106)   7.   In a therapeutic relationship, interaction between the nurse and the patient should

_____.

Student Name_____

(106) 8. Four characteristics of the nurse that facilitate a therapeutic nurse-patient relationship are:

  a. _____

  b. _____

  c. _____

  d. _____

(110) 9. When calling a physician regarding a patient, you should assess the patient before the call. What data should you have on hand in case the physician asks for it?

  _____

  _____

  _____

(110) 10. List three tasks you as a nurse might have to perform by computer during a shift.

  a. _____

  b. _____

  c. _____

(108) 11. To communicate more successfully with the elderly patient, it is best to:

  a. _____

  b. _____

  c. _____

  d. _____

(108) 12. When communicating with a young child, the best techniques are to:

  _____

  _____

  _____

(108) 13. Three specific actions to increase success when trying to communicate with an aphasic person are:

  a. _____

  b. _____

  c. _____

(108) 14. When communicating with a hearing-impaired patient, four specific actions that enhance success are:

  a. _____

  b. _____

  c. _____

  d. _____

NCLEX-PN® EXAM REVIEW

*Directions: Choose the **best** answer(s) for each of the following questions.*

(101) 1. Within the communication process, active listening is very important. However, in order for the initiator of the communication to know that the message was received,
1. an answer must be given.
2. feedback must be received.
3. words must be spoken by each person.
4. the listener's expression must indicate comprehension.

(101) 2. Greater comprehension of what a person is saying will occur if the nurse also pays attention to the
1. timbre of the voice.
2. level of the vocabulary used.
3. body language displayed.
4. degree of enthusiasm expressed.

(101) 3. The "active listener" (Select all that apply)
1. maintains eye contact.
2. give cues that show interest.
3. blocks out distractions.
4. doesn't interrupt.

(102) 4. The use of silence in therapeutic communication is to encourage
1. verbalization of feelings or thoughts.
2. a nonthreatening atmosphere.
3. expression of concerns.
4. expression of innermost thoughts.

(104-105) 5. There are therapeutic techniques for communication and some that are nontherapeutic. Nurses do a lot of patient teaching, but giving advice is considered _____ _____ to therapeutic communication. (Fill in the blank)

(106) 6. A nonjudgmental attitude is essential for
1. effective communication.
2. a therapeutic nurse-patient relationship.
3. adequate comprehension of patient teaching.
4. collaboration regarding patient care.

(109) 7. Giving a shift report is a daily nursing task. A thorough report on an average patient should take about
1. 3–5 minutes.
2. 30–60 seconds.
3. 1–3 minutes.
4. 1 1/2–2 minutes.

(103) 8. Touch can be therapeutic and must be used judiciously. It may be used to signify
1. agreement with what is being said.
2. caring and comfort.
3. the need to listen closely.
4. the need to gain the person's attention.

(104) 9. The best way to encourage elaboration when interacting with a patient is to say,
1. "I'm not certain that I follow what you mean."
2. "The treatment caused pain?"
3. "I'll listen if you will tell me more."
4. "We'll continue after the doctor checks you over."

(105) 10. An example of offering false reassurance would be to say,
1. "We'll have the report back in 3 days."
2. "The pathologist is very good."
3. "The results only take 24–48 hours."
4. "I'm sure the pathology report will be just fine."

Student Name _____

(106)   11.   Empathy is
1. feeling concerned about how another is feeling.
2. showing you care about the other person.
3. placing oneself in another's position to understand how she or he feels.
4. making sympathetic statements to someone who has had a loss.

(108)   12.   When communicating with an elderly person who is slightly hard of hearing it is important to (Select all that apply)
1. speak normally, but distinctly.
2. eliminate other noise in the room.
3. speak in low tones.
4. face the listener.

(108)   13.   One action that enhances communication success with a hearing-impaired person is to
1. sit within 5 feet of the person.
2. be sure the area is well-lit.
3. be certain to face the person when speaking.
4. use higher tones when speaking.

(101)   14.   Which one of the following is a nonverbal communication?
1. a giggle
2. shouting
3. smiling
4. "yes"

(108)   15.   When obtaining a history from an elderly patient, you should
1. allow sufficient time to answer a question.
2. anticipate the person's answers and fill in for him or her.
3. quickly ask another question to keep him or her on topic.
4. tell the person, "Just answer the question."

MATCHING

Directions: Match the therapeutic technique in Column II with the statement/question in Column I.

(102)

Column I		Column II
1. _____	"…won't do it?"	a. Offering self
2. _____	"…go on…"	b. Clarifying
3. _____	"He said you couldn't go home until Saturday."	c. Restatement
4. _____	"I'll come quickly if you call."	d. Summarizing
5. _____	"So you have pain when you move, but it isn't very bad."	e. Using silence
6. _____	Leaning forward, nodding head.	f. Giving information
7. _____	"How do you feel about that?"	g. Open-ended question
8. _____	"Tell me what the doctor said."	h. General lead
9. _____	"You think it was the coffee that kept you awake?"	i. Reflection
10. _____	"Your surgery is scheduled for 10:00 A.M."	j. Seeking information

APPLICATION OF COMMUNICATION TECHNIQUES

Directions: For each of the following communication exchanges, indicate the technique being used. Label the exchange "therapeutic" or "nontherapeutic." If the exchange is nontherapeutic, give an alternative statement that would have been more therapeutic.

1. Patient: "I can't believe what that doctor said to me!"
   Nurse: "He didn't mean it the way it sounded."

   _____

   _____

2. Patient: "I'm really scared about this surgery."
   Nurse: "Is it the idea of anesthesia that bothers you?"

   _____

   _____

3. Patient: "It's so hard to watch him die."
   Nurse: "It's time to do your exercises now."

   _____

   _____

4. Patient: "It's been a really rough year for me."
   Nurse: "I'd like to hear more about that."

   _____

   _____

5. Patient: "I wonder if the chemotherapy will work."
   Nurse: "I'm sure it will and you'll be fine."

   _____

   _____

6. Patient: "I had a really hard time with the medication last time."
   Nurse: "Tell me more about that experience."

   _____

   _____

7. Patient: "I'm trying to decide if I should have the colonoscopy."
   Nurse: "If I were you, I would have it done."

   _____

   _____

8. Patient: "Then he started shouting at me."
   Nurse: "Ummmmm…"

   _____

   _____

9. Patient: "I know the bone marrow aspiration is going to really hurt."
   Nurse: "It won't hurt for long."

   _____

   _____

10. Patient: "I really tossed and turned last night."
    Nurse: "You had a really hard time sleeping?"

    _____

    _____

CRITICAL THINKING ACTIVITIES

1. List three instances in which communication would be important to the collaborative process (with other health care workers).

2. From the following scenario, underline the information that should be included in the end-of-shift report.

   B.F., room 328, states he is in pain and wants his medication. At 8:30 A.M. he is given a Vicodin. The pain is relieved by 9:15 A.M. He is interrupted by three phone calls during his assisted bath. His IV site is clean and dry; the doctor discontinues the IV when he makes afternoon rounds. The dressing over the abdominal incision is clean and dry. B.F.'s wife comes to visit at noon. He is cooperative with his coughing and deep-breathing exercises. He walks in the hall three times. He has been taking fluids and a clear liquid diet without signs of nausea.

MEETING CLINICAL OBJECTIVES

Directions: The following suggested activities will help you meet the stated clinical practice objectives for the chapter. Review your school's clinical objectives for the week and outline a plan of activities that will help you meet them. If you are unsure how to meet them, consult with your instructor at the beginning of the clinical day.

1. Listen carefully to various nurses give report. Determine which one gives the best report and try to figure out why you feel this report is the best.

2. When you come home from your clinical experience, take the information you have on your worksheet for the patients you cared for, and using a tape recorder, practice giving report.

3. Plan a specific interaction with a patient or family member and practice using therapeutic communication techniques.

4. During lunch, practice "attentive" listening with a classmate.

5. Interview a patient and compile an admission assessment.

6. Seek assignment to a hearing-impaired person for practice in communication with such a person.

7. Review your interactions with patients on the way home at the end of the clinical day. Pick out any instances where you felt your communication was ineffective and by using therapeutic techniques, see what you could have said that might have made the outcome of the interaction better.

STEPS TOWARD BETTER COMMUNICATION

VOCABULARY BUILDING GLOSSARY

Term	Pronunciation	Definition
A. Individual Terms		
abrupt	a BRUPT	sudden, quick, short
ambivalent	am BIV a lent	uncertain, especially between two choices
closure	CLO sure	a satisfactory ending or conclusion
concisely	con CISE ly	in a few words, briefly
conveyed	con VEYed	to make known, to communicate something; carried or transferred from one place to another
discount (verb)	dis COUNT	to not pay attention to, to disregard; to not consider valuable
elaborating	e LAB or a ting	explaining in more detail
elicit	e LI cit	bring out
format	FOR mat	an arrangement or order
gesture	GES ture	a movement, especially of the hands or arms
hunched	HUNCHed	shoulders pulled forward and down, forming a hump with the back
intonation	in to NA tion	rising and falling level of the voice in speech
judiciously	ju DI cious ly	carefully; in small amounts
lead (noun)	LEAD	something to get you started
mood	MOOD	an emotional state or feeling that lasts for a period of time
optimal	OP ti mal	the best possible
pry	PRY	to force by continual pressure
ramble	RAM ble	to go around in different directions without making connections; off of the point
refrain	re FRAIN	to stop oneself, to avoid doing something
side-tracked	SIDE-tracked	get away from the main track or issue
strive	strive	try
transpired	tran SPIR ed	occurred
verify	VER i FY	make sure
wincing	WIN cing	a facial expression of pain
B. Phrases and Idioms		
all walks of life	all walks of life	all levels and conditions of society
being defensive	BE ING de FEN sive	defending oneself against criticism, sometimes where none is intended
closed body stance	closed BOD y stance	a way a person holds his or her body with arms close to the body or crossed over the chest, legs crossed or pulled up, in a protective way; may even turn away from others.
issue at hand	IS sue at HAND	the topic being discussed

Student Name _____

nonjudgmental attitude	NON judge men tal AT ti tude	accepting, not criticizing
open ended	O pen END ed	something for which there is no definite answer or decision
personal space	PER son al SPACE	the amount of space around a person that feels comfortable in communication with others, such as the distance between speakers or people in an elevator
put oneself in another's shoes	put ONE self in an O ther's shoes	to think about how another person would feel in this situation
seen through their eyes	seen through their eyes	see things as the other person would, with his or her beliefs and circumstances
take personally	take PER son ally	interpret that another's emotions, words, or actions (especially negative ones) are directed toward or caused by oneself

COMPLETION

Directions: Fill in the blank(s) with the correct word(s) from the Vocabulary Building Glossary to complete the sentence.

1. The patient was _____ from his room to the O.R. on a stretcher.

2. While she was _____ about the care needed for the wound, the patient took notes on the steps involved.

3. When surgery is performed, all concerned hope for a(n) _____ outcome.

4. Never _____ the family's input as it is often very valuable.

5. The medication is to be used _____ on the skin lesions; a little bit is better than a lot.

6. The nurse checks the patient's armband when administering medications to _____ the patient's identity.

7. The fact that the patient worked in a metal foundry gave the nurse a(n) _____ regarding the possible cause of his symptoms.

8. Each nurse must _____ to do the best job possible for every patient.

VOCABULARY DIFFERENCES

Directions: Note the difference in the following similar words.

elicit vs. illicit

Elicit means to bring out information from another person.
Illicit means something is illegal.

Consider the difference between two meanings of *discount*.

DIS count (noun)—means an amount of money taken off the full price.
dis COUNT (verb)—means to disregard; to not consider valuable.

COMMUNICATION EXERCISE

Certain expressions used in English show the other person that you are listening and that you want him or her to continue to talk. Some of these expressions (from the informal to the more formal) are:

Yeah. Mmmmm. Uh-huh. Right. Go on. Yes. I see.

Nonverbal behavior is another important way to show you are listening. Looking the speaker in the eye is a way of showing you are paying attention. Leaning forward in a chair toward the person indicates that you are really interested in what is being said. Nodding your head up and down and changing the expression on your face according to what is being said also show attention and interest. The following is an example of delegating a task to a nurse's aide.

Directions: After studying the example, write out a conversation on a separate sheet of paper where you delegate to the aide taking vital signs for several patients.

Nurse: "Jim, I want you to shower Ms. B. and change her bed. After you are finished showering and performing her hygiene care, take her for a walk in the hall down to the solarium and back."

Jim: "Does she have any special problems I need to know about?"

Nurse: "She does have a PRN lock in place and that needs to be covered with plastic before showering like I have shown you. She has dentures that need to be cleaned and she may need help with the adhesive. She uses a cane for ambulation. Check her skin before helping her dress and let me know if there are any new lesions. She has a reddened area on the sacrum."

Jim: "OK."

Nurse: "Jim, what do you understand that you are to do?"

Jim: "I'm to shower Ms. B. and make her bed. I help her with her hygiene care and then take her for a walk to the solarium and back."

Nurse: "Yes, that is right. And please check her skin and let me know if there are any new lesions. Be sure to have her use her cane for walking."

Jim: "I've got it."

CULTURAL POINTS

1. The chapter points out that it is considered impolite in some cultures to maintain eye contact when speaking to a person. If this is true in your culture, can you explain to your peers the rationale and how another person knows you are paying attention to what he or she is saying when eye contact is not maintained?

2. With your classmates or a partner, discuss personal space. How much space do you need around you to feel comfortable when talking to others or in an elevator? Americans generally prefer not to be touched in such situations, and will apologize if they touch or bump another, but other cultures take touching as normal. What differences have you noticed about touch within various cultures?

3. What about intentional touching, such as shaking hands or holding hands, or patting someone on the shoulder, or hugging another person? Are these the same or different in your country, and how do these instances of touching make you feel?

4. Do people in your culture have difficulty taking orders from someone younger or someone of the opposite sex? Give an example of a situation in which you might feel uncomfortable acting as a nurse for another person.

Review the chapter key points, answer the study questions, and complete the
critical thinking activities at the end of the chapter in the textbook.

CHAPTER 9

Patient Teaching for Health Promotion

Answer Key: Textbook page references are provided as a guide for answering selected questions. A complete answer key was provided for your instructor.

TERMINOLOGY

Directions: Fill in the blank(s) with the correct term(s) from the terms list in the textbook chapter to complete the sentence.

(113) 1. Learning through lecture or discussion is termed _____ learning.

(113) 2. One teaching method used for _____ learners is to show a videotape.

(113) 3. Performing procedures step by step in the laboratory promotes _____ learning.

(115) 4. A(n) _____ is a statement that represents the desired changes or additions to current behaviors and attitudes.

(118) 5. Obtaining _____ from the patient regarding what was taught assures that he or she understands.

(118) 6. Obtaining a(n) _____ of the technique of changing a dressing is a good way to evaluate the success of your teaching on that subject.

SHORT ANSWER

Directions: Write a brief answer for each question.

(114) 1. When assessing learning needs of a patient, you would consider the following areas:

_____

_____

_____

(114) 2. When preparing a teaching plan for a 78-year-old patient, you should consider physical factors that might affect learning, such as:

_____

_____

(114)   3.   Situational factors that indicate it may not be a good time to begin teaching a patient are:

_____

_____

_____

(115, 117)   4.   Three types of resources for patient teaching and meeting patient learning needs are:

a.   _____

b.   _____

c.   _____

(115)   5.   When teaching the elderly patient, it is important to be certain that:

a.   _____

b.   _____

c.   _____

d.   _____

COMPLETION

Directions: Fill in the blank(s) with the correct word(s) to complete the sentence.

(114)   1.   For teaching to be successful, it is necessary to work within the patient's

_____ and _____

system.

(114)   2.   To build confidence in the patient's ability to perform a task, break the task down into

_____.

(114)   3.   _____ techniques are very successful when teaching

children.

(115)   4.   When preparing a teaching plan that includes written materials, never assume that the pa-

tient is _____; find out.

(115)   5.   The nursing diagnosis utilized for patients who have learning needs is

"_____" followed by the specifics such as "related to

self-administration of insulin."

(115)   6.   In order for the patient to master and retain new information,

_____ of teaching is important.

(117)   7.   During a teaching session, it is wise to frequently ask if there are

_____.

(118)   8.   When a patient is performing a return demonstration as a method of feedback, allow the pa-

tient to perform at his or her own _____.

(113)   9.   Discharge teaching begins at the time of _____.

(113)   10.   A teaching moment is when a patient is at an optimal level of

_____ to learn and

_____ a particular piece of information.

Student Name _____

(113) 11. Learning to draw up a medication is an example of
_____ learning.

(114) 12. When teaching the elderly, the pace is slowed to allow more time for
_____ the information.

(114) 13. Advanced age of the learner may interfere with _____
or strength for performing certain tasks.

(115) 14. The reason for assessing what the patient knows about the topic to be taught is so that you
can build upon the current _____.

(115) 15. One aspect of preparing a patient for teaching is to show him or her the
_____ of learning what he or she needs to know.

(115) 16. When several people are involved in the care and teaching of a patient,
_____ in teaching is important.

(117) 17. During a teaching session it is important to frequently ask for
_____.

(118) 18. Each ongoing teaching session should begin with a(n)
_____ of what has been previously learned.

(118) 19. The best type of feedback for a psychomotor skill is a(n)
_____.

(118) 20. At discharge it is very helpful to send a(n) _____ plan
home with the patient.

NCLEX-PN® EXAM REVIEW

*Directions: Choose the **best** answer(s) for each of the following questions.*

(113) 1. There are several modes of learning including auditory, visual, and kinesthetic learning. The person who learns best by practicing a skill, such as drawing up medication for injection, is a(n) _____ _____ learner.
(Fill in the blank)

(115) 2. When considering a teaching plan, the knowledge base is what the patient
1. needs to know about a subject.
2. is taught about a subject.
3. expresses a desire to learn.
4. already knows about a subject.

(114) 3. Which of the following would be considered a "situational" block to learning? (Select all that apply)
1. pain
2. blindness
3. fatigue
4. illiteracy

(118) 4. Which one of the following would be the best feedback that the patient has mastered the material taught? The patient
1. presents a written outline of the material.
2. demonstrates the task that was taught.
3. has questions regarding the specifics of performing the task.
4. reads all of the written material the nurse presented.

(115) 5. An appropriate behavioral objective for a teaching plan to teach the patient to give his own insulin would be: The patient will
1. explain the purpose of insulin.
2. identify the signs of hypoglycemia.
3. draw up the correct dose for each injection.
4. identify the complications of diabetes.

(115) 6. An initial step in formulating a teaching plan is to
1. evaluate the patient's knowledge base.
2. locate resources for teaching.
3. write out the behavioral objectives.
4. plan times when teaching can be accomplished.

(117) 7. Learning will be enhanced by (Select all that apply)
1. a very specific teaching plan.
2. a relaxed, quiet atmosphere.
3. teaching aids appropriate to the patient's learning style.
4. use of one mode of learning.

(117) 8. A very important part of the teaching process is
1. the type of materials used.
2. the expertise of the teacher.
3. documenting the teaching session.
4. reinforcement of the material taught.

(115) 9. A patient's ability to learn would most likely be enhanced by his or her
1. illness.
2. anxiety.
3. readiness.
4. knowledge.

(115) 10. One way to increase motivation to learn is to
1. make the environment comfortable.
2. use a variety of learning tools.
3. give timely feedback.
4. explain the advantage of the learning.

(115) 11. A learning objective should contain
1. performance criteria and conditions.
2. encouragement and motivation.
3. data and behaviors.
4. learning activity and long-term need.

(114) 12. Affective learning is directed at a change in
1. knowledge.
2. skills.
3. values.
4. practices.

(115) 13. When several disciplines are involved in the care and teaching of a patient,
1. collaboration on the plan is important.
2. each discipline teaches one aspect of care.
3. the nurse always oversees the teaching plan.
4. the patient is not consulted.

(115) 14. A female patient is readmitted with a foot ulcer, a complication of her diabetes. She has received diabetic teaching in the past. When formulating her teaching plan, you should first
1. tell her what she is doing wrong.
2. assess her present knowledge base.
3. determine her insulin requirements.
4. write learning objectives.

Student Name _____

(114) 15. A factor in the failure of the patient to carry out the foot care teaching she had before might be
   1. a sedentary lifestyle.
   2. poor eyesight.
   3. family responsibilities.
   4. financial difficulties.

16. When the patient gives you a return demonstration of the correct way to dry her feet, she does not dry between all her toes as you had instructed. The best comment would be
   1. "That's fine, you are making good progress."
   2. "You are reaching the bottom of the foot well, but you forgot to dry between your toes."
   3. "Oh oh, you forgot to dry between your toes."
   4. "Good, you've dried the top and bottom of the foot. What parts of the foot are still damp?"

(113-114) 17. The patient is an auditory learner. Besides attending lecture, which of the following would be the best way for her to learn material?
   1. Read the chapters in the textbook.
   2. Listen again to the lectures on tape.
   3. Use flash cards to memorize facts.
   4. Practice the steps of the skills in the laboratory.

CRITICAL THINKING ACTIVITIES

1. List which modes of learning are best for you.

2. Considering your best mode of learning, what techniques might make learning nursing content easier for you?

3. Devise a general teaching plan outline for teaching patients about their medications.

MEETING CLINICAL OBJECTIVES

Directions: The following suggested activities will help you meet the stated clinical practice objectives for the chapter. Review your school's clinical objectives for the week and outline a plan of activities that will help you meet them. If you are unsure how to meet them, consult with your instructor at the beginning of the clinical day.

1. Consider the most frequent types of teaching needed on the unit to which you are assigned. Prepare teaching outlines for those topics.

2. Evaluate the learning needs of each patient to whom you are assigned.

3. Prepare a complete teaching plan and perform the teaching for a patient.

4. Practice teaching with a peer and obtain feedback.

5. Evaluate your teaching and revise the plan as needed.

STEPS TOWARD BETTER COMMUNICATION

VOCABULARY BUILDING GLOSSARY

Term	Pronunciation	Definition
admonishment	ad MON ish ment	scolding, criticizing, warning
cognition	cog NI tion	the process of thinking or perceiving
detach	de TACH	to remove, separate
deficit	DEF i cit	to lack, to be missing
dexterity	dex TER i ty	skill or ability, especially with the hands
domains	do MAINS	areas
frame of reference	FRAME of REF er ence	the knowledge and beliefs that affect one's understanding of new information
goes a long way	goes a LONG way	is very helpful
intact	in TACT	all in one piece, not broken
literate	LIT er ate	the ability to read and write
patient teaching	PA tient TEACH ing	teaching a patient
taut	TAUT	tight
teaching moments	TEACH ING MO ments	times that are best for teaching because of the situation, mood, and condition of the learner

COMPLETION

Directions: Fill in the blank(s) with the correct word(s) from the Vocabulary Building Glossary to complete the sentence.

1. Teaching a patient how to self-catheterize requires some degree of _____ on the part of the patient.

2. It is necessary to know whether the patient is _____ before using written materials as part of the teaching process.

3. The patient has a(n) _____ in regard to knowledge about the side effects of his medication.

4. While administering the patient's medications after his afternoon rest, a good _____ appeared for teaching information about the side effects of the medication.

5. Learning usually takes longer when the subject matter is outside of the patient's _____.

Student Name _____

VOCABULARY EXERCISES

Look at these two words which have the same sound and spelling, but have two different meanings and are used differently. Can you explain the meanings and uses?

patient vs. patient

1. _____

2. _____

These next two words sound the same, but are spelled differently. What is their relationship to the words above?

patients vs. patience

3. _____

4. _____

WORD ATTACK SKILLS

Directions: Look at the words below and think about how they relate to one another.

1. The root, CO +GNOSCERE, means to come to know.
   cognition (noun)—the process of thinking or perceiving
   cognitive (adj)—involving thought and knowledge; knowing
   cognizant (adj)—having knowledge; aware
   recognize (verb)—to see again and know or remember
   recognition (noun)—remembering someone or something when you see or hear it

   Example: The patient was not cognizant of his surroundings, but he recognized his family.

2. detach/attach (soft *ch* as in chair) mean to unfasten or separate/to fasten to.

   Example: She detached the call light from the bed rail and attached it to the pillowcase.

COMMUNICATION EXERCISES

1. Read the dialogue with a partner, giving feed back about pronunciation and comprehensibility (how easy it is to understand).

   Nurse: "Mr. O., I need to teach you how to cleanse your wound."

   Mr. O.: "I need to do that myself?"

   Nurse: "Yes, unless you can convince your granddaughter to come over and do it for you."

   Mr. O.: "She's awfully busy with school and work."

   Nurse: "OK then. First you wash your hands and then put on the gloves. Next, you remove the old dressing and put it into a sealable plastic bag. Then, use some of this saline solution on a gauze pad to cleanse around the wound. You need to cleanse from the inside of the wound outward first on one side and then with another moistened gauze pad on the other side."

   Mr. O.: "Do I have to cleanse down in the wound?"

   Nurse: "No, that might disrupt the healing tissue. Then apply the new dressing and tape it in place."

Mr. O.:   "Can I do the cleaning tomorrow before I go home so that you can watch to see if I do it correctly?"

Nurse: "Certainly. That is a good idea."

2. With a partner, write a short dialogue teaching a patient how to empty a Foley catheter leg drainage bag. Correct and practice your dialogue, then join another pair and teach them, using your dialogue.

3. Tell how you could use each of the three ways of teaching to teach a patient to develop a weight reduction diet.

CULTURAL POINTS

1. What teaching methods were used in your elementary and high school? Were they different than the methods used in schools today? Share your experience in a group with people of different ages and from different countries. How do your experiences differ?

2. Has your learning style changed through the years? Do you learn in the same way you did as a child, or have you learned a different way?

3. Are you aware of any traditional medicines or healing techniques that were/are used in your culture or your family? Any "folk" medicines or traditions your grandparents used? Share these in small groups, and talk about why they may have worked.

Review the chapter key points, answer the study questions, and complete the critical thinking activities at the end of the chapter in the textbook.

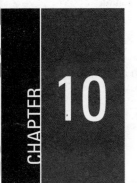

10 Delegation, Leadership, and Management

CHAPTER

Answer Key: Textbook page references are provided as a guide for answering selected questions. A complete answer key was provided for your instructor.

TERMINOLOGY

Directions: Match the leadership style in Column I with the descriptions in Column II.

	Column I	**Column II**
(120) 1. _____ laissez-faire		a. Seek participation from staff
(120) 2. _____ autocratic		b. Little direction
(121) 3. _____ democratic		c. Close supervision

COMPLETION

Directions: Fill in the blanks with the appropriate words from the chapter to complete the sentences.

(121) 1. A key factor in delivering cost-effective patient care is _____ with all other health team members.

(122) 2. A feeling of confidence in one's clinical ability allows a leader to readily admit when _____.

(124) 3. Efficient _____ is essential to the organized running of a nursing unit.

(122) 4. A good problem-solver first _____.

(122) 5. When delegating, you are _____ for the tasks you delegate.

(122) 6. _____ of unlicensed assistive personnel must be documented before tasks are delegated to them.

(122) 7. It is essential to be familiar with the UAP's _____ before delegating a task.

(122) 8. Effective communication to the UAP means _____ messages and _____ to feedback.

(122)   9. When delegating a task effectively, the nurse includes communication about the
_____ and the
_____ for completion.

(122)   10. When you delegate, you do not give up _____ for the task.

(122)   11. A good delegator obtains _____ about how the task was done.

(122)   12. If it is necessary to give criticism to someone to whom you have delegated a task, it is essential to provide _____ beforehand.

(123)   13. When giving constructive criticism, begin by tactfully acknowledging
_____ and expressing
_____.

(123)   14. When delegating a variety of tasks to the UAP, you should help him or her to
_____ the order in which to do them.

(123)   15. When performance of a UAP is poor, _____
_____ must be done.

SHORT ANSWER

Directions: Write a brief answer for each of the following.

(122)   1. List four things that one must know to delegate appropriately.

    a. _____
    b. _____
    c. _____
    d. _____

(123)   2. What are six functions of a team leader?

    a. _____
    b. _____
    c. _____
    d. _____
    e. _____
    f. _____

(120)   3. List seven points that a new nurse should know regarding the appropriate "chain of command."

    a. _____
    b. _____
    c. _____
    d. _____

Student Name _____

e. _____

f. _____

g. _____

(122) 4. List the five steps in problem-solving.

a. _____

b. _____

c. _____

d. _____

e. _____

(126) 5. For the health care agency to obtain reimbursement for equipment used in the care or treatment of a patient, what criteria must be met?

_____

_____

_____

_____

(121) 6. Name six attributes of a good leader that you think are the most important.

_____

_____

_____

NCLEX-PN® EXAM REVIEW

*Directions: Choose the **best** answer(s) for the following questions.*

(121) 1. Elements of good communication include (Select all that apply)
1. directness.
2. firmness.
3. nonthreatening manner.
4. abruptness.

(122) 2. When delegating a task, directions should be
1. given in great detail.
2. thorough but concise.
3. written for later reference.
4. itemized for clarity.

(122) 3. A good problem-solver, after defining the problem,
1. considers the outcomes.
2. determines if other problems exist.
3. looks at alternative solutions.
4. decides on one solution.

(122) 4. Good work organization and time management requires (Select all that apply)
1. making a daily "to do" list.
2. considering all tasks that must be accomplished.
3. setting a few goals for the day.
4. consulting each of the staff members.

CRITICAL THINKING ACTIVITIES

1. Determine what tasks you might delegate to a UAP from the patient assignment you receive for the next clinical shift.

2. Set priorities of care and create a time organization sheet for a two- or three-patient clinical assignment.

MEETING CLINICAL OBJECTIVES

Directions: The following suggested activities will help you meet the stated clinical practice objectives for the chapter. Review your school's clinical objectives for the week and outline a plan of activities that will help you meet them. If you are unsure how to meet them, consult with your instructor at the beginning of the clinical day.

1. Pick a nurse who you think displays good leadership qualities and ask to work with the patients assigned to that nurse for a day so that you can closely observe how this nurse communicates, delegates, and obtains the cooperation of others.

2. Make out a time and work organization plan for each clinical shift. Include all of the tasks and assessments for which you are responsible. Consult with other nurses about how they organize their work.

3. Observe various nurses delegating tasks to UAPs. Decide which ones use the best delegation techniques. Speak with some of the UAPs and ask them which nurses they prefer to work with. Ask them if they can tell you why they prefer those nurses.

STEPS TOWARD BETTER COMMUNICATION

VOCABULARY BUILDING GLOSSARY

The meanings of words and phrases used in special situations (contexts) often cannot be found in regular dictionaries. Health care is one of these situations, but there are many others. These special words are called *terminology* (as in medical terminology) or sometimes *jargon.* Much of the terminology used in this chapter has special meanings in the area called *human relations*—how people communicate and work together.

Term	Pronunciation	Definition
collaboration	co LAB or a tion	working together with other team members
chain of command	chain of com MAND	structure of an organization; who is above whom in authority
laissez-faire	LAIS sez faire	permissive; to leave alone; no interference
cost-effective	cost e FFEC tive	getting the most for the money; worth its cost
feedback	FEED back	response to ideas or actions; may be positive or negative
eye contact	EYE CON tact	a look directly at the eyes of another person (Usage: In American culture, a person who does not use eye contact might be considered rude or dishonest, while someone who looks you in the eye is believed to be honest and truthful.)
conflict resolution	CON flict res o LU tion	a method of settling differences in a friendly way

Student Name _____

domain	do MAIN	area of responsibility or knowledge
delegate	del e GATE	give a task or job to another person
competent	COMP e tent	able and qualified to do something
constructive criticism	con STRUCT ive CRIT I cis m	helpful evaluation of accomplishments or actions
reimbursement	re im BURSE ment	payment for services or money given
active listener	AC tive LIST ner	a person who focuses attention and reacts to the ideas and feelings of a speaker
instills	in STILLS	puts into a person's mind gradually
fosters	FOS ters	encourages
concise	con CISE	short and clear
enlists	en LISTS	gets someone to help or support
domain	do MAIN	area
discern	dis CERN	figure out, understand
expedite	EX pe DITE	to make faster, speed up an action
grid	GRID	a kind of chart with squares (like a calendar page)
jot	JOT	write a quick short note
adverse	AD verse	negative
mitigate	MIT i gate	minimize, make less serious

VOCABULARY EXERCISES

Directions: The following words relate to emotions or a person's abilities. Pronounce the word. Match the word with its meaning. Ask a native speaker or use your dictionary if you are not sure of the meaning.

1. _____ wise, careful
2. _____ unhappy, upset
3. _____ knowledge and experience
4. _____ understanding what another person feels
5. _____ skilled, able to do well

a. Empathy (EM path y)
b. Expertise (ex per TISE)
c. Prudent (PRU dent)
d. Proficient (pro FI cient)
e. Disgruntled (dis GRUN tled)

COMPLETION

Directions: Fill in the blanks with the appropriate words from the Vocabulary Building Glossary to complete the sentence.

1. When conveying instructions to a UAP, it is best to first establish _____ .

2. When disagreements occur between administration and staff, some method of _____ is called for.

3. A(n) _____ leader gives little direction to the members of the staff.

4. To be a good leader in nursing, one must be _____ in the skills of the profession.

5. Every health care agency in the nation is trying to devise more _____ measures for patient care.

6. Accurate charting of equipment used and documentation of the need for the equipment is essential for _____.

7. When going to work for a health care agency, the nurse should gain an understanding of the _____.

8. To delegate well, the nurse must be a good communicator and a(n) _____.

9. After delegating a task to a UAP, the nurse should seek _____ the patient about how the task was performed.

10. To delegate to others effectively, the nurse must understand what is within the _____ of the person.

11. The nurse should always provide privacy for the individual before giving _____.

12. An important part of being a team leader is the ability to _____ tasks to others.

VOCABULARY EXERCISES

Word Families

Some words are in "families" that have the same "name" or root word but different forms and meanings depending on their functions (how they are used).

Verb:	**compete:** to try to do something better than someone else
Nouns:	**competence:** degree of ability to do something
	competency: what a person is able to do (often used in the plural)
	competitor: person trying to do something better than someone else
Adjective:	**competent:** having the ability to do something well
Adverb:	**competently:** doing something well, with ability

Directions: Fill in the blank with the correct form of the word from the list above to complete the sentence.

1. She performs skills well and is a _____ nurse.

2. When we are on the unit for clinical experience, we often have to _____ for the instructor's time.

3. I really want to be able to perform as a nurse _____.

Student Name _____

Polite and Effective Communication

The following are important examples of polite and effective communication:

> "I don't know, but I will find out."
> "Would you help the nurse turn the patient in room 309, please?"
> "Thank you for taking the extra shift for Janice."
> "Please be sure to get your time cards in by noon on Wednesday."

Communication is important in the art of delegating. Write out the words you would use to delegate the task of obtaining daily weights for three patients to LuAnn.

4. _____

_____

_____

_____

_____

_____

_____

_____

_____

_____

_____

_____

_____

ABBREVIATION IDENTIFICATION

Directions: Write the meaning of each abbreviation and then pronounce the words.

1. MAR _____
2. UAP _____
3. STAT _____
4. ASAP _____

COMMUNICATION EXAMPLE

Giving constructive criticism requires tact and empathy as well as a concerned manner. The following dialogue is one example of how a nurse might give constructive criticism to a nursing assistant or UAP.

An aide was delegated to safely ambulate Mr. Thompson, age 80, who has had pneumonia and is still weak. When the nurse passed the two in the hallway, he noticed that the aide was simply walking by the side of Mr. Thompson, talking to him, as he unsteadily walked back to his room. The nurse entered the room after them and quickly helped the aide place Mr. Thompson in the chair.

"Helen, when you finish here would you touch base with me for a minute?"

"Sure, John. I'll be out shortly."

(*Later*)

"What is it, John?"

"Helen, it seems as if Mr. Thompson is still very weak. I'm glad you got his morning ambulation in because that will help him build strength. You can prevent him from possibly falling if you will use a gait belt when he is up ambulating until he is stronger. If you don't have one, physical therapy will provide one for you. Would you like to try that this afternoon?"

"That's a good idea, John. It made me nervous watching him walk that unsteadily."

COMPLETION SENTENCES

Directions: Fill the blanks in the sentences with the correct words from the glossary or vocabulary exercise above.

1. The job called for someone who could _____ the problems and then _____ them.

2. The new LVN was very _____ in her work.

3. Be sure to _____ the orders in pen in the correct square on the _____.

4. A good teacher _____ good work habits in her students.

SPECIAL USE

Immediate—In addition to the usual meaning, "occurring at once, right now," *immediate* also means "the next or nearest; with nothing in between."

EXAMPLE: The person on my immediate right is my sister.

IDIOMATIC PHRASES

effective utilization	to use in the best way
chain of command	the order in a series of positions of authority
establish eye contact	look at a person's eyes or face as you talk to them
actively listen	pay attention and try to understand what the person is saying
weigh the consequences	consider or think about the result of an action
define the problem	figure out what the problem is
track down	look for and find
take precedence over	come first or before something else
get a feel for	obtain a general idea, begin to understand

Directions: Fill in the blank for each statement using the phrases listed above.

1. When talking to someone you should _____.

2. Emergencies should _____ routine duties.

3. The nurse tried to _____ the missing order.

Student Name _____

COMMUNICATION EXERCISES

Directions: With another student, practice asking the person to do each of the following:

1. Demonstrate a skill and then

2. Do the task

> ***Review the chapter key points, answer the study questions, and complete the critical thinking activities at the end of the chapter in the textbook.***

11 Growth and Development: Infancy Through Adolescence

CHAPTER

Answer Key: Textbook page references are provided as a guide for answering selected questions. A complete answer key was provided for your instructor.

TERMINOLOGY

A. Matching

Directions: Match the terms in Column I with the definitions in Column II.

	Column I		Column II
(137)	1. _____ bonding	a.	Knowledge and thinking processes
(136)	2. _____ cephalocaudal	b.	Union of ovum and sperm
(129)	3. _____ cognitive	c.	Male or female
(129)	4. _____ conception	d.	Brothers or sisters
(138)	5. _____ egocentric	e.	Fertilized egg
(131)	6. _____ gender	f.	Periods of 3 months
(134)	7. _____ neonate	g.	Able to survive outside the womb
(139)	8. _____ peers	h.	Newborn
(142)	9. _____ puberty	i.	Instinctive protective actions
(135)	10. _____ reflexes	j.	Sense of attachment between two people
(131)	11. _____ siblings	k.	Feeling that I am the center of the world
(134)	12. _____ trimesters	l.	Others of similar age and background
(134)	13. _____ vernix caseosa	m.	Sexual maturation
(134)	14. _____ viable	n.	Cheesy, waxy substance that protects fetal skin
(133)	15. _____ zygote	o.	Proceeding from head to tail

B. Completion

Directions: Fill in the blank(s) with the correct word(s) from the terms list in the chapter in the textbook to complete the sentence.

(131)   1.   Theory about human development and behavior is based primarily on

_____.

(131)   2.   Ordinal position, the _____ in which siblings are born into a family, is thought to be a factor in growth and development by some people.

(135)   3.   The _____ reflex is elicited by making a loud noise near the baby.

(138)   4.   Children learn _____ during Erikson's stage of Initiative.

(139)   5.   The development of _____ is learning about what is right and wrong.

(141)   6.   _____ is a combination of verbal ability, reasoning, memory, imagination, and judgment.

(141)   7.   During the middle years of childhood, children begin developing _____ competence.

(145)   8.   By the end of adolescence, _____ should be fairly well-established and this includes a moral code.

(133)   9.   The chromosomes contained in the _____ inherited from one's parents carry the blueprints of development for the child.

(138)   10.   A(n) _____ is a method of discipline where the child spends quiet time alone without toys.

(134)   11.   A woman who is planning on becoming pregnant should be certain her intake of _____ is at least _____ mcg per day to help prevent neural tube defects in the infant.

(135)   12.   The first regular checkup for an infant should occur at _____ months of age.

(135)   13.   One nutrition objective for *Healthy People 2010* is aimed at increasing the number of women who _____ their infants.

(137)   14.   Regular checkups to assess growth and development should occur every _____ years.

REVIEW OF STRUCTURE AND FUNCTION

Directions: Write a brief answer for each question.

(130)   1.   In the germinal stage of prenatal development, how soon does cell division occur?

_____

(130)   2.   When does the blastocyst attach to the uterine wall and how does this occur?

_____

(130)   3.   When does the embryonic stage begin?

_____

(130)   4.   At what point does the heart begin beating?

_____

(130)   5.   At what point in time are 95% of the body's parts already formed?

_____

(130)   6.   What is the approximate size of the fetus by the fifth month?

_____

Student Name_____

(130) 7. What causes multiple births?

_____

(130) 8. At what average age does puberty for a female occur?

_____

(130) 9. What is the average age of puberty in the male?

_____

IDENTIFICATION

Directions: For the following developmental milestones, identify the age at which they generally occur.

a. 0–1   b. 2–3   c. 4–5   d. 6–9   e. 10–12   f. 13–18

(137)	1. _____	Full set of deciduous teeth
(137)	2. _____	Toilet trained (bladder)
(138)	3. _____	Knows 8,000–14,000 words
(138)	4. _____	Develops some autonomy
(145)	5. _____	Sexual preference is developed
(142)	6. _____	Sexual maturation has occurred
(138)	7. _____	Gender roles have been learned
(142)	8. _____	Seeks friendships and experiences outside the home
(140)	9. _____	May show signs of prepuberty
(138)	10. _____	Begins to want to accomplish things
(142)	11. _____	Denial of privileges becomes a more effective discipline
(143)	12. _____	Begins Piaget's stage of Formal Operations
(135)	13. _____	Grows 10–12 inches in 12 months
(136)	14. _____	Develops object permanence
(138)	15. _____	Begins to engage in pretend play

SHORT ANSWER

Directions: Write a brief answer for each question.

(131) 1. Erik Erikson's theory of development defined eight psychosocial stages that lead to a healthy ego. Each stage is identified by:

_____

_____

(131) 2. Jean Piaget developed a theory about how children learn based on the need to adapt to the environment. He stressed two principles, which are:

a. _____

b. _____

(131)   3.   Lawrence Kohlberg developed a theory of moral development. Identify a behavior that belongs in each of the following three stages of moral development.

   a.   Preconventional reasoning: _____

   _____

   b.   Conventional reasoning:_____

   _____

   c.   Postconventional reasoning:_____

   _____

(131)   4.   Basic principles of growth and development are:

   a.   _____

   b.   _____

   c.   _____

   d.   _____

   e.   _____

(132)   5.   List one behavior that indicates positive accomplishment for each of the following stages of childhood according to Erikson:

   a.   Trust vs. Mistrust:_____

   _____

   b.   Autonomy vs. Shame and Doubt:_____

   _____

   c.   Initiative vs. Guilt: _____

   _____

   d.   Industry vs. Inferiority: _____

   _____

   e.   Identity vs. Role Confusion: _____

   _____

(136)   6.   Six safety factors for care of an infant are:

   a.   _____

   b.   _____

   c.   _____

   d.   _____

   e.   _____

   f.   _____

Student Name _____

(143)   7. Two safety points that should be taught to adolescents are:

a. _____

b. _____

(141)   8. A *Healthy People 2010* objective related to nutrition that is especially pertinent in preventing obesity in young people and cutting down on the amount of "junk" food consumed is:

_____

_____

(134)   9. Two *Healthy People 2010* objectives related to pregnancy are:

a. _____

b. _____

COMPLETION

Directions: Fill in the blank(s) with the correct word(s) to complete the sentence.

(131)   1. The rate of growth and development is _____.

(131)   2. According to Kohlberg, moral values are not internalized until about age _____.

(131)   3. According to Kohlberg, children begin using conventional reasoning at about age _____.

(131)   4. Growth occurs in orderly and _____ ways.

(129)   5. Development is multidimensional and involves _____, _____, and _____ aspects.

(133)   6. Each child has _____, half from the mother and half from the father.

(134)   7. A full pregnancy lasts _____ weeks.

(134)   8. It is best if a woman is well- _____ before becoming pregnant.

(134)   9. It is considered healthiest for a woman to gain about _____ pounds during pregnancy.

(134)   10. Prolonged stress in the pregnant woman interferes with adequate _____ and _____ to the fetus.

(134)   11. Infancy is the period from birth through _____.

(135)   12. A typical newborn sleeps for _____ hours a day.

(135)   13. Most babies can be given table food at _____ of age.

(135)   14. Permanent eye color develops in the infant by _____ months.

(135)   15. Brain growth is very rapid during the _____ year.

NCLEX-PN® EXAM REVIEW

*Directions: Choose the **best** answer(s) for each of the following questions.*

(135) 1. If physical growth is normal, a child will
   1. double the birth weight by 2 months of age.
   2. gain 10–12 inches in length by 6 months of age.
   3. triple the birth weight by 1 year of age.
   4. double head size by 6 months of age.

(136) 2. Normal motor development results in a child being able to
   1. draw before he can walk.
   2. coordinate small muscles before large ones.
   3. lift the chest before being able to lift the head.
   4. sit before being able to stand.

(136) 3. Different skills develop at different times in the infant. The cognitive skill of object permanence occurs at about _____ months. (Fill in the blank)

(137) 4. Initially infants usually do not have security issues when picked up by a stranger. Insecurity with strangers begins at about _____ months. (Fill in the blank)

(137) 5. The primary environmental influence on physical growth is
   1. nurturing.
   2. attention.
   3. nutrition.
   4. heredity.

(140) 6. A positive function of day care for the child is that it
   1. promotes socialization skills.
   2. helps build immunity to childhood illness.
   3. prevents separation anxiety.
   4. builds self-esteem.

(141) 7. It is important that the 6–12-year-old child receive
   1. strict discipline when misbehavior occurs.
   2. encouragement and praise for tasks accomplished.
   3. lots of guidance when performing a task.
   4. opportunities to make his or her own decisions.

(143) 8. A major reason that adolescents need more sex education is that (Select all that apply)
   1. adolescents often pretend to know more about sex than they actually do.
   2. adolescents are maturing physically earlier.
   3. statistics indicate that 50% of girls and 66% of boys have had intercourse by age 18.
   4. they don't think pregnancy will happen to them if they are sexually active.

(144) 9. Conflict between the young adolescent and parents is partly influenced by
   1. growth in intelligence as the child matures.
   2. major hormonal shifts that occur at this time.
   3. the many activities in which the adolescent participates.
   4. the need for strong attachment to the parents while spending more time with peers.

Student Name _____

(145) 10. A sign of anorexia nervosa in an adolescent girl might be
1. spending all her time in her room.
2. eating little and exercising a lot.
3. refusing to participate in family activities.
4. cutting classes and getting poor grades.

(133) 11. According to Piaget, the child starts seeing him- or herself as separate from others at age
1. 4–8 months.
2. 8–12 months.
3. 18–24 months.
4. 2–4 years.

(133) 12. A child cannot be expected to logically manipulate abstract and unobservable concepts until about age
1. 4.
2. 6.
3. 8.
4. 11.

(137) 13. Bonding is important for the infant because it helps the person develop
1. relationships with others throughout life.
2. a good relationship with its parents.
3. interest in other people.
4. full growth and development.

(137) 14. A milestone in motor development for the toddler is
1. climbing stairs without holding on.
2. becoming toilet trained.
3. throwing a ball accurately.
4. increasing height by 3–5 inches.

(145) 15. Signs of adolescent depression include (Select all that apply)
1. expressions of feeling sad or blue.
2. anger at parents.
3. alcohol or other drug use.
4. declining school grades.

TABLE ACTIVITY

Directions: Fill in the table with the changes that occur to males and females during puberty.

Physical Changes of Puberty

(143) Male	Female
_____	_____
_____	_____
_____	_____
_____	_____
_____	_____
_____	_____
_____	_____
_____	_____
_____	_____

CRITICAL THINKING ACTIVITIES

1. What ways can you think of to assist adolescents with the areas of concern listed in the chapter?

2. What do parents need to know about the growth and development of their new infant?

MEETING CLINICAL OBJECTIVES

Directions: The following suggested activities will help you meet the stated clinical practice objectives for the chapter. Review your school's clinical objectives for the week and outline a plan of activities that will help you meet them. If you are unsure how to meet them, consult with your instructor at the beginning of the clinical day.

1. Visit a preschool and observe the types of play occurring among the children.

2. Teach a newly pregnant female about the type of prenatal care that she needs.

3. Perform a Denver Developmental Screening on a child.

4. Assist parents to develop consistent methods of discipline for children of various ages.

STEPS TOWARD BETTER COMMUNICATION

VOCABULARY BUILDING GLOSSARY

Term	Pronunciation	Definition
A. Individual Terms		
cyanotic	cy a NOT ic	bluish color of the skin
deciduous	de CID u ous	related to shedding or falling off of the old (later replaced by the new); i.e., deciduous trees lose their leaves in the winter and children lose their teeth at certain ages
direly	DIRE ly	urgently
erupt	e RUPT	come out, break through, such as teeth erupting through the gums
resilient	re SIL i ent	able to recover its original shape, recover from difficulty
suffer	SUF fer	to undergo pain, loss, or disadvantage
B. Phrases		
baby fat	BA by FAT	the layer of fat under a healthy infant's skin, not the fat of overweight people
bounce back	BOUNCE back	come back to an original position or condition (like a ball bounces)
gender stereotypes	gen der STER e o types	certain actions or roles are automatically assumed for a gender/sex
growth spurt	growth SPURT	a period during which growth happens very rapidly

Student Name_____

COMPLETION

Directions: Fill in the blank(s) with the correct word(s) from the Vocabulary Building Glossary to complete the sentence.

1. The bluish tint to the skin indicates that the newborn is _____.

2. Babies often become fussy when a tooth begins to _____.

3. Although children can become very sick quite quickly, they are usually
    _____ and get well just as fast.

4. The _____ on an infant is partly what makes it so soft and cuddly.

5. The idea that only boys become heavy equipment operators is a(n)
    _____.

6. Children frequently stay the same size for weeks at a time and then have a(n)
    _____ where they increase height by a half an inch or more.

VOCABULARY EXERCISES

1. English often has many words that mean basically the same thing, and can be used interchangeably with only slight difference in meaning. It is often thought to be good literary style to use different words rather than repeat the same one. Below is one example of words with similar meanings found in this chapter:

    resilient/flexible/bounce back

    Can you give two words that mean the same thing as the words below?
    a. vital   b. helping

2. Give examples of abilities a person might have related to the following kinds of intelligence:

    Linguistic   Bodily kinesthetic

    Mathematical   Interpersonal

    Spatial   Intrapersonal

    Musical

COMMUNICATION EXERCISES

1. With a partner, write a dialogue of a nurse helping the parents of a 2–4-year-old child develop a consistent method of discipline. Among your classmates or friends, find a mother of young children and ask if the dialogue is realistic or useful.

2. Write and practice a dialogue with a partner, showing a parent or health care worker talking with a child about his feelings when he has to go to the hospital for surgery.

CULTURAL POINTS

1. Compare the raising of children as suggested in the chapter and the way children are raised in your native country. What are the similarities? What are the differences? Discuss these in a small group. How do you learn to parent in your country? How do people learn here?

2. Physical punishment, for the most part, is no longer considered an acceptable method for disciplining children. Many people, in this country as well as other countries and cultures, were raised with physical punishment and may resort to it as parents in moments of stress. Can you recall stories of how your parents were disciplined or do you have memories of physical punishment yourself? What is your feeling about its effectiveness versus the new methods? How would you help a person adapt to the new cultural norms?

3. Some language theorists say that people learn a second language in much the same way they learned their first language as children. First, they listen and begin to understand but do not speak, then they respond to questions with brief answers, and learn to communicate to make their needs known. Later, they become more fluent as they have need and opportunity to interact with other speakers of the language they are learning. They learn and speak better in a supportive, nonthreatening environment than when they are nervous and afraid. How do you feel about this? Is this the way you experienced learning a language? Share your experience with a first language speaker. How do they feel about the languages they have learned?

Review the chapter key points, answer the study questions, and complete the
critical thinking activities at the end of the chapter in the textbook.

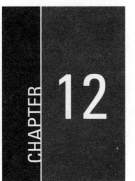

CHAPTER

12

Adulthood and the Family

Student Name _____

Answer Key: Textbook page references are provided as a guide for answering selected questions. A complete answer key was provided for your instructor.

TERMINOLOGY

A. Matching

Directions: Match the terms in Column I with the definitions in Column II.

	Column I		Column II
(154)	1. _____ baby boomers	a.	Being fully developed
(148)	2. _____ career	b.	Work which requires specific training
(156)	3. _____ empty nest syndrome	c.	Trade, professional, or occupational
(149)	4. _____ intimacy	d.	People born between 1946 and 1964
(155)	5. _____ libido	e.	Decreased flexibility of the eye lens
(150)	6. _____ maturity	f.	Loss of hearing
(156)	7. _____ mentor	g.	The sex drive
(154)	8. _____ presbycusis	h.	Children have left the home causing a sense of
(154)	9. _____ presbyopia		loss
(152)	10. _____ vocational	i.	Teacher or coach
		j.	Close, meaningful relationship

B. Completion

Directions: Fill in the blank(s) with the correct word(s) from the terms list in the chapter in the textbook to complete the sentence.

(148) .   1. According to Schaie, the young adult stage of cognitive development is the

_____.

(148-149)   2. The _____ stage, concerned with real-life problems, occurs in middle adulthood.

(151)   3. The young adult should be encouraged to maintain weight within normal limits and to reduce fat to _____ percent of caloric intake.

(149)   4. Some middle adults who have multiple responsibilities are in the

_____.

(156) 5. In Erikson's stage of _____, the middle adult guides the lives of younger people.

(149) 6. _____ occurs if the middle adult is engaged in inactivity and self-absorption.

(152) 7. Offspring who return to the parental home for a period of time are termed
_____.

(156) 8. Middle adults who find themselves with both dependent children and dependent parents needing care giving are in the _____.

(154) 9. Screening for osteoporosis for those women with a family history of the disease should begin at age _____.

(154) 10. Calcium intake in adult women before menopause should be _____ mg per day. After menopause, calcium intake should be increased to _____ mg per day.

(155) 11. Ideal blood pressure for an adult is _____.

SHORT ANSWER

Directions: Write a brief answer for each question.

(148) 1. The first stage of cognitive development according to Schaie is the Achievement stage. List three goals of young adults in this stage.

a. _____
b. _____
c. _____

(148-149) 2. List three types of responsibilities middle adults encounter when they enter the Responsibility stage according to Schaie.

a. _____
b. _____
c. _____

(149) 3. Three functions of those middle adults who are in the Executive substage according to Schaie are:

a. _____
b. _____
c. _____

(149) 4. In Erikson's stage of Intimacy vs. Isolation, a young adult who adjusts positively might exhibit the following behaviors:

a. _____
b. _____
c. _____

Student Name_____

(149)   5. When a middle adult is in the stage of Generativity vs. Stagnation, behaviors indicating a positive adjustment might be:

_____

_____

_____

(149)   6. List three functions of families.

      a. _____

      b. _____

      c. _____

(150)   7. List three possible outcomes for the people involved in divorce.

      a. _____

      b. _____

      c. _____

(151)   8. Risky behaviors of young adults that may affect health are:

      a. _____

      b. _____

      c. _____

      d. _____

      e. _____

(155)   9. The major health problems of middle adults include:

_____

_____

_____

(155)   10. Activities that stimulate the mind and help a person maintain mental crispness are:

_____

_____

_____

_____

TABLE ACTIVITY

Physical Changes

Directions: Fill in the table with the typical physical changes of young- and middle adults.

Physical Changes of Young- and Middle Adults

(151, 154) **Young Adult**	**Middle Adult**

COMPLETION

Directions: Fill in the blank(s) with the correct word(s) to complete the sentence.

(151) 1. Stress-related illnesses begin to be common after age _____.

(152) 2. Personality development continues throughout the _____.

(153) 3. Approximately _____ percent of adults of all ages live alone.

(153) 4. By age _____, a woman is statistically at high risk during a pregnancy.

(154) 5. The average age for menopause is _____.

(155) 6. Creativity is believed to peak during _____.

(155) 7. Leisure activities can be healthy ways to reduce _____.

(156) 8. It is vital to the marriage that middle adults develop mutual _____ and _____.

(156) 9. Throughout adulthood, close _____ are very important.

(154) 10. Physical changes related to aging begin in the _____.

(149-150) 11. A factor that has greatly affected relationships among extended family members is _____.

(150) 12. Nearly _____% of two-parent families have two wage earners.

(150)   13.   Divorce ends approximately _____% of marriages.

(150)   14.   The increasing incidence of divorce is seen as a major cause of
_____ among women.

(151)   15.   Biannual mammograms are recommended for all women beginning at age
_____.

(151)   16.   A Pap test is recommended for women to screen for
_____ cancer.

(152)   17.   The earning power of women continues to be _____ of
what men earn in similar work.

(154)   18.   Noisy work settings and _____ contribute to eventual
hearing loss.

(156)   19.   _____ with others is the focus of psychosocial development in middle adults.

(156)   20.   Middle adults who have centered their lives around their children may experience the
_____ when the children leave home.

NCLEX-PN® EXAM REVIEW

*Directions: Choose the **best** answer(s) for each of the following questions.*

(149)   1.   A 22-year-old female who has a back injury is assigned to you. You recall that a major developmental task for this age is
1. establishing trust relationships.
2. establishing close personal relationships.
3. guiding other young people.
4. balancing work with a multitude of other roles.

(151)   2.   Major factors that will impact the health of young adults when they become older adults is (Select all that apply)
1. engagement in a regular exercise program.
2. compliance with recommended physical exams.
3. lack of attention to good nutrition.
4. degree of affluence that they will attain.

Situation (questions 3–6): The patient is 26 years old. She is married, has an executive position and works 50–60 hours a week. She gets little exercise and does not eat many balanced meals, often eating fast food between meetings. She complains of fatigue and insomnia.

(151)   3.   The patient has come into the clinic for a Pap smear. At this time you would reinforce teaching regarding (Select all that apply)
1. planning for child bearing, if children are desired.
2. the need to do monthly breast self-examination.
3. prevention of sexually transmitted diseases.
4. the necessity for practicing birth control.

(152)   4.   You suspect her fatigue is partly caused by stress, and to combat it you recommend
1. a daily walk.
2. increased protein.
3. changing jobs.
4. a midday nap.

(151) 5. If the patient continues her pattern of poor nutrition and eating lots of fast food, she will be at risk for (Select all that apply)
1. obesity.
2. loss of energy.
3. hypercholesterolemia
4. malnutrition.

(149) 6. At this stage of her life, it is important that this patient spend time maintaining
1. activities that ensure a promotion at work.
2. her intimate relationship with her husband.
3. an efficient and tidy household.
4. her heavy schedule of overtime at work.

Situation (questions 7–10): The patient is 54. He has a wife and two children. He has been employed in his present job for 15 years.

(149) 7. An activity that would indicate that the patient is engaged in the stage of generativity is
1. membership in the local golf club.
2. time spent quietly working on his stamp collection.
3. participation as a youth counselor at his church.
4. taking his wife out to dinner at least once a week.

(154) 8. The patient should have his eyes examined every 2–3 years at this age because
1. decreasing hormone levels affect vision.
2. nutritional problems may cause vision changes.
3. lack of exercise may affect vision.
4. presbyopia may affect near vision.

(155) 9. As a healthy individual, the patient at this age can count on
1. intellect remaining stable.
2. a stable level of strength and endurance.
3. an increased libido.
4. a decline in responsibilities.

(154) 10. A physical change that this patient might have is
1. steadily decreasing body fat.
2. graying of the hair on the head.
3. increasing muscle mass.
4. a need for increasing amounts of sleep.

(149) 11. A blended family consists of
1. a parent and child and a new parent.
2. a mom, dad, and children.
3. a single parent, a child, and a step-child.
4. mom and her children, dad and his children.

(150) 12. A risk factor for divorce among couples is (Select all that apply)
1. one or both partners did not finish high school.
2. only one partner is employed.
3. one partner's parents are deceased.
4. both partners are under age 20.

(150) 13. A behavior indicating maturity is
1. ability to earn a living.
2. being respectful of elders.
3. being able to tolerate frustration.
4. continuing to pursue education.

Student Name_____

CRITICAL THINKING ACTIVITIES

1. Determine which of your activities show that you are in a positive state of development according to Erikson.

2. Think about what health risks you face at this stage of your life. What can you alter in your lifestyle to decrease those risks?

MEETING CLINICAL OBJECTIVES

Directions: The following suggested activities will help you meet the stated clinical practice objectives for the chapter. Review your school's clinical objectives for the week and outline a plan of activities that will help you meet them. If you are unsure how to meet them, consult with your instructor at the beginning of the clinical day.

1. Assess an assigned patient's developmental stage.

2. Assess assigned patients for signs of the problems for which they are at the highest risk for within their age group.

3. Develop a teaching plan for the young adult to promote a healthy lifestyle that may help avoid health problems later in life.

4. Teach the middle adult about the preventive health care and diagnostic testing needed at this stage of life.

STEPS TOWARD BETTER COMMUNICATION

VOCABULARY BUILDING GLOSSARY

Term	Pronunciation	Definition
A. Individual Terms		
boomerang	BOOM e RANG	a curved stick that returns to the person who throws it (the children return home to live with their parents after living away for a while)
confidant/e	CON fi DANT	a person with whom you share close personal feelings and information
down-sizing	DOWN siz ing	when companies decrease their size and expenses by letting employees go
family-friendly	FAM i ly FRIEND ly	a situation that is positive or encouraging for the well-being of a family
hot flashes	HOT flashes	a sudden sensation of extreme warmth, often accompanied by perspiration and reddening of the face caused by the hormonal changes of menopause, not external temperatures
juggle	JUG gle	keep many things happening at the same time
menopause	MEN o pause	the time when a woman ceases to have monthly menstrual periods

parenting	PAR en ting	the qualities and skills used in raising children
peak (verb)	PEAK	to be at a high point
skeptical	SKEP ti cal	not sure something is true or right, doubtful
susceptible	sus CEP ti ble	easily affected or influenced by
urbanization	ur ban i ZA tion	becoming more like a city than the country
volunteering	vol un TEER ing	helping others on a voluntary basis, not for pay

B. Phrases

biological clock	bi o LOG i cal CLOCK	the natural growth and aging pattern of the human body, especially used about the period during which a woman can get pregnant
family ties	FAM i ly TIES	family relationships
life is all downhill	life is All DOWNhill	the best or highest part of life has been reached, and the rest of life will be worse, or going down
opposites attract	OPP o sites at TRACT	a saying that means a person is attracted to someone with opposite characteristics or qualities: a quiet person is attracted to an outgoing person, blondes to dark-haired people, etc.

COMPLETION

Directions: Fill in the blank(s) with the correct word(s) from the Vocabulary Building Glossary to complete the sentence.

1. Young adult females often have a(n) _____ with whom they can share problems and concerns.

2. P.T. lost his job due to _____ of his company.

3. Women often have a difficult time learning to _____ the responsibilities of both career and child-raising.

4. Many middle-aged couples have the problem of _____ children who return home after being gone for a few years.

5. Unfortunately for middle-aged women, _____ often occurs at the same time that there are teenagers at home.

6. Once children leave the home, adults have more time for _____ in the community.

7. The couple did not want the transfer the company was offering because they have _____ in the area and do not wish to be far away from all their relatives.

Student Name _____

VOCABULARY EXERCISES

Directions: List some opposite types that might attract each other.

Example: urban vs. rural

1. quiet _____
2. blonde _____
3. athletic _____
4. tall _____
5. large _____

PRONUNCIATION AND STRESS

In the Vocabulary Building Glossary, we have indicated where the stress or accent falls in a word as it is normally used. For understanding, using the correct stress pattern is more important than using the correct sounds. There are a few basic rules for placing stress in words in English:

1. Not counting verbs, 90% of two-syllable words are stressed on the first syllable; for example: healthy, lifestyle, caring, people, spinal, column.

2. In words with three or more syllables, one syllable gets the main stress (indicated by capital letters in the glossary), and sometimes there is a secondary stress.

3. There also are certain pronunciation patterns that can be found. In words with certain endings, like those below, the stress is on the syllable that comes before the ending.

Directions: Underline the stressed syllable, then practice the pronunciation aloud. Add other words to the list as you find them, and notice any that are different from the pattern.

-tion/-sion	-ic/-ical	-omy	-ogy	-ity
urbanization	pelvic	economy	biology	maturity
generation	chronic	autonomy	sociology	infidelity
question	biological		gerontology	validity
maturation	skeptical			flexibility
tension	physical			obesity
stagnation	cervical			promiscuity
				generativity
				personality

-ery	-edy	-istry
delivery	remedy	dentistry
grocery	tragedy	chemistry
nursery	comedy	
surgery		

COMMUNICATION EXERCISES

1. Read the following conversation. Discuss it with your classmates or a friend. Practice reading it aloud with a partner. How do you think Ms. L. will feel? What do you think she will do? Was this a good way to handle the problem?

Nurse:	"Thank you for coming in today, Ms. L. I want to talk to you about your son."
Ms. L.:	"Has he gotten into trouble again?"
Nurse:	"No, but the kindergarten teacher brought him into the office because he has bruises on his upper arms. Do you know how he might have gotten them?"
Ms. L.:	"No, not unless he got in a fight with the boys."
Nurse:	"These look like an adult held him very tightly. Do you know when that could have happened?"
Ms. L.:	"Well, 2 days ago when he wouldn't sit down and be quiet, I grabbed him and gave him a good shaking. But I didn't hurt him. That boy just won't listen!"
Nurse:	"I know you think you didn't hurt him, but he is bruised. Did you know that severe shaking can cause brain damage and even death in young children?"
Ms. L.:	"No! But I am sure I didn't hurt him that much."
Nurse:	"It doesn't take very much when they are small. And we are required to report any suspected physical abuse—like repeated shaking, slapping, and hitting—to the authorities."
Ms. L.:	"But how am I supposed to get him to listen? That is the way our parents treated us, and it didn't hurt us any!"
Nurse:	"We know more now about the damage it can cause, and at any rate, there are laws about it now. Let me give you this pamphlet on discipline and make an appointment for you and your husband to come back so we can talk about other ways that you can use to discipline your son."
Ms. L.:	"Well, I guess I had better do something. I don't want to hurt my son and I don't want to get in trouble with the law."

2. Discuss with a group whether you think opposites attract. Can you think of some examples? Why do you think it might be true?

CULTURAL POINTS

1. How do people in your native country learn about parenting? Are classes available or do they learn from their families? How have you learned? How do you feel about a different way of learning? What methods of discipline are common? Do you think they are effective? Would they be acceptable in the U.S.?

2. Do the three stages of adulthood follow the same pattern in your native country? In a group, talk about how they are the same or different.

Review the chapter key points, answer the study questions, and complete the critical thinking activities at the end of the chapter in the textbook.

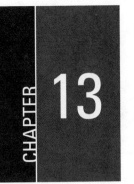

CHAPTER 13
Promoting Healthy Adaptation to Aging

Answer Key: Textbook page references are provided as a guide for answering selected questions. A complete answer key was provided for your instructor.

TERMINOLOGY

A. Matching

Directions: Match the terms in Column I with the definitions in Column II.

Column I

(164)	1. _____	ageism
(161)	2. _____	centenarians
(162)	3. _____	dementia
(161)	4. _____	demographic
(159)	5. _____	gerontologist
(160)	6. _____	longevity
(164)	7. _____	reminiscence
(163)	8. _____	wisdom

Column II

a. Length of life
b. Statistics about populations
c. People over 100 years old
d. Degeneration of brain tissue
e. Having good judgment based on accumulated knowledge
f. Discrimination because of age
g. Reviewing one's life
h. Specialists in the study of aging people

B. Completion

Directions: Fill in the blank(s) with the correct term(s) from the terms list in the chapter in the textbook to complete the sentence.

(161)   1. _____, the normal changes of aging, begin in early adulthood.

(160)   2. Ways to look at the physical aging process are based on _____ theories.

(164)   3. Erikson's stage of development for older adults is called _____ vs. Despair.

(165)   4. A nurse must legally report _____ to a law enforcement agency.

(160)   5. The _____ for human beings is 115–120 years.

(160)   6. The disengagement theory, a _____ theory, states that it is normal for older people and society to withdraw from each other.

SHORT ANSWER

Directions: Write a brief answer for each question.

(160)   1.   Identify five biologic theories on the aging process.

a. _____

b. _____

c. _____

d. _____

e. _____

(160)   2.   Give a probable response of an aging adult considering the following psychosocial theories of aging:

a.   Disengagement theory _____

_____

_____

b.   Activity theory _____

_____

_____

c.   Continuity theory_____

_____

_____

(160)   3.   Four factors that contribute to longevity are:

a. _____

b. _____

c. _____

d. _____

(162)   4.   Indicate one physical change that occurs with aging for each body system.

a.   Cardiovascular:_____

b.   Respiratory: _____

c.   Musculoskeletal: _____

d.   Integumentary:_____

e.   Urological: _____

f.   Neurological: _____

g.   Endocrine: _____

h.   Gastrointestinal: _____

i.   Reproductive: _____

Student Name_____

(163) 5. Describe the essence of Shaie's theory for cognitive development in the older adult.

_____

_____

(164) 6. Give two examples of behaviors that would indicate a person is in the stage of Ego Integrity.

a. _____

b _____

(163) 7. Give three examples of activities that might help older adults maintain cognitive health.

a. _____

b. _____

c. _____

(166) 8. Identify five signs that an older person needs assistance.

a. _____

b. _____

c. _____

d. _____

e. _____

(162-163) 9. Ways to physically prepare the older adult to prevent falls are to encourage:

_____

_____

(162-163) 10. Four ways to promote health in the older adult are:

a. _____

b. _____

c. _____

d. _____

COMPLETION

Directions: Fill in the blank(s) with the correct word(s) to complete the sentence.

(160) 1. The average life span according to the U.S. Census Bureau is _____ years.

(160) 2. Two lifestyle factors, a healthy _____ and regular _____, are crucial to longevity.

(160) 3. A person's _____ seems to affect the length of life as well as the quality.

(160) 4. Heredity seems to account for only _____ percent of longevity.

(161) 5. Nearly 75% of the population over age _____ has some hearing loss.

(161) 6. _____ is the most common chronic health problem in those over age 75.

(162) 7. About 10% of older adults are clinically _____.

(163) 8. Others often think that older adults cannot continue to learn simply because they _____ more slowly; they can and do continue to learn.

(163) 9. More severe memory losses and dementias of aging are often the result of _____ changes.

(164) 10. Having a(n) _____ attitude is very important to successful aging.

(164) 11. Active involvement in the community through _____ work is a good way for an older adult to stay active and involved.

(165) 12. Older adults need to feel _____ as this contributes to their self-concept and emotional health.

(163) 13. Regular exercise of at least 30 minutes 5 times a week is thought to decrease mental decline by _____ percent.

NCLEX-PN® EXAM REVIEW

*Directions: Choose the **best** answer(s) to each of the following questions.*

Situation: The patient is 78 years old. She is a widow and lives alone. She has hypertension which is controlled and some rheumatoid arthritis that is worsening.

(160) 1. The arthritis in the patient's knees could possibly be explained by which of the following biologic theories of aging?
1. Biological clock theory
2. Free-radical theory
3. Immune system failure theory
4. Autoimmune theory

(160) 2. The continuity theory explains why this patient
1. copes as she has coped before.
2. is more withdrawn than in younger years.
3. wants to stay as active as possible.
4. makes no effort to contribute to the community.

(162) 3. One reason the patient might feel cold in rooms where younger people feel warmer is that
1. her thyroid function has declined.
2. she is not as active as she used to be.
3. she has less subcutaneous fat at this age.
4. the skin thins with advanced age.

(162-163) 4. The patient's appetite has waned. Her appetite might be improved by (Select all that apply)
1. sharing meals with others.
2. using a microwave oven to heat meals.
3. adding additional seasonings to foods.
4. increasing the amount of fresh vegetables at meals.

Student Name _____

5. Patient teaching includes using various methods for instruction. A variety of teaching aids can also be utilized. When teaching the older adult, in addition to going over things orally and demonstrating any skill, it is wise to give the patient _____ _____ as well. (Fill in the blank)

(163) 6. The older patient is having trouble with recent memory. One technique that can assist with remembering things is to
   1. repeat what she needs to remember out loud.
   2. concentrate on what needs to be remembered for 10 seconds.
   3. tell someone else to remind her of what she needs to remember.
   4. make written lists or mark appointments on a calendar.

(164) 7. One factor that may contribute to ego integrity for the older adult is
   1. setting goals for the future.
   2. being proud of the children she raised.
   3. regretting that she did not go to college.
   4. wishing that she had had a career.

(164) 8. The older patient has a better chance of adjusting to continued aging in positive ways if he or she
   1. remains actively involved with others.
   2. curtails her activities to prevent fatigue.
   3. depends on her daughter to do her errands.
   4. has a living will in place with her doctor.

(166) 9. It would be wise for an older patient's daughter to speak about
   1. how he or she wishes to distribute her estate when death occurs.
   2. granting power of attorney before becoming really ill.
   3. how various crises that may occur should be handled.
   4. having someone come and live with him or her now.

(166) 10. The patient's daughter would know that her mother needs more assistance if
   1. the dishes are not done before noon.
   2. the clothes she is wearing are often soiled.
   3. she starts spending all her time at the senior center.
   4. she repeats stories about the trips she has made.

CRITICAL THINKING ACTIVITIES

1. Create an educational program to assist older adults to maintain physical and mental health. Points to cover are:

2. Identify problems that will occur if an older adult mentally deteriorates.

MEETING CLINICAL OBJECTIVES

Directions: The following suggested activities will help you meet the stated clinical practice objectives for the chapter. Review your school's clinical objectives for the week and outline a plan of activities that will help you meet them. If you are unsure how to meet them, consult with your instructor at the beginning of the clinical day.

1. Assess an older adult for physical signs of aging.

2. Take a psychosocial history on an older adult and identify areas that contribute to ego integrity.

3. Assess an older adult who has a chronic disease and determine how this, along with the changes attributed to aging, affects the quality of life.

4. Identify problems related to psychosocial health in an elderly patient with a chronic health problem.

5. Using possible community resources, try to help an older adult improve the quality of his or her life.

6. Design a general educational program to assist older adults maintain physical and cognitive health.

STEPS TOWARD BETTER COMMUNICATION

VOCABULARY BUILDING GLOSSARY

Term	Pronunciation	Definition
benign	be NIGN	harmless, gentle
elder hostel	ELD er HOS tel	relatively low-cost programs where elders can travel or live in dormitories for a short period of time, and take classes and attend lectures or programs
irrelevant	ir REL e vant	not important, not connected with what is happening
lifestyle	LIFE style	the manner and habits of a person's life
myth	MYTH	a story told by many people as true, but without proof
nest egg	NEST egg	some money put aside for future use, such as retirement

COMPLETION

Directions: Fill in the blank(s) with the correct word(s) from the Vocabulary Building Glossary.

1. The fact that there was a senior center in town was _____ to C.S., as she had no way to get there.

2. It is hoped that each elderly person will not outlive his or her _____ and have to rely on community and government services to survive.

3. It is a(n) _____ that elderly people have no power in this country.

4. One must put aside considerable money throughout life in order to maintain the same _____ after retirement.

VOCABULARY EXERCISES

Myth versus Theory versus Fact

A fact is something that has been proven to be true. Neither myths nor theories are proven facts; but a theory is based on facts, while a myth is based on tradition or on beliefs that may not be true.

Student Name _____

Directions: Indicate whether the following statements are Myth (M), Theory (T), or Fact (F).

1. Gerontologists say heredity plays a part in determining longevity. _____

2. Older people cannot learn new things. _____

3. Heart and lungs are usually less efficient in the older adult. _____

PRONUNCIATION AND STRESS

In the Vocabulary Building Glossary, we indicated where the stress or accent falls in a word as it is normally used. Using the correct stress pattern is often more important for people's understanding than using the correct sounds. Equally important for clear understanding of meaning is where the stress falls in a sentence or a phrase.

In English, the content words are usually given extra emphasis. Content words are words which have the most information. Even if you only heard those words you would have some idea of what was being said. You can emphasize a word by giving extra length to the stressed syllables.

She ATE all her MEAL.

Stress can change the meaning in the following phrases:

YOU did excellent work. (But your friend did not.)
You DID excellent work. (But this week, your work is not so good.)
You did EXCELLENT work. (It was very, very good.)
You did excellent WORK. (But your attitude was not very good.)

COMMUNICATION EXERCISE

Directions: Put a line in the sentence under the words that receive stress, then practice reading it aloud. With a partner read the following dialogue:

Mr. H. has hypertension, high cholesterol, and diabetes mellitus and his doctor has prescribed medications. The nurse is doing a regular home visit with him.

Nurse: "Good morning, Mr. H. How are you feeling?"

Mr. H.: "Pretty good for an old guy my age."

Nurse: "Now, what medications are you taking?"

Mr. H.: "Oh, I don't know. There are some pink ones and some red ones. There were some big horse pills too, but I stopped taking them."

Nurse: "Why? Did the doctor tell you to stop?"

Mr. H.: "No, but they weren't doing me any good and they stuck in my throat."

Nurse: "How do you know they weren't doing you any good?"

Mr. H.: "Well, I don't feel any different when I take them."

Nurse: "Mr. H., some medications don't make any difference in how you feel, but they are doing their job in your body. Your cholesterol and hypertension pills help keep the blood vessels open to your heart and brain so you won't have a stroke or heart attack. You don't want your wife to have to take care of you if you can't talk or feed yourself, do you?"

Mr. H.: "Oh gosh, no! Is that what will happen?"

Nurse:	"Well, the medication helps prevent those types of complications. If you have some side effects or other problems taking those pills, talk to the doctor and maybe he can change the prescription. But you should continue taking them until you talk to the doctor."
Mr. H.:	"Well, OK, but I sure don't like those horse pills!"
Nurse:	"You know the old saying, 'healthy as a horse.' Maybe that's how they stay healthy! Seriously, let's see if the pills can be cut in half."

Review the chapter key points, answer the study questions, and complete the critical thinking activities at the end of the chapter in the textbook.

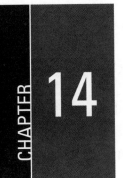

CHAPTER 14

Cultural and Spiritual Aspects of Patient Care

Answer Key: Textbook page references are provided as a guide for answering selected questions. A complete answer key was provided for your instructor.

TERMINOLOGY

A. Matching

Directions: Match the terms in Column I with the definitions in Column II.

Column I

(169)	1. _____	agnostic
(169)	2. _____	atheist
(169)	3. _____	beliefs
(174)	4. _____	bias
(175)	5. _____	egalitarian
(174)	6. _____	ethnocentrism
(169)	7. _____	faith
(174)	8. _____	generalization
(171)	9. _____	kosher
(175-176)	10. _____	matriarchal
(175-176)	11. _____	patriarchal
(173)	12. _____	race
(169)	13. _____	rituals
(168)	14. _____	values
(173)	15. _____	transcultural

Column II

a. Ceremonial acts or practices
b. Conviction or opinion considered to be true
c. Belief which cannot be proven
d. Person who does not believe in the existence of God
e. Person who doubts the existence of God
f. Biologic way of categorizing people
g. Positive or negative attitude or opinion that inhibits impartial judgment
h. Female-dominated
i. Male-dominated
j. Equal authority between male and female
k. Tendency of humans to think that their way of thinking, believing, and doing things is the only way
l. Identifies common trends, patterns, and beliefs of a group
m. Ideas and perceptions seen as good and useful
n. Recognizing cultural diversity
o. Way of ritually slaughtering, preparing, and packaging food

B. Completion

Directions: Fill in the blank(s) with the correct term(s) from the terms list in the chapter in the textbook to complete the sentence.

(173)   1. Respecting accepted patterns of communication and refraining from speaking in ways that are disrespectful of a person's cultural beliefs displays cultural

_____.

(174)   2. Nurses must not _____ a patient by applying an overall opinion of a cultural group to that individual.

(174)   3. Different _____ of a language reflect regional variations with different pronunciation, grammar, or word meanings.

(168)   4. The shared values, beliefs, and practices shared by a majority of a group of people is termed their _____.

(168)   5. A group's _____ is the way in which they explain life events and view life's mysteries.

(169)   6. An element of religion, _____, concerns the spirit, or soul.

(169)   7. _____ is a formalized system of belief and worship.

(173)   8. _____ groups are differentiated by geographic, religious, social, or language differences.

(176)   9. Many Asians/Pacific Islanders believe that health is dependent on the flow of _____, the universal life force.

(176) 10. Many Asians also believe that the forces of _____ and _____ must be in balance in order to be in good health.

(176) 11. Some Hispanic Americans may seek the services of a _____ when ill.

(177) 12. Many American Indians will wish to consult a _____ when ill.

(171) 13. In the Jewish religion, _____, removal of the penile foreskin, is performed on the eighth day of life.

(174) 14. The distance from each other at which people are comfortable when conversing is called _____ space.

COMPARISONS

Directions: List three beliefs or values affecting health care for each cultural group.

(176)

Cultural Group	Beliefs or Values
Hispanic American	
Asian American	

Student Name _____

American Indian	
African American	
European American	

SHORT ANSWER

Directions: Write a brief answer for each question.

(173)   1. List three ways in which poverty often impedes adequate health care in our country.

  a. _____

  b. _____

  c. _____

2. Identify one dietary/nutritional practice or belief that is pertinent to the nursing care of each of the following cultural/religious groups:

  a. Hispanic American _____

    _____

    _____

  b. Muslim _____

    _____

    _____

  c. Jewish _____

    _____

    _____

  d. Hindu _____

    _____

    _____

(173-174)   3.   Identify ways in which you can achieve cultural competence.

_____

_____

_____

_____

(173)   4.   Cultural awareness involves:

_____

_____

_____

(174)   5.   Areas in which cultural difference is evident are:

a.   _____

b.   _____

c.   _____

d.   _____

e.   _____

f.   _____

COMPLETION

Directions: Fill in the blank(s) with the correct word(s) to complete the sentence.

(169)   1.   Both spirituality and culture have to do with attempting to understand one's place in the world and life's _____ or _____.

(169)   2.   During illness or when facing death are times when religious and spiritual beliefs may be strengthened, questioned, or _____.

(169)   3.   Religious beliefs and rituals are interwoven into a group's _____.

(169)   4.   For Christians, death is viewed as a(n) _____ to a life with God.

(171)   5.   The religious book of Muslims is the _____.

(172)   6.   Circumcision of the Jewish male infant is to be done on the _____ day of life.

(172)   7.   Many Hindus are _____ and this must be considered when planning the diet.

(172-173)   8.   Buddhists believe that liberation from _____ through following Buddha's teachings is important in promoting health and recovery.

Student Name _____

(173)   9. Taoists believe that illness or disease is due to an imbalance in
_____ and _____.

(173)   10. Within cultures, the homeless are considered a(n) _____
with distinct problems of their own.

(173)   11. Dr. M.M. Leninger claims that _____ is what all people
need most to grow, remain well, avoid illness, and survive or face death.

(174)   12. Care must be taken not to let _____ affect one's attitude toward a patient.

(174)   13. The Vietnamese patient may avoid eye contact when talking with someone
they consider an _____ figure or who is
_____.

(174)   14. In European American culture, _____ is the usual
space between people that is comfortable when they are talking together.

(174)   15. An orientation toward the future is a(n) _____ domi-
nant cultural trait in the United States, but not of the African American or the Hispanic
American cultures.

(176)   16. The Hispanic American family is essentially _____ in
structure, while the African American family is _____.

(176)   17. Foods considered "hot" or "cold" within some cultures are based on characteristics other
than _____.

(175)   18. All cultures have an element of _____ medicine that is
handed down through families for treatment of common illnesses.

(178)   19. Keloid formation is more common among _____.

(178)   20. Diabetes is more common among the _____ and
_____ population due to a genetic susceptibility.

APPLICATION OF THE NURSING PROCESS

Directions: Write a brief answer for each question.

1. Without looking in the textbook, list four assessment questions regarding culture and spirituality you
would ask your patient.

   a. _____

   b. _____

   c. _____

   d. _____

2. List three common nursing diagnoses related to cultural and spiritual problems.

   a. _____

   b. _____

   c. _____

3. Write an expected outcome for each nursing diagnosis related to spirituality and culture.

   a. _____

   b. _____

   c. _____

4. List three general ways in which you could individualize nursing actions for a patient's culture while meeting basic needs.

   a. _____

   b. _____

   c. _____

5. Identify how you would evaluate care to determine if the expected outcomes were met.

   _____

   _____

   _____

   _____

NCLEX-PN® EXAM REVIEW

*Directions: Choose the **best** answer(s) for each of the following questions.*

(174) 1. Assuming that all African Americans like grits with their breakfast is an example of
   1. ethnocentrism.
   2. stereotyping.
   3. values.
   4. culture.

(170) 2. A religious group that does not believe in using the services of physicians in most instances is
   1. Muslims.
   2. Jews.
   3. Taoists.
   4. Christian Scientists.

(171) 3. The Jewish religious leader is called a(n)
   1. imam.
   2. priest.
   3. rabbi.
   4. minister.

(172) 4. Orthodox Jews should never be served which two items at the same meal?
   1. milk and meat
   2. meat and bread
   3. milk and bread
   4. fruit and meat

(172) 5. Many Hindus believe that
   1. Christ was a prophet.
   2. what happens to them is the will of God.
   3. eating meat is necessary to keep healthy.
   4. praying will bring a favorable response from God.

(173) 6. A group within a larger culture that holds different beliefs, values, and attitudes is called a(n)
   1. subculture.
   2. diversity.
   3. sect.
   4. ethnic group.

Student Name_____

(175) 7. A group that does not view punctuality at all times to be of high value is
   1. European Americans.
   2. Arab Americans.
   3. Hispanic Americans.
   4. Asian Americans.

(176) 8. A cultural group in which families are often matriarchal is
   1. Hispanic American.
   2. European American.
   3. Asian American.
   4. African American.

(178) 9. Diabetes is more common among
   1. European Americans.
   2. Arab Americans.
   3. Asian Americans.
   4. Hispanic Americans.

(175) 10. Cultures that view foods as "hot" or "cold" based on their effect in the body are (Select all that apply)
   1. European American.
   2. Arab American.
   3. Asian American.
   4. Hispanic American.

(168) 11. Culture is the
   1. language, food preferences, and habits of a group.
   2. values, beliefs, and practices of a people.
   3. rituals, language, and traditions of a people.
   4. ethnicity, religion, and values of a people.

12. Knowing who is the dominant person in the family is important because the dominant person
   1. determines the family value system regarding health practices.
   2. is the main health care provider for the family.
   3. tends to make health care decisions.
   4. is the family member designated to communicate to the nurse.

(178) 13. Certain groups tend to have a genetically based lactase deficiency. Lactase deficiency is prevalent among _____ _____. (Fill in the blank)

(178) 14. Sickle-cell disease is a genetically transmitted disorder. Sickle-cell trait is most prevalent among _____ _____. (Fill in the blank)

(175) 15. A family with equality between the man and the woman is considered
   1. egalitarian.
   2. patriarchal.
   3. matriarchal.
   4. ethnocentric.

CRITICAL THINKING ACTIVITIES

1. Compare your own cultural beliefs toward health care with those of a peer from a different culture.

   Your beliefs:_____

   Peer's beliefs: _____

2. Plan how you would help meet the spiritual needs of a Hindu, a Buddhist, and a Muslim.

   Hindu:_____

   Buddhist: _____

   Muslim:_____

MEETING CLINICAL OBJECTIVES

Directions: The following suggested activities will help you meet the stated clinical practice objectives for the chapter. Review your school's clinical objectives for the week and outline a plan of activities that will help you meet them. If you are unsure how to meet them, consult with your instructor at the beginning of the clinical day.

1. Ask to be assigned to patients from different cultural groups.

2. Ask to be assigned to a patient whose language you do not speak.

3. Locate the health facility chapel so that you can offer its solace to family members when appropriate.

4. Contact a religious leader for a patient to whom you are assigned.

5. Identify spiritual distress in assigned patients and plan interventions to relieve it.

6. Discuss how to protect patients' rights when they wish to refuse a medical treatment because of cultural or religious beliefs.

STEPS TOWARD BETTER COMMUNICATION

VOCABULARY BUILDING GLOSSARY

Term	Pronunciation	Definition
A. Individual Terms		
attire	at TIRE	what people wear; clothing
impede	im PEDE	to slow down; get in the way of
prevalent	PREV a lent	common, observed frequently
refrain from	re FRAIN from	to avoid, or not do, something
sustained	sus TAINed	continued, constant
B. Phrases		
a wealth of information	a WEALTH of in for MA tion	a very large amount of information or facts
keep an open mind	keep an OPEN mind	to listen for new information before making a decision about something or someone

COMPLETION

Directions: Fill in the blank(s) with term(s) from the Vocabulary Building Glossary to complete the sentence.

1. She tried to _____ making a quick judgment about the person from his appearance.

2. Her _____ was that of a Hindu woman.

3. African Americans are very _____ in our hospital population.

4. The nurse made a(n) _____ effort to perform a cultural assessment on every patient.

5. The old chart contained a(n) _____ about the patient's medical history and psychosocial needs.

PRONUNCIATION OF DIFFICULT TERMS

Remember that even if all the sounds in a word are correctly pronounced, placing the stress incorrectly can cause misunderstanding.

Directions: Practice pronouncing the following words.

agnostic	ag NOS tic
atheist	A the ist
egalitarian	e GAL i TAR i an
ethnocentricity	ETH no cen TRI ci ty
matriarchal	MA tri ARCH al
patriarchal	PA tri ARCH al

WORD ATTACK SKILLS

Directions: Find five words in the chapter in each of the following categories and underline the stressed syllable.

1. Accent or stress on the first syllable:

    _____

    _____

2. Accent or stress on the second syllable:

    _____

    _____

3. Accent or stress on the third syllable:

    _____

    _____

4. Accent or stress on the fourth syllable:

    _____

    _____

COMMUNICATION EXERCISES

1. With a native speaker, read the words you found in the exercise above to make sure you have the correct stress.

2. Number practice: Stress makes a great difference in understanding numbers. Two different stress patterns are possible with numbers, but native speakers usually choose the one that makes the meaning clear. THIRty and THIRteen are possible, but when you are trying to distinguish or contrast the two, the stress changes: THIRty, not thirTEEN, or twenty-THREE, not twenty-FOUR.

3. Complete the following chart with a partner. Look only at your chart. Ask your partner questions to help you fill in the blanks in your chart, and answer your partner's questions.

STUDENT A		
Room Number	**Date of Birth**	**Time of Admission**
790	?	10:31 A.M.
?	3/16/70	?
231	?	7:17 P.M.
?	8/15/80	?
STUDENT B		
Room Number	**Date of Birth**	**Time of Admission**
?	7/13/50	?
314	?	12:15 P.M.
?	11/30/19	?
240	?	5:14 P.M.

CULTURAL POINTS

While it is important to be sensitive and observe all the considerations and precautions that are mentioned in the textbook, it may be somewhat reassuring to realize that most of the patients you will encounter have been living in this culture for some time and will be used to the predominant way of interacting. However, it is still respectful and caring, especially in a time of illness, to treat them with as much sensitivity and understanding as possible.

Review the chapter key points, answer the study questions, and complete the critical thinking activities at the end of the chapter in the textbook.

CHAPTER 15

Loss, Grief, and the Dying Patient

Answer Key: Textbook page references are provided as a guide for answering selected questions. A complete answer key was provided for your instructor.

TERMINOLOGY

A. Matching

Directions: Match the terms in Column I with the definitions in Column II.

Column I			Column II
(192)	1.	_____ autopsy	a. Philosophy of care for the dying
(183)	2.	_____ bereavement	b. Study of death
(192)	3.	_____ coroner	c. Treatment provided solely for comfort
(185)	4.	_____ hospice	d. Person with legal authority to determine cause of death
(190)	5.	_____ obituary	
(187)	6.	_____ palliation	e. Examination of body tissues to determine cause of death
(192)	7.	_____ postmortem	
(193)	8.	_____ rigor mortis	f. A notice of death published in the newspapers
(193)	9.	_____ shroud	g. State of having suffered a loss by death
(186)	10.	_____ thanatology	h. Cover with which body is wrapped after death
			i. After death
			j. Stiffening of a dead body

B. Completion

Directions: Fill in the blank(s) with the correct term(s) from the terms list in the chapter in the textbook to complete the sentence.

(183)   1. _____ refers to no longer possessing or having an object, person, or situation.

(183)   2. The emotional feeling of pain and distress in response to a loss is termed

_____.

(183)   3. _____ may occur before a loss actually happens.

(183)   4. Dysfunctional grieving would be that which falls outside

_____.

(187)   5. Hope can be described as a feeling that what is desired is

_____.

(191)   6. _____ spell out the patient's wishes for health care at that time when the person may be unable to indicate his or her choice.

SHORT ANSWER

Directions: Write a brief answer for each question.

(184)   1. In the high-tech hospital environment where equipment and medications can sustain a patient's breathing and heartbeat, what is necessary for death to be declared?

_____

(185)   2. Today, a hospice is: _____

_____

(187)   3. Identify three common fears a patient is likely to experience when dying.

a. _____

b. _____

c. _____

(191)   4. What is euthanasia?

_____

_____

(191)   5. Describe the difference between active and passive euthanasia.

_____

_____

_____

_____

(191)   6. How does assisted suicide differ from active euthanasia?

_____

_____

_____

_____

(191)   7. What parts of the ANA Position Statements make it a violation for a nurse to participate in active euthanasia or assisted suicide?

_____

_____

_____

_____

Student Name_____

(185) 8. Which portion of the Rights of the Dying Patient guide the nurse's behavior regarding the patient's right to have treatment to extend life withheld?

_____

(188-189) 9. Give one nursing intervention for comfort care particular to the dying patient for each of the following problems.

a. pain_____

_____

b. nausea_____

_____

c. dyspnea_____

_____

d. anxiety _____

_____

e. constipation _____

_____

f. incontinence_____

_____

g. thirst _____

_____

h. anorexia _____

_____

(191) 10. Describe a health care proxy.

_____

_____

(189) 11. It is essential to monitor bowel patterns daily in terminally ill patients because they tend to develop constipation due to:

a. _____

b. _____

c. _____

(189) 12. The bad taste in the mouth that many terminal patients develop can be improved by _____.

(189) 13. A medication that can ease the secretions in the terminal patient that cause noisy respirations and a "death rattle" is _____.

(189) 14. Encouraging a life review allows a patient to put his or her life in perspective. When doing this it is more important to _____ than to _____.

(183)   15.   List five specific signs or symptoms of grief.

a. _____

b. _____

c. _____

d. _____

e. _____

CORRELATION

Directions: Correlate the behavior in Column I with Kubler-Ross's stages of dying in Column II.

(186)

Column I   **Column II**

1. _____ Stays in bed most of the time.   a. Denial
2. _____ Tells God, "I'll quit smoking if I can   b. Bargaining
             just live until after my daughter's   c. Anger
             wedding."   d. Depression
3. _____ "My family will be fine after I'm   e. Acceptance
             gone."
4. _____ "My stomach is just easily upset; I
             don't have cancer."
5. _____ "Go away, I don't want company."
6. _____ Thinks "If Mom will just be OK,
             I'll do my homework every day."
7. _____ "I'm going to sue that doctor for
             telling him that."
8. _____ "She'll soon be at peace."
9. _____ "She's not that sick!"
10. _____ "I feel so hopeless about Mom's
             condition."

APPLICATION OF THE NURSING PROCESS

Directions: Write a brief answer for each question.

(187-188)   1.   Four other areas to specifically assess in addition to gathering a history and performing a physical assessment for a terminally ill patient would be:

a. _____

b. _____

c. _____

d. _____

Student Name_____

(188) 2. List three nursing diagnoses you feel would be common at some point to most dying patients.

    a. _____

    b. _____

    c. _____

(188) 3. During the planning process, a first priority is to _____.

4. Write a realistic expected outcome for each of the nursing diagnoses listed above.

    a. _____

    b. _____

    c. _____

(188) 5. Interventions regarding pain control for the terminally ill often require adding prn medication for _____.

(189) 6. A(n) _____ and _____ program can be used to alleviate problems of constipation.

(189) 7. A point to remember when considering nutritional intake for the terminal patient is that decreased intake is _____ for the patient than having _____.

(190) 8. Evaluation of success of the nursing care plan is based on _____.

NCLEX-PN® EXAM REVIEW

*Directions: Choose the **best** answer(s) for each of the following questions.*

1. A major focus for the nurse in caring for the terminally ill patient should be
   1. assisting the patient to interact with family members.
   2. advocating medications and treatments that can prolong life.
   3. providing comfort measures that promote well-being.
   4. assuring the patient that things will get better.

(191) 2. Advance directives usually do NOT
   1. direct disposition of the patient's belongings.
   2. state what measures the patient wishes to be used to prolong life.
   3. direct which organs may be donated after death.
   4. express whether resuscitation should be attempted.

(186) 3. There are several stages of grief that a patient may go through when given a terminal prognosis. When a patient who is dying continues to make concrete plans for next summer's vacation, it indicates he is in the stage of _____.

(Fill in the blank)

(186)   4. Likewise, family members often go through the stages of grief. A family member who is argumentative and rude to the dying patient may be going through the stage of

_____. (Fill in the blank)

(190)   5. The nurse sometimes can tell when the terminal patient nears death because there is
   1. elevation of the blood pressure.
   2. a period of quiet acceptance.
   3. mottling of the dependent extremities.
   4. cyanosis around the mouth.

(190)   6. As death approaches in the terminally ill patient, there is often a change in
   1. facial color.
   2. patient behavior.
   3. skin odor.
   4. respiratory pattern.

(185)   7. Hospice care focuses on (Select all that apply)
   1. prolonging life as long as possible.
   2. supporting the family through the patient's last illness.
   3. providing support and comfort measures.
   4. ending illness and hastening death.

(183)   8. Nurses may have a difficult time dealing with patient deaths if they
   1. did not foresee that the illness was terminal.
   2. have no friends among the unit staff.
   3. have not come to terms with their own mortality.
   4. cared for the patient for several days.

(187)   9. During assessment of the dying patient, it is good to ask
   1. "How did this illness come about?"
   2. "What are your concerns?"
   3. "Isn't your family coming to see you?"
   4. "How long do you think you will live?"

(188) 10. A continuing problem in caring for the dying patient is that
   1. families want the patient to die in the hospital.
   2. physicians expect nurses to tell them what the patient needs.
   3. narcotic regulations prevent adequate treatment of pain for the terminal patient.
   4. more than half of terminally ill patients die with uncontrolled pain.

CRITICAL THINKING ACTIVITIES

1. Your patient who suffered head trauma in an accident is on life support and expected to die at any time. Write out what you would say to the family regarding organ or tissue donation.

2. L.S., age 46, is dying of metastatic breast cancer. She becomes weaker every day and suffers from pain, constipation, incontinence, dyspnea, and anxiety. How can you support or instill hope in this patient and her family?

Student Name _____

MEETING CLINICAL OBJECTIVES

Directions: The following suggested activities will help you meet the stated clinical practice objectives for the chapter. Review your school's clinical objectives for the week and outline a plan of activities that will help you meet them. If you are unsure how to meet them, consult with your instructor at the beginning of the clinical day.

1. Imagine you have just been diagnosed with a terminal illness. Think about what you would want to do with your remaining days. How would you go about getting your "affairs in order"?

2. Devise a will and plan your own funeral.

3. Accompany a nurse who is going to give postmortem care.

4. Role play with a peer measures to support a grieving family member.

5. Explain to a patient how to complete an advance directive and what the terms *health care proxy* and *DNR* mean in lay terms.

6. Devise a plan of care for a dying patient that includes comfort measures for the problems of pain, nausea, dyspnea, anxiety, constipation, incontinence, thirst, and anorexia.

STEPS TOWARD BETTER COMMUNICATION

VOCABULARY BUILDING GLOSSARY

Term	Pronunciation	Definition
A. Individual Terms		
anticipatory	an tic i pa tor y	looking ahead at what might happen
clichés	cli CHES	sayings so common, or untrue, that they lose any meaning
closure	CLO sure	a condition where things are completed; a conclusion
collaboratively	col LAB or a tive ly	working together, sharing ideas and plans
commonalities	COM mon AL i ties	elements that are the same among a set of things
culmination	cul mi NA tion	final and total result
eradicate	e RAD i cate	to remove, to get rid of
enhance	en HANCE	to improve; add to
fluctuating	FLUC tu A ting	moving up and down; changing
grapple	GRAP ple	struggle; try hard to solve a problem
impending	im PEND ing	coming soon
inevitability	in EV i ta BIL i ty	happening no matter what action is taken
obituary	o BIT u ar y	an article in the paper announcing the death and describing the life of a person
proactive	PRO act ive	actively doing something for another person, **not** just standing by
prompted	PROMP ted	caused
proxy	PROX y	acting for another person

respite	RES pite	relief; rest
shielded	SHIELD ed	protected
validating	VAL i da ting	giving worth or value to something

B. Phrases

anticipating the likelihood	an TIC i PAT ing the LIKE li hood	expecting that something will happen
first and foremost	FIRST and FORE most	put the most important thing first
have a chilling effect	have a CHILL ing e FFECT	make something difficult, dangerous, or frightening

COMPLETION

Directions: Fill in the blank(s) with the correct term(s) from the Vocabulary Building Glossary to complete the sentence.

1. When the daughter heard about her father's metastatic cancer, she went into a state of _____ grief.

2. The nurse worked _____ with the respiratory therapist, the dietitian, and the occupational therapist to make the patient's remaining days as comfortable as possible.

3. Attending to the patient's problems with bowel function can _____ his or her comfort level and quality of life during a terminal illness.

4. Active listening on the part of the nurse can assist a patient to _____ with the issues facing him or her at the end of life.

5. The nurse needs to be _____ in working with the physician to alleviate the patient's pain.

6. The daughter was designated the patient's _____ regarding end-of-life care and desires.

7. Mr. O.'s wife badly needed a(n) _____ from the almost 24-hour-a-day care she was providing during his terminal illness.

8. Reviewing with Mr. O. his life accomplishments and major milestones was _____ for him.

VOCABULARY EXERCISE

Directions: Read the short paragraph about cloning which uses the phrases in the Vocabulary Building Glossary. Then, write a similar paragraph about euthanasia, using the same phrases.

"Scientists are anticipating the likelihood of the cloning of the human embryo. Even if ethical and moral considerations are first and foremost, the idea has a chilling effect on most people."

Student Name_____

WORD ATTACK SKILLS

Directions: Find the words in the Vocabulary Building Glossary that have more than four syllables and write them below, underlining the stressed syllable. Next, write the root word you find in the glossary word. What is its meaning?

Glossary Word	Root Word	Meaning

COMMUNICATION EXERCISES

Role Play

1. Write out what you would say to a family regarding organ or tissue donation. Role play that dialogue with a partner until you feel comfortable with the words and the emotions.

2. Look at your answers for Critical Thinking Activity #1c in the chapter in the textbook. Write two short dialogues, one with the patient and one with her family, of what you might say for support and comfort. Role play the dialogues with a partner.

CULTURAL POINTS

1. Customs around death vary from culture to culture and are very important to families, as they mark an important passage in life. Most cultures and religions have rules and rites dealing with death and the disposal of the body. In the United States, people are often very removed from death, as it usually occurs in hospitals, and health and funeral professionals handle the body. Some people do not even wish to view the body of a friend or loved one. In other cultures, such as Islam, the family is expected to wash the body and prepare it for burial according to custom and ritual. Be sure you know the family's wishes and needs if death is approaching.

2. Some euphemisms (a more agreeable expression used in place of an unpleasant one) used in English to refer to death are death, passed away, expired, deceased.

    He died/passed away/expired an hour ago.

    My mother is dead/deceased/departed/gone to be with God.

    She is at peace/at rest/in no more pain/with God.

3. Words of sympathy or condolence you might use to the family and friends are:

"I am sorry." "I am sorry for your loss." "You have my sympathy." "I'm so sorry this has happened to your family." "I'm so sorry things have ended like this." "I'm sorry that in spite of all efforts, we couldn't prevent his death." "I am sorry for your loss; is there someone I can call for you?"

Review the chapter key points, answer the study questions, and complete the critical thinking activities at the end of the chapter in the textbook.

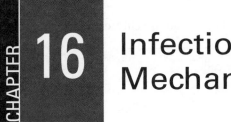

Student Name _____

CHAPTER 16
Infection, Protective Mechanisms, and Asepsis

Answer Key: Textbook page references are provided as a guide for answering selected questions. A complete answer key was provided for your instructor.

TERMINOLOGY

A. Matching

Directions: Match the terms in Column I with the definitions in Column II.

Column I

(198)	1. _____	antibiotic
(208)	2. _____	antimicrobial
(218)	3. _____	antiseptic
(207)	4. _____	asepsis
(201)	5. _____	contaminate
(203)	6. _____	debris
(217)	7. _____	disinfectant
(197)	8. _____	microorganism
(201)	9. _____	sterile
(201)	10. _____	sterilization

Column II

a. Organism only visible with a microscope
b. Chemical substance that can kill microorganisms
c. Process of destroying all microorganisms
d. Make unclean
e. Without pathologic organisms
f. Freedom from pathogenic microorganisms
g. Dead tissue or foreign matter
h. Killing or suppressing growth of microorganisms
i. Chemical compound used on skin or tissue to inhibit growth of microorganisms
j. Agent that destroys microorganisms

B. Completion

Directions: Fill in the blank(s) with the correct word(s) from the terms list in the chapter in the textbook to complete the sentence.

(198)   1. _____ organisms can only grow when oxygen is absent.

(197)   2. A single-celled organism lacking a nucleus that reproduces about every 20 minutes is a(n) _____ .

(199)   3. _____ can only grow and replicate within a living cell.

(199)   4. _____ are one-celled organisms that belong to the animal kingdom.

(199)   5. _____ are rod-shaped microorganisms that are transmitted by the bites of insects that act as _____ .

(199)   6. Tiny primitive organisms of the plant kingdom that contain no chlorophyll and reproduce by means of spores are _____.

(199)   7. Roundworm and tapeworm are parasitic and are called

_____.

(197)   8. _____ is a poisonous protein produced by certain bacteria.

(203)   9. A(n) _____ infection is one that is acquired in the hospital.

(197) 10. Microorganisms that are capable of causing disease are called

_____.

(198) 11. In order to determine which antibiotic will eradicate an infection, it is necessary to _____ the bacteria.

(207-208) 12. One of the most effective ways to prevent the transfer of microorganisms from one person to another is to _____.

(212, 216) 13. Handwashing is performed before _____ and immediately after _____ as they are not 100% protective.

(208) 14. When soap and water are not conveniently available, hands may be decontaminated with a(n) _____ hand rub.

(208) 15. When washing hands with soap and water, the scrub should last a minimum of _____ seconds.

(209) 16. Nail tips should be kept no longer than _____ inch long to prevent harboring of microorganisms.

(209) 17. When providing direct patient care you should not wear artificial _____ or extenders.

(217) 18. Disposable sharp instruments such as syringes, scalpel blades, and suture needles are often called _____.

(217) 19. Contaminated waste such as soiled dressings is disposed of in sealed plastic bags marked

_____.

1995) 20. Prions cause _____ disease, also known as "mad cow disease."

SHORT ANSWER

Directions: Write a brief answer for each question.

(201)   1. Characteristics that affect the virulence of microorganisms are the abilities to:

    a. _____

    b. _____

    c. _____

    d. _____

    e. _____

Student Name_____

(200-203) 2. Give one example for each of the links of the chain of infection.

      a. Causative agent_____

      b. Reservoir_____

      c. Portal of exit_____

      d. Mode of transmission_____

      e. Portal of entry _____

      f. Susceptible host _____

(207) 3. Describe the difference between medical asepsis and surgical asepsis.

_____

_____

_____

_____

(212) 4. Personal protective equipment (PPE) items include:

_____

_____

_____

(218) 5. The most effective means for destroying viruses and all other kinds of microorganisms is to:

_____

(205) 6. Four factors that may place an elderly patient at higher risk of infection compared to the younger adult are:

      a. _____

      b. _____

      c. _____

      d. _____

(203) 7. The first line of defense against infection is:

_____

(203) 8. The five defense mechanisms that destroy pathogens via the second line of defense are:

      a. _____

      b. _____

      c. _____

      d. _____

      e. _____

(204) 9. Phagocytes consist of _____ and _____ and work to remove cellular debris, destroy bacteria and viruses, and remove metabolic waste products by _____.

(206) 10. Briefly describe the inflammatory process.

_____

_____

_____

_____

_____

(207) 11. Naturally acquired immunity occurs when:

_____

_____

(207) 12. To develop passive acquired immunity, a person must be given a(n) _____ or _____ that contains _____.

(207) 13. Artificially acquired immunity is achieved through:

_____

_____

(212) 14. Considering standard precautions, a gown is to be worn _____.

(212) 15. A mask is worn when there is a chance of contact with _____ or _____.

(212) 16. Protective eyewear is worn whenever there is a possibility of _____.

(217) 17. To clean visibly soiled instruments or other items that are washable, gloves are always used and the following steps are taken:

a. _____

b. _____

c. _____

d. _____

e. _____

Student Name _____

NCLEX-PN® EXAM REVIEW

*Directions: Choose the **best** answer(s) for each of the following questions.*

(218)   1.   In the home care setting, contaminated dressings should be handled by _____ before disposal.
1.   boiling them for ten minutes
2.   treating them with a 1:10 chlorine solution
3.   securing them in plastic zip-closure bags
4.   washing in hot soapy water

(218)   2.   The hospital patient considered at high risk for nosocomial infection is the one who has
1.   been there more than 3 days.
2.   pneumonia.
3.   an indwelling catheter.
4.   just delivered a baby.

(201)   3.   Considering the chain of infection and the way pathogens are spread, contaminated water is considered a
1.   reservoir.
2.   portal of exit.
3.   susceptible host.
4.   causative agent.

(198)   4.   Many gram-negative bacteria are more dangerous than gram-positive bacteria because they
1.   multiply more rapidly.
2.   produce a dangerous endotoxin.
3.   cause severe diarrhea.
4.   are more virulent.

(203)   5.   The liver participates in protection of the body against infection by
1.   phagocytic action in the liver tissue.
2.   action of bile inactivating bacteria.
3.   flushing bacteria from the blood.
4.   destroying bacteria via the Kupffer's cells.

(203)   6.   Another body defense occurs in the gastrointestinal system as the
1.   hydrochloric acid in the stomach destroys pathogens.
2.   bile in the stool kills bacteria.
3.   digestive enzymes in the small intestine kill bacteria.
4.   peristaltic action of the intestines eliminates pathogens.

(204)   7.   Fever helps fight infection because heat
1.   kills most pathogens.
2.   slows the growth of pathogens.
3.   causes diaphoresis and flushing out of bacteria.
4.   causes more water consumption and urine production.

(206)   8.   The redness and warmth in an inflamed area is due to
1.   dilation of blood vessels and increased blood flow.
2.   increased temperature in the affected tissues.
3.   phagocytosis and chemical action against pathogens.
4.   formation of debris, causing tissue swelling.

(207)   9.   Normally, the immune system does not attack the self because
1.   only microorganisms cause antibody production.
2.   macrophages never attack one's own cells.
3.   cellular antigens help in distinguishing self from nonself.
4.   only foreign proteins cause antibody reaction.

(218)   10.   Effective disinfection of surfaces contaminated with blood and possible HIV is accomplished by
1.   scrubbing with soap and hot water for 3 minutes.
2.   soaking with 70% alcohol solution for 10 minutes.
3.   washing with iodine solution and then swabbing with alcohol.
4.   cleansing with a solution of 1:10 chlorine bleach and water.

(198)   11.   Performing a culture and sensitivity test when a patient has a wound infection is important because
1.   antibiotics will kill the bacteria.
2.   different organisms are killed by specific antibiotics.
3.   some wound infections should not be treated.
4.   cleansing alone will not cure the infection.

(199)   12.   Various microorganisms cause different problems. Diarrhea is often caused by
1.   *Rickettsia.*
2.   fungi.
3.   protozoa.
4.   helminths.

(199)   13.   Various types of organisms cause different disorders. Vaginal *Candidiasis* is caused by _____
_____.
(Fill in the blank)

(203)   14.   Nurses pay great attention to skin care for patients because (Select all that apply)
1.   cleanliness reduces the chance of infection.
2.   dirty skin predisposes to skin breakdown.
3.   everyone should have a bath every day.
4.   the skin is the first line of defense against infection.

(207)   15.   Giving a patient a serum immune globulin injection will provide
1.   passive acquired immunity.
2.   naturally acquired passive immunity.
3.   artificially acquired immunity.
4.   passive artificially acquired immunity.

(209)   16.   Considering handwashing as a measure to prevent infection, important guidelines are that (Select all that apply)
1.   a 5-minute scrub is always appropriate.
2.   handwashing time should be adjusted to the amount of contamination of the hands.
3.   hands should be washed in running water to wash away any bacteria.
4.   only special antimicrobial soap will sufficiently kill the bacteria on the hands.

(212)   17.   Standard precautions were developed by the CDC to
1.   protect patients.
2.   protect health care workers.
3.   break the chain of infection.
4.   prevent hospital-acquired infection.

(212, 216) 18.   Handwashing after removing gloves is necessary because
1.   powder from the gloves remains on the hands.
2.   gloves are not 100% protective.
3.   contamination occurs when removing the gloves.
4.   otherwise the gloves irritate the hands.

Student Name_____

(201) 19. Which one of the following could be a vector capable of transmitting pathogens?
1. tick
2. eating utensil
3. human
4. water

(217) 20. Before sterilizing instruments, you should
1. rinse off all visible matter with cool water.
2. soak them in cool water.
3. soak them in alcohol.
4. soak them in hot water.

CRITICAL THINKING ACTIVITIES

1. Give specific examples of the methods of medical asepsis and surgical asepsis used in the health care setting.

2. Explain to a family member how the body's protective mechanisms work to prevent infection.

3. Explain to a patient why the use of standard precautions is essential to both the health care worker's and the patient's protection.

MEETING CLINICAL OBJECTIVES

Directions: The following suggested activities will help you meet the stated clinical practice objectives for the chapter. Review your school's clinical objectives for the week and outline a plan of activities that will help you meet them. If you are unsure how to meet them, consult with your instructor at the beginning of the clinical day.

1. Interview the infection control officer regarding how infection is prevented and tracked in the clinical facility.

2. Observe 10 health care workers giving patient care and washing their hands. How many are following accepted protocols?

3. Teach a home care patient with a wound infection how to prevent the spread of infection to family members.

STEPS TOWARD BETTER COMMUNICATION

VOCABULARY BUILDING GLOSSARY

Term	Pronunciation	Definition
A. Individual Terms		
aerosolization	A er o sol i ZA tion	particles become suspended in a gas (air)
caustic	CAUS tic	able to burn or dissolve
commode	com MODE	toilet
impede	im PEDE	to get in the way, obstruct
impermeable	im PER me a ble	nothing can go through it
oozing	OO zing	coming out slowly

prevalent	PREV a lent	common
render	REN der	make
replicate	REP li cate	produce exact copies of
scrupulously	SCRUP u lous ly	carefully, perfectly
stringent	STRIN gent	strict, severe
vectors	VEC tors	carriers
virulent	VIR u lent	very harmful and rapidly spreading

B. Phrases

| wall off | wall off | to isolate |

COMPLETION

Directions: Fill in the blank(s) with the correct word(s) from the Vocabulary Building Glossary to complete the sentence.

1. Bacteria can be very _____ and their spread must be prevented.

2. A blood spill must be _____ cleaned up to prevent the spread of blood-borne pathogens.

3. A dressing over a wound will _____ the transfer of microorganisms.

4. When there is likely to be splashing of body fluids, health personnel must wear a(n) _____ gown.

5. Autoclaving instruments should _____ them free of microorganisms.

6. Unfortunately, nosocomial infection is _____ in the hospital setting.

7. Mosquitoes are a(n) _____ for several diseases including encephalitis and malaria.

WORD ATTACK SKILLS

Directions: Match the word part with its meaning.

1. _____ -cyte   a. white
2. _____ -osis   b. cell
3. _____ leuk-   c. abnormal condition

Student Name_____

PRONUNCIATION OF DIFFICULT TERMS

Directions: With a partner, practice pronouncing the following words.

immunosuppressive	im mu no sup press ive
leukocytosis	leu ko cy to sis
macrophage	mac ro phage
mucous	mu cous
mucosal	mu co sal
nosocomial	nos o co mi al
phagocytosis	pha go cy to sis
secrete	se crete
streptococcal	strep to coc cal

COMMUNICATION EXERCISE

With a partner, write a dialogue teaching a home care patient with a wound infection how to prevent the spread of infection to family members (Clinical Activity #3 above). Explain in simple terms how infection occurs (infectious agents enter the body), and steps to prevent its spread in the home (handwashing, treatment and disposal of contaminated material, cleaning of surfaces, etc.). Include questions the patient might ask. Practice the dialogue with your partner until you feel comfortable with it.

CULTURAL POINTS

1. In modern cities, the government departments of public health and sanitation take much of the responsibility for infection control and sanitation. Some of these are garbage and trash collection, monitoring and purification of the water system, requiring inoculation of children before entrance to school, restaurant inspection, requiring permits for food service, and maintaining sewage treatment plants. These are necessary in densely populated areas with a concentration of people that can include hosts and carriers of disease. In a rural area with few people and less interaction among them, so many precautions might not be necessary.

2. How is infection control handled in your home country?

Review the chapter key points, answer the study questions, and complete the critical thinking activities at the end of the chapter in the textbook.

CHAPTER 17

Infection Control in the Hospital and Home

Answer Key: Textbook page references are provided as a guide for answering selected questions. A complete answer key was provided for your instructor.

TERMINOLOGY

A. Completion

Directions: Fill in the blank(s) with the correct term(s) from the terms list in the chapter in the textbook to complete the sentence.

(222) 1. The _____ is the time from invasion of the body by the microorganisms to the onset of symptoms.

(222) 2. The _____ is the time from the onset of nonspecific symptoms to the beginning of specific symptoms of an infection.

(222) 3. Elevated temperature and _____ may occur during the prodromal period.

(223) 4. A systemic sign of infection is _____ where the white blood cells increase in number.

(223) 5. When symptoms begin to subside, the _____ period begins.

(223) 6. When a patient has a highly contagious infection, placing the patient in _____ helps prevent the spread of the infection.

(224) 7. _____ are the guidelines established by the CDC to prevent the transmission of infection by one of two methods.

(224) 8. Standard precautions are an outgrowth of measures to prevent the spread of the _____.

(225) 9. _____ require the use of a gown when entering the room if there is a possibility of contact with infected surfaces or items.

(224) 10. The transfer of microorganisms by _____ from the patient's wound to the nurse's hands can occur if the nurse does not wear gloves when cleansing a wound.

SHORT ANSWER

Directions: Write a brief answer for each question.

(222-223)   1.   The four stages of an infectious process are:

a.   _____

b.   _____

c.   _____

d.   _____

(223)   2.   Five ways to decrease the incidence of nosocomial infection are:

a.   _____

b.   _____

c.   _____

d.   _____

e.   _____

(224)   3.   The main reason transmission-based precautions have taken the place of previous isolation procedures is:

_____

_____

_____

(229)   4.   The difference in procedures between airborne precautions and droplet precautions is:

_____

_____

_____

(231)   5.   Three examples of nursing measures to meet the psychosocial needs of patients in an isolation room are:

a.   _____

b.   _____

c.   _____

(230)   6.   In what ways do infection control procedures in the home differ from those in the hospital?

_____

_____

_____

_____

Student Name_____

(229)   7. Special requirements for airborne precautions when the patient has tuberculosis and needs to leave the isolation room for diagnostic tests are:

_____

_____

(230)   8. When a patient is immunocompromised, protective (neutropenic) isolation is required and everyone entering the room must:

_____

_____

_____

(224)   9. The three main modes of occupational exposure to blood-borne pathogens through skin, eye, mucous membrane, or parenteral route are:

    a. _____

    b. _____

    c. _____

(231)   10. The four rules of surgical asepsis are:

    a. _____

    b. _____

    c. _____

    d. _____

(223)   11. For the following situations, indicate ways to prevent nosocomial infection.

    a. C.O. is recovering from a colon resection. He has a Foley catheter, IV line, and a wound dressing.

_____

_____

_____

_____

_____

_____

    b. L.M. is admitted with urinary retention and requires the insertion of an indwelling catheter.

_____

_____

_____

_____

_____

_____

   c.   R.C. had a hip replacement 3 days ago. He tends to dribble urine and needs assistance with turning.

_____

_____

_____

_____

_____

(232)   12.   Considering the principles of aseptic technique, explain why the following are considered breaks in sterile technique.

   a.   Turning your back to a sterile field:

_____

_____

   b.   Talking to the patient while performing a sterile dressing change:

_____

_____

   c.   Spilling sterile saline on the package wrapper that is used as your sterile field:

_____

_____

   d.   Placing unopened packages of sterile 4 x 4 gauze on the sterile field for a sterile dressing change:

_____

_____

MATCHING

Directions: Match the type of infection in Column I with the required type of precautions in Column II (may require more than one answer).

(224)

Column I		Column II
1. _____	pneumonia	a. Standard precautions
2. _____	diarrhea from *E. coli*	b. Airborne precautions
3. _____	*Haemophilus influenzae* infection	c. Droplet precautions
4. _____	measles	d. Contact precautions
5. _____	herpes simplex virus	
6. _____	tuberculosis	
7. _____	impetigo	
8. _____	*Varicella* (chickenpox)	
9. _____	streptococcal pharyngitis	
10. _____	viral influenza	

Student Name_____

APPLICATION OF THE NURSING PROCESS

Directions: Write a brief answer reflecting application of the nursing process.

(225)   1.   Assessment—Indicate four signs or symptoms in a patient that might indicate a need for transmission precautions.

      a.   _____

      b.   _____

      c.   _____

      d.   _____

(225)   2.   Nursing diagnosis—The correct nursing diagnosis for a patient with an open wound regarding possible infection is:

    _____

(225)   3.   Besides writing expected outcomes for the patient, planning for the patient requiring transmission precautions includes:

    _____

    _____

    _____

(225)   4.   Implementation—The types of teaching required for the patient with an infection are:

    _____

    _____

    _____

(225)   5.   Disposable soiled equipment and supplies from the room of a patient under transmission precautions are handled by:

    _____

    _____

    6.   Evaluation—Evaluation of the patient who has had an infection includes:

      a.   _____

      b.   _____

NCLEX-PN® EXAM REVIEW

*Directions: Choose the **best** answer(s) for each of the following questions.*

1. For most nurses, one of the difficult things to remember to do regarding standard precautions is to always
   1. turn gloves inside out when removing them.
   2. instruct the patient when to use gloves.
   3. wash hands after removing gloves even when no contamination occurred.
   4. wash hands before gloving.

(228) 2. A sharps container should be replaced whenever it is
   1. completely full.
   2. 1/2 full.
   3. filled to an inch from the top.
   4. 2/3 full.

3. When changing the bed of an incontinent patient, you should wear both gloves and a gown because
   1. contamination of the uniform is likely.
   2. feces stains are hard to remove.
   3. the uniform will carry an odor after this task.
   4. urine will soak through the uniform to the skin.

(224) 4. When working with a patient who is under droplet precautions, you should
   1. talk to the patient over the intercom frequently.
   2. gather all needed equipment before entering the room.
   3. refrain from entering the room more than four times in a shift.
   4. avoid tiring the patient with a lot of conversation.

(223) 5. The goal of nursing actions is the same for surgical asepsis and for protective isolation; that is, to
   1. confine the organisms to the infected patient.
   2. protect the nurse from infection.
   3. protect other people from the microorganism.
   4. reduce the microorganisms in the vicinity of the patient.

(231) 6. You are assigned to the operating room to assist with a minor surgical procedure. When performing the surgical scrub, you do the following. (Select all that apply)
   1. Use continually running water.
   2. Use an antiseptic agent and scrub brush or pad.
   3. Scrub to an inch above the elbow.
   4. Scrub to 2 inches above the elbow.

(235) 7. When working with a sterile field, you should (Select all that apply)
   1. always face the sterile field.
   2. keep the hands above the waist.
   3. use only one hand within the field.
   4. open sterile packages away from your body.

(238) 8. When pouring a sterile liquid, you should
   1. pour it in short batches so as not to splash.
   2. pour with the label away from the palm of the hand.
   3. pour with the label toward the palm of the hand.
   4. place the cap open side down on a sterile surface.

Student Name _____

(234)   9.   If your hand touches the sink faucet while performing a surgical scrub, you must
1. rescrub the area that touched the faucet.
2. begin the entire scrub process over.
3. rescrub the entire hand and arm.
4. resoap the area and continue the scrub.

(235)   10.   When opening a sterile package, you should
1. open it toward your body.
2. hold it down with one hand while opening it.
3. drop the contents onto the sterile field without touching them.
4. pull the package apart equally with each hand.

(236)   11.   Some parts of a sterile field are not considered sterile. When working with a sterile field you know that the area within _____ inch(es) of the edge is not sterile. (Fill in the blank)

(223)   12.   You know that nosocomial infection often occurs because an opportunistic organism is more likely to cause infection when
1. the patient's resistance is high.
2. the patient's resistance is low.
3. in the hospital environment.
4. present in small numbers.

(222)   13.   You wash your hands frequently because you realize that
1. soap kills pathogens.
2. patients expect it.
3. it is required as part of standard precautions before gloving.
4. it is the best method of preventing nosocomial infection.

(223)   14.   The emphasis of protective (neutropenic) isolation is to
1. protect the health care worker from infectious organisms.
2. prevent the transfer of microorganisms outside of the patient's environment.
3. protect the patient from microorganisms in the hospital environment.
4. build up the patient's immunity to normal flora.

       15.   For which of the following procedures would sterile technique be *unnecessary*?
1. surgical wound dressing change
2. insertion of a Foley catheter
3. insertion of a nasogastric tube into the stomach
4. changing a solution bag on an intravenous infusion

CRITICAL THINKING ACTIVITIES

1. Decide how you would handle the situation if you were participating in a surgical procedure and you noticed the surgeon contaminate one glove.

2. Describe how to assess the psychosocial needs of a patient under transmission precautions and how you could plan to meet them.

MEETING CLINICAL OBJECTIVES

Directions: The following suggested activities will help you meet the stated clinical practice objectives for the chapter. Review your school's clinical objectives for the week and outline a plan of activities that will help you meet them. If you are unsure how to meet them, consult with your instructor at the beginning of the clinical day.

1. Ask to be assigned to patients under different types of transmission precautions.

2. Teach a home care patient and family how to dispose of used needles and syringes and how to sterilize implements used for dressing changes.

3. Practice the surgical scrub in the skill lab, or home-simulated situation, until you are comfortable with the procedure. Have a peer observe your technique.

4. Practice setting up a sterile field, opening sterile packages, and sterile gloving. Have a peer observe your technique.

5. Observe for breaks in asepsis when working with other nurses and decide how you would have avoided the break and how to remedy it.

STEPS TOWARD BETTER COMMUNICATION

VOCABULARY BUILDING GLOSSARY

Term	Pronunciation	Definition
affixed	af FIXed	fastened, attached, put on
curtail	cur TAIL	decrease, make less
enhance	en HANCE	improve
immunocompromised	IM mu no COM pro mised	poor immune response
impervious	im PER vi ous	nothing can go through it
intact	in TACT	whole, unbroken
integrity	in TEG ri ty	completeness, strength
muster	MUS ter	to collect, summon
onset	ON set	beginning
premise	PREM ise	a basis for reasoning, assumption
prudent	PRU dent	showing carefulness
residual	re SID u al	left over, remaining
rectified	REC ti fied	corrected, changed
scalding	SCALD ing	extremely hot, almost boiling
sensory deprivation	SEN so ry DEP ri va tion	a situation with little stimulation for the senses, like a dark, quiet room with no visitors
surveillance	sur VEIL lance	continually watching, looking for
tiers	TIERS	levels

Student Name _____

COMPLETION

Directions: Fill in the blank(s) with the correct word(s) from the Vocabulary Building Glossary to complete the sentence.

1. The patient who has undergone radiation treatment or chemotherapy for cancer is _____.

2. A sterile package is only sterile if the package's _____ is unbroken.

3. The _____ urine on the spout of a catheter bag can form a breeding area for bacteria.

4. One form of disinfection in the home is to pour _____ water over dishes and utensils.

5. The patient who is in an isolation room may experience _____ because people only enter when they have to perform some function and there is little social interaction.

6. A good handwashing program will _____ infection control in any agency.

VOCABULARY EXERCISES

Directions: Underline the word from the Vocabulary Building Glossary and fill in the blank.

1. What is the premise for handwashing? _____

2. What is affixed to the hospitalized patient's wrist? _____

3. What is a sign of the onset of infection? _____

4. We need to muster enough _____ to safely transfer the totally dependent 250 lb. patient.

5. If we curtail the noise, the halls will be _____.

6. If you line out and note your _____ over the error in your nurse's notes, the error will be rectified.

7. If the skin is not broken, is it intact or enhanced? _____

8. A prudent nurse would maintain surveillance over a patient. True or false? _____

9. The disposable gown was impervious to _____.

10. The tiers of nursing administration end with the _____.

PRONUNCIATION OF DIFFICULT TERMS

Directions: Practice pronouncing the following words with a partner.

adenovirus	ad en o vir us
antimicrobial	an ti mi CRO bi al
epidemiology	EP i de mi OL o gy
epiglottitis	ep i glot TI tis

hemorrhagic	hem or rhAG ic
immunodeficiency	IM mu no de FI cien cy
leukocytosis	leu ko cy TO sis
Neisseria meningitidis	NES ser i a me NIN gi tid is
pharyngeal	pha ryn ge al
serosanguineous	ser o SAN gui ne ous
staphylococcal	STAPH y lo COC cal
furunculosis	fur UN cu los sis
streptococcal pneumonia	strep to CO cal pneu mon ia

COMMUNICATION EXERCISES

Directions: With a partner, write one of these dialogues and practice it together.

1. Describe to the patient's wife or husband how to remove contaminated gloves.

2. Explain to your home care patient's spouse why and how to keep the patient's room clean.

3. Explain to an extended family who wants to gather around the bed of their grandfather who has active tuberculosis why they must gown and mask when visiting him.

CULTURAL POINTS

Many of the procedures used for infection control are commonly known and accepted by the general public, even if they are not always followed: handwashing after using the toilet and before handling food, covering the mouth and nose when sneezing and coughing, disposing of soiled tissues in the trash, isolating oneself from people when contagious, not spitting or cleaning the nose with fingers.

However, in some cultures it is common and accepted practice for the family and friends to gather around the sick person. They may prefer to be very close to each other when they talk, and may commonly share drinking vessels and dishes. They may not have facilities for handwashing, or have a way to keep themselves and their belongings washed, and may not consider it important. They may not put used toilet paper in the toilet because they have not had modern plumbing or have been trained that it will clog the pipes. Some people commonly spit on the ground, and reuse the same dirty handkerchiefs.

Where have you observed these behaviors? Can you think of others? Do you think it affects those people's health? How would you explain to them the need for a change in behavior during illness, without offending them or saying anything negative about their culture?

Review the chapter key points, answer the study questions, and complete the critical thinking activities at the end of the chapter in the textbook.

CHAPTER 18

Lifting, Moving, and Positioning Patients

Answer Key: Textbook page references are provided as a guide for answering selected questions. A complete answer key was provided for your instructor.

TERMINOLOGY

A. Matching

Directions: Match the anatomical terms in Column I with the definitions in Column II.

	Column I	
(245)	1. _____ bone	
(245)	2. _____ bursa	
(245)	3. _____ cartilage	
(245)	4. _____ joint	
(245)	5. _____ ligament	
(245)	6. _____ tendon	

Column II

a. Cords of fibrous connective tissue connecting muscle to bone that are necessary for movement
b. Fibrous connective tissue that acts as a cushion
c. Supports and strengthens the bones of joints
d. Small, fluid-filled sacs that provide a cushion in movable joints
e. Union of two or more bones in the body
f. Dense and hard type of connective tissue

B. Completion

Directions: Fill in the blank(s) with the correct term(s) from the terms list in the chapter in the textbook to complete the sentence.

(244) 1. When a patient is positioned in bed, the body should be kept in proper _____ to prevent strain on joints and promote comfort.

(248) 2. A(n) _____ movement, when moving a patient from bed to chair, will help prevent twisting of the body and possible injury to the nurse.

(248) 3. A(n) _____ ulcer is one that forms from a local interference with circulation.

(248) 4. Unrelieved pressure on an area can cause death of tissue referred to as _____.

(248) 5. When a patient slides down while sitting in a chair, a(n) _____ force can occur which may cause a pressure ulcer.

(248)   6.   During musculoskeletal assessment, observe for muscle weakness, paralysis, and _____ of the extremities.

(249)   7.   When assessing ability to perform activities of daily living (ADLs), assess the patient's ability to _____ and change position independently.

(249)   8.   The style of walking, called _____, is assessed to see if it is even and unlabored.

(257)   9.   The _____ method is used to turn patients in bed who have spinal injuries.

(262)   10.   Positioning the patient on the side of the bed with the legs and feet over the side is called having the patient _____.

(268)   11.   A device that makes ambulating or transferring a patient much safer for both the nurse and the patient is a _____.

(248)   12.   If the arm is not placed in correct alignment and exercised regularly, the complication of elbow _____ may occur.

(244)   13.   The study of movement of body parts and positioning is called _____.

SHORT ANSWER

Directions: Write a brief answer for each question.

(244, 246)   1.   Give two reasons that correct body alignment and body mechanics are important:

     a.   _____

     b.   _____

(249)   2.   Changing the patient's position accomplishes four things:

     a.   _____

     b.   _____

     c.   _____

     d.   _____

(246)   3.   Principles of body mechanics to be used when transferring or repositioning a patient are (*complete the sentences*):

     a.   Keep your feet _____.

     b.   Use smooth _____.

     c.   Keep your elbows and work _____.

     d.   Work at the same _____.

     e.   Pull and _____.

     f.   Face in the direction _____.

Student Name _____

4. Give an example of use of each of the principles in question #3 above.

a. _____
_____

b. _____
_____

c. _____
_____

d. _____
_____

e. _____
_____

f. _____
_____

(248) 5. The three main hazards of improper alignment and positioning are:

a. _____

b. _____

c. _____

6. Indicate ways to help maintain correct alignment and position for each of the following patients.

a. A 26-year-old male with a head injury who is on bed rest. He is in the supine position and is comatose.

_____

_____

_____

_____

_____

b. A 76-year-old female with congestive heart failure and shortness of breath. She is in high Fowler's position and is very weak.

_____

_____

_____

_____

_____

(263) 7. Describe the steps you would take to transfer a patient from the wheelchair to the bed.

_____

_____

_____

_____

_____

_____

(248) 8. Pulling is easier than pushing because:

_____

_____

(247) 9. How do you provide lateral stability when reaching?

_____

(268-270) 10. Describe ways to decrease the risk of a patient falling while ambulating.

_____

_____

_____

(259) 11. When performing passive ROM exercises, all muscles over a joint are
_____ to achieve or maintain
_____.

(259) 12. Each set of movements for ROM exercises should be performed a minimum of
_____ times.

(259) 13. When performing passive ROM exercises, it is important always to support the
_____ above and below the joint.

14. Pick up your heaviest book or a similar object and hold it out at arm's length for at least 30 seconds. Now bring it close to your body for the same length of time. What difference did you notice in its apparent weight?

_____

_____

Student Name_____

MATCHING

Directions: Match the position in Column I with its description in Column II.

	Column I		**Column II**
(249)	1. _____ supine	a.	Lying face down
(250)	2. _____ side-lying	b.	On left side with left arm behind the body and the right knee and thigh up above the left lower leg
(250)	3. _____ prone		
(249)	4. _____ Fowler's		
(249)	5. _____ semi-Fowler's	c.	Resting on the back
(250)	6. _____ Sims'	d.	On back with head of bed between 30–60 degrees
		e.	Weight on side of body
		f.	On back with head of bed between 60–90 degrees

APPLICATION OF THE NURSING PROCESS

Directions: Write a brief answer for each question.

(248)   1. When assessing the patient's position in bed for correct alignment you would check:

_____

_____

_____

_____

(249)   2. The main or most common nursing diagnosis for patients who have a problem with body movement is _____.

(249)   3. An expected outcome for the nursing diagnosis in question #2 above is:

_____

(258)   4. When implementing ROM exercises, you know that they should be performed

_____.

(262)   5. When a patient has been lying in bed and is to ambulate or sit in a chair, the patient should be _____ before arising from the bed.

(263)   6. When moving a patient in or out of a wheelchair it is extremely important to first

_____.

(271)   7. Evaluation should include your own use of _____.

(271)   8. Write two evaluation statements that would indicate that the above expected outcome is being met.

a. _____

b. _____

NCLEX-PN® EXAM REVIEW

*Directions: Choose the **best** answer(s) for each of the following questions.*

(247) 1. To ensure good stability of the base of support of the body, the feet should be positioned
   1. parallel and very close together.
   2. about 8" apart, one a little ahead of the other.
   3. about 6" apart with toes pointed slightly laterally.
   4. parallel and about shoulder-width apart.

(248) 2. Areas that should be checked for problems due to pressure when the patient has been in the supine position are (Select all that apply)
   1. hip and shoulder.
   2. scapula and sacrum.
   3. elbows and the heels.
   4. hips and ankles.

(250) 3. The position most commonly used for inserting a rectal suppository is the
   1. prone position.
   2. Sims' position.
   3. side-lying position.
   4. knee-chest position.

4. A 67-year-old male suffered a stroke 3 days ago. He has left arm and leg weakness (hemiparesis) and aphasia. His speech is limited to "boler," "soup," and "no." He is conscious and quite depressed. While performing passive ROM to his affected extremities, he says, "Boler, boler, boler." You don't understand what he is trying to say. What would you do now?
   1. Report to the charge nurse that he is crying and might be having pain or discomfort.
   2. Go ahead and carry out the bath and exercises, since he must be confused.
   3. Ask the patient to nod his head for "yes" and shake his head for "no," then explain again and ask questions to see if he understands what you mean.
   4. Tell him not to cry and reassure him that everything will

5. A stroke patient's tray arrives with his lunch. As you feed him, you hand him a piece of bread, which he holds in his unaffected hand. As he moves his hand to his mouth to eat, what movement does he use?
   1. flexion of the wrist
   2. external rotation of the shoulder
   3. internal rotation of the shoulder
   4. pronation of the wrist

Student Name _____

(260) 6. When performing ROM exercises for a stroke patient, you raise the left arm straight out from the side to shoulder height. This movement is called
1. flexion.
2. abduction.
3. extension.
4. adduction.

(263) 7. Before transferring a stroke patient from the bed to a wheelchair, the most important step is to
1. position the chair so you can pivot him into it.
2. engage the lock on the wheelchair.
3. assist him with putting on his robe and slippers.
4. raise the head of the bed to Fowler's position.

(262) 8. The stroke patient has made very good progress in physical therapy. An order has been written to ambulate him with assistance. Before you assist him to walk for the first time, you help him to dangle his legs. The reason(s) for this could be to (Select all that apply)
1. strengthen his leg muscles before he stands.
2. improve the circulation of the paralyzed leg and foot.
3. help him recover from any dizziness.
4. help him adjust to the change of position.

(268-270) 9. You are going to walk the stroke patient in his room for the first time with the assistance of another nurse. Which of the following will you do?
1. Use a gait belt and walk on his weaker side.
2. Provide support by having one walk in front of the patient and the other behind him.
3. Hold him at the waist, walk backwards in front of him with the other nurse at his side.
4. each support one arm and match his steps.

10. Considering the stroke patient's state of weakness, when planning to ambulate him it is important to (Select all that apply)
1. ambulate after a meal when he is strongest.
2. remember to plan the distance for a 'round trip.'
3. use a gait belt for safety and stability.
4. have someone follow with a wheelchair in case of weakness.

CRITICAL THINKING ACTIVITIES

1. If your patient is in leg traction, what can you do to try to prevent pressure ulcers that often occur when a patient is in a supine position?

2. An unconscious patient does not move voluntarily at all. If you place him in Sims' position, which areas would need to be closely watched for signs of undue pressure?

3. Which positioning devices would be useful for the patient who is unconscious?

MEETING CLINICAL OBJECTIVES

Directions: The following suggested activities will help you meet the stated clinical practice objectives for the chapter. Review your school's clinical objectives for the week and outline a plan of activities that will help you meet them. If you are unsure how to meet them, consult with your instructor at the beginning of the clinical day.

1. Practice principles of body alignment and movement when performing daily tasks such as carrying groceries, reaching for things on high shelves, vacuuming, picking up a child, carrying your school books, and so forth.

2. With a peer or family member, practice placing the body in the various positions used for positioning the bed patient.

3. Work with another nurse on the unit to which you are assigned and learn how pillows and other aids are used to position patients.

STEPS TOWARD BETTER COMMUNICATION

VOCABULARY BUILDING GLOSSARY

Term	Pronunciation	Definition
alleviates	al LE vi ates	reduces
dispersed	dis PERSed	spread out over an area
hyperflex	HY per FLEX	bend too much
inertia	in ER tia	lack of movement or change
predisposes	pre dis POS es	makes vulnerable, more likely to happen
striated	STRI a ted	having long streaks, composed of long bands
sway	SWAY	move back and forth

VOCABULARY EXERCISE

Directions: Using terms from the Vocabulary Building Glossary, fill in the sentences in the following paragraph.

The _____ muscle works to move the extremities. _____ for long periods tends to make the muscles atrophy. When muscles are not exercised and joints are not moved, the joints are _____ to contractures. Exercising the joints also _____ the pain that can occur with inactivity. Proper positioning insures that the weight of the body is _____ over a broad area. When performing ROM exercises, it is best not to _____ a joint, as that may cause injury. When transferring a patient from the bed to a chair, a wide base of support is used so that you do not _____ while moving the patient.

Student Name_____

WORD ATTACK SKILLS

Abduction versus Adduction

1. "Ab" means away from, so *ab*duction would mean movement away from the body. Think of a hand open with the fingers spread away from each other.

2. "Ad" means toward, so *ad*duction would mean movement toward the body. Think of a hand that is open but with the fingers touching each other.

3. *Flex* means to bend.

4. A *flexion* position would mean a bent neck, elbow, knee, etc. Think of a hand with the fist closed.

5. *Extend* means to stretch out. Therefore, an extension position would be one where joints (the elbow, knee, neck, or wrist and finger) are not bent. Think of a hand held open and straight.

PRONUNCIATION OF DIFFICULT TERMS

Directions: Practice pronouncing the following words.

alignment   ligament

When the consonant combination "gn" falls in the same syllable, the "g" is silent. Examples: sign (SIgN), ma-lign (ma LIgN), gnaw (gNAW)

When the two consonants fall in different syllables, they are both pronounced. Examples: ignore (ig NORE), ignite (ig NITE), designation (des ig NA tion), dignitary (DIG ni tary)

Directions: Mark the syllables in these words and pronounce them:

prognosis   design   aligned   magnificent

COMMUNICATION EXERCISE

Write a short dialogue explaining to O.B. (Questions 4-10 in the multiple choice section) what you are doing as you prepare to ambulate him/move him to a wheelchair. O.B. has very limited speech.

Review the chapter key points, answer the study questions, and complete the critical thinking activities at the end of the chapter in the textbook.

19 Assisting with Hygiene, Personal Care, Skin Care, and the Prevention of Pressure Ulcers

CHAPTER

Answer Key: Textbook page references are provided as a guide for answering selected questions. A complete answer key was provided for your instructor.

TERMINOLOGY

A. Matching

Directions: Match the terms in Column I with the definitions in Column II.

	Column I	Column II
(276)	1. _____ blanch	a. System of skin hair, nails, and sweat and seba-
(275)	2. _____ integumentary	ceous glands
(276)	3. _____ maceration	b. Outer, thicker layer of skin
(275)	4. _____ cerumen	c. Substance secreted by sebaceous glands
(275)	5. _____ dermis	d. Substance secreted by ceruminous glands in the
(275)	6. _____ epidermis	ear
(289)	7. _____ halitosis	e. Practice of cleanliness
(274)	8. _____ hygiene	f. Foul-smelling breath
(277)	9. _____ induration	g. Turn white or become pale
(275)	10. _____ sebum	h. Hardening of an area
		i. Softening of tissue
		j. Inner, thinner layer of the skin

B. Completion

Directions: Fill in the blank(s) with the correct term(s) from the list of terms in the chapter in the textbook to complete the sentence.

(276)   1. The redness that occurs at the beginning of a pressure ulcer is caused by _____ and vasodilation.

(276)   2. A patient who is experiencing _____ is at risk of skin breakdown from the excess moisture.

(278)   3. Stage IV pressure ulcers often have dry, black, necrotic tissue called _____ within them.

(289)   4. If teeth are not brushed regularly, _____ may form.

(275)   5. Skin color is determined by the amount of _____ se- creted by the melanocytes in the epidermis.

(275) 6. Sebum is an oily substance secreted by the _____ glands.

(287) 7. When assisting a patient out of a very warm bath, the patient should move slowly to avoid dizziness and _____.

REVIEW OF STRUCTURE AND FUNCTION

Directions: Note the structure that fits with the function listed.

(275) 1. _____ absorbs light and protects against ultraviolet rays.

(275) 2. _____ helps regulate temperature by dilating and constricting blood vessels.

(275) 3. _____ make skin waterproof.

(275) 4. _____ lubricates the skin and hair.

(275) 5. _____ help maintain homeostasis of fluid and electrolytes.

(275) 6. _____ protect against bacterial invasion, secrete mucus, and absorb fluid and electrolytes.

(275) 7. _____ contains sensory organs for touch, pain, heat, cold, and pressure.

(275) 8. _____ is the first line of defense in protecting the body from invading organisms.

SHORT ANSWER

Directions: Write a brief answer for each question.

(274) 1. List the five factors that affect hygiene practice:

    a. _____

    b. _____

    c. _____

    d. _____

    e. _____

(276) 2. List the five risk factors for pressure ulcers and give one rationale for each factor.

    a. _____
    _____

    b. _____
    _____

    c. _____
    _____

Student Name_____

        d.   _____

               _____

        e.   _____

               _____

(276)   3. What are the other factors that may contribute to pressure ulcer formation?

         _____

         _____

(279)   4. List five nursing interventions that you feel are most important in preventing pressure ulcers.

        a. _____

        b. _____

        c. _____

        d. _____

        e. _____

(277)   5. For each of the following positions, list pressure points to be checked when the patient's position is changed.

        a. Sitting in a wheelchair:

         _____

         _____

        b. Supine in semi-Fowler's position:

         _____

         _____

        c. Sims' position:

         _____

         _____

(276)   6. A thorough skin assessment should be done upon admission and every _____ thereafter.

(278)   7. A reddened area caused by pressure should subside within _____ _____ when the patient's position is changed.

(279)   8. Give three characteristics of each stage of pressure ulcer.

        a. Stage I:

         _____

         _____

        b. Stage II:

         _____

         _____

    c. Stage III:

_____

_____

    d. Stage IV:

_____

_____

(279)   9. Older adults have an increased risk of developing impaired skin integrity because:

_____

_____

_____

(281)   10. The four basic purposes for bathing are:

    a. _____

    b. _____

    c. _____

    d. _____

(281)   11. A partial bath done by a patient alone consists of washing the:

_____

(289)   12. Whirlpool baths are therapeutically used to:

    a. _____

    b. _____

    c. _____

(289)   13. A sitz bath is used to promote _____ by applying moist heat which increases circulation in the perineal area.

(289)   14. Sitz baths are used after _____ or _____ surgery and after childbirth.

(289)   15. A back rub is essential for patients who are _____.

(290)   16. Full mouth care for the unconscious patient should be provided at least once every _____ hours.

(292)   17. When not in the mouth, dentures should be cared for by placing them in _____.

(297)   18. Nail care is important, but a physician's order is needed to cut the toe-nails of the _____ patient or one with _____ of the lower extremities.

(298)   19. A contact lens should be cleansed by moistening and rubbing gently between the fingers while holding over a _____.

(298)   20. A hearing aid should never be cleaned by _____ it in water.

(276)   21. In the older adult, dry and itchy skin is caused by the decreased activity of the _____.

Student Name_____

APPLICATION OF THE NURSING PROCESS

Directions: Write a brief answer for each question.

(274)　　1.　Two primary areas to assess when considering hygiene needs and problems are:

　　　a.　_____

　　　b.　_____

(280)　　2.　Most patients with a problem of mobility or who are on bed rest will have the following nursing diagnosis related to hygiene:

　　_____

(280-281)　3.　Write an expected outcome for the above nursing diagnosis:

　　_____

(287)　　4.　When implementing a bed bath for an elderly patient, you would alter your bath procedure by:

　　_____

　　_____

(299)　　5.　Write an evaluation statement that would indicate that the expected outcome, "patient will maintain intact skin while on bed rest" is being met.

　　_____

NCLEX-PN® EXAM REVIEW

*Directions: Choose the **best** answer(s) for each of the following questions.*

(287)　1.　A 76-year-old patient is hospitalized with dehydration and pneumonia. She also has peripheral vascular (circulatory) disease of the lower extremities. She has been confused and in bed for several days before admission. An especially important aspect of giving a bed bath to an elderly patient is to (Select all that apply)
1. move very slowly to prevent agitating the patient.
2. seek assistance in order to finish the bath quickly.
3. keep the patient covered well to prevent chilling.
4. lubricate the skin with lotion after bathing.

(283)　2.　When washing a patient's face you wash the eye area from the inner to the outer canthus with separate parts of the washcloth to
1. promote circulation.
2. prevent infection.
3. avoid getting soap in the eye.
4. prevent visual obstruction.

(283)　3.　When washing this patient's arm, you use long, firm strokes, moving from the hand to the axilla to
1. fully assess the skin on all sides of the arm.
2. improve circulation in the extremity.
3. prevent infection by cleansing from dirty to clean.
4. provide range-of-motion exercise for the joint.

(289) 4. The patient refuses perineal care. You know that this is probably because she
1. can do it well by herself.
2. has no vaginal secretions and does not need it.
3. is embarrassed to have someone else perform it.
4. prefers to do this only once a week.

(292) 5. When preparing to store the patient's dentures in a denture cup, you must be certain to
1. label the cup with her name and room number.
2. place denture solution in the cup.
3. line the cup with a paper towel.
4. send the dentures home with the family.

(276) 6. When turning the patient, you provide skin care by (Select all that apply)
1. assessing now-visible portions of the skin.
2. providing a back massage after turning.
3. rubbing all areas that were against the mattress.
4. checking all bony prominences that were dependent for reddening.

(279) 7. The patient has a reddened, slightly abraded area on the inner aspect of her right knee. This would be considered a _____ pressure ulcer.
1. Stage I
2. Stage II
3. Stage III
4. Stage IV

(279) 8. Because of a pressure area, it would be best to position the patient with a reddened, slightly abraded area on the inner aspect of her right knee
1. on her back or right side.
2. on her back or left side.
3. supine in Semi-Fowler's only.
4. in Sims' position or supine.

(276) 9. There are many factors that contribute to pressure ulcer formation. A contributing factor for pressure ulcers for this patient is _____

_____.

(Fill in the blank)

(297) 10. The patient who has vascular insufficiency has toenails in need of trimming. You would
1. ask the family to bring clippers from home.
2. ask her daughter to perform this function for her.
3. call her podiatrist to come and trim them.
4. seek an order from the physician to cut her toenails.

CRITICAL THINKING ACTIVITIES

1. What should you do if your patient refuses to bathe?

2. Your male patient normally shaves with an electric razor. He was admitted as an emergency patient and does not have his razor with him. You would like to shave him. How would you plan to do this?

MEETING CLINICAL OBJECTIVES

Directions: The following suggested activities will help you meet the stated clinical practice objectives for the chapter. Review your school's clinical objectives for the week and outline a plan of activities that will help you meet them. If you are unsure how to meet them, consult with your instructor at the beginning of the clinical day.

1. Practice the bed bath procedure at home on a family member or friend until you are comfortable and efficient with the procedure.

2. Practice shaving the face of a male family member or friend to decrease initial anxiety and awkwardness when performing the procedure in the health care agency.

3. Accompany another nurse when she gives hygiene care to an unconscious patient. Pay particular attention to the technique of giving safe mouth care.

4. When observing hygiene care being given by other nurses, notice how the patient's privacy is protected or invaded. Discuss this issue in clinical conference.

5. Assist another nurse in giving a bed shampoo in order to become more familiar and comfortable with this task.

6. Provide personal care for a patient.

7. Attempt to stage a pressure ulcer and describe appropriate care.

STEPS TOWARD BETTER COMMUNICATION

VOCABULARY BUILDING GLOSSARY

Term	Pronunciation	Definition
acuity	a CU i ty	sharpness of perception
adipose	AD i pose	containing fat
débridement	de BRIDe ment (day breed maw) (French pronunciation)	removal of foreign, contaminated, or dead tissue from a wound
don	DON (verb)	to put on
exacerbation	ex a CER bA tion	increase in severity of symptoms
mottled	MOT tled	irregular patches of color
nick	NICK (verb)	very small cut, usually accidental
slough off	SLOUGH (pronounced "sluff") off	to shed, to drop off
stratified	STRA ti fied	in layers
subside	sub SIDE (verb)	to gradually go away, become less

COMPLETION

Directions: Fill in the blank(s) with the correct word(s) from the Vocabulary Building Glossary to complete the sentence.

1. Sometimes using soap on a patient's skin causes a(n) _____ of a dry skin condition.

2. When shaving a patient with a safety razor, be careful not to _____ the skin.

3. While bathing the patient, she noticed that the skin around the ankle was

    _____.

4. It is essential to _____ gloves before cleansing the perineal area.

5. The patient who has sustained a deep burn often must undergo

    _____ of the burned area.

VOCABULARY EXERCISES

Directions: Match the following words in Column I with their meanings in Column II.

Column I		Column II	
1.	_____ blanched	a.	Hardened
2.	_____ mottled	b.	Blocked
3.	_____ occluded	c.	Softened
4.	_____ macerated	d.	Covered with patches of color
5.	_____ indurated	e.	Lost color

WORD ATTACK SKILLS

Directions: Match the following words with their meanings.

1. If <u>dermis</u> is the inner layer of the skin, and <u>epidermis</u> is the outer, thicker layer of the skin, what does *epi*- mean? _____

2. What does *derm*- mean? _____

3. If <u>induration</u> means hardening, and <u>durable</u> means sturdy or long-lasting, what does *dur*- mean?

    _____

PRONUNCIATION OF DIFFICULT TERMS

Directions: Practice pronouncing the following terms.

débridement	day breed MAW
decubitus	de CU bi tus
diaphoresis	di a pho RE sis
eschar	ES kar; ESC har

Student Name_____

mottled	MOT ulled (this word is pronounced with a quick stop of breath between the two "t"s, and sounds almost like "modeled")
phimosis	phi mo sis
sebaceous	se BA ceous
syncope	SYN co pe

COMMUNICATION EXERCISE

What would be some things you could talk about as you give your patient a bath? Or should you talk?

CULTURAL POINTS

Americans today are very concerned about cleanliness and bathing often, usually every day, and about how they smell. Any natural body odor is usually considered bad. Perhaps this has been influenced by an over-application of the theory of health hygiene. On the other hand, as the public health environment has become "cleaner" we may have become lax about such things as handwashing.

What habits of hygiene are different here in the U.S. than they were in your country? Which ones make a difference for health, and which are only cosmetic—for looks or comfort?

Why would sociocultural or economic background affect hygiene? In what ways?

Is there a difference between personal hygiene and community hygiene? Can you think of ways in which hygiene makes a difference for the health of people in your native country?

Discuss these issues with your peers.

Review the chapter key points, answer the study questions, and complete the critical thinking activities at the end of the chapter in the textbook.

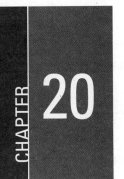

CHAPTER 20 Patient Environment and Safety

TERMINOLOGY

Directions: Fill in the blank(s) with the correct term(s) from the terms list in the chapter in the textbook to complete the sentence.

(301) 1. Room temperature, furniture arrangement, neatness of the area, and lighting are all part of the patient _____.

(301) 2. When a person is ill, _____ of the room is even more important as fresh air is essential.

(301) 3. A very low _____ dries respiratory passages and the skin.

(314) 4. A(n) _____ is a substance that may cause functional or structural disturbances if it is ingested, inhaled, absorbed, injected, or developed within the body.

(312) 5. A biological agent or condition that can be harmful to a person's health, such as a contaminated needle, is called a(n) _____.

SHORT ANSWER

Directions: Write a brief answer for each question.

(301) 1. The goal in caring for the patient environment is to provide _____ while making the patient as _____ as possible.

(301) 2. The patient's room temperature should be kept at _____ to _____.

(302) 3. Lighting should meet these three requirements:

a. _____

b. _____

c. _____

(302) 4. Two important measures that can assist in reducing odors that seem unpleasant to patients are to:

a. _____

b. _____

(302) 5. Since the major source of noise is people, staff can assist in reducing the problem by:

_____

_____

_____

(302) 6. To maintain neatness in the patient unit, the area should be straightened whenever:

_____

_____

(303) 7. For safety, whenever a bed is not being moved, it is important to make certain that the

_____.

(310) 8. Principles of body mechanics used when making a bed are:

a. _____

b. _____

c. _____

d. _____

e. _____

(310) 9. A measure to prevent falls for the ill patient is to prevent attempts to get out of bed unassisted by _____

_____.

(310) 10. List four measures to be used in the home environment that you consider to be most important in preventing patient falls.

a. _____

b. _____

c. _____

d. _____

(311) 11. Extra vigilance to prevent burns is essential for these four types of patients:

a. _____

b. _____

c. _____

d. _____

(311) 12. Smoking is never allowed when oxygen is in use as _____

_____.

Student Name_____

(312)   13.   For fire safety, each staff member must know:

         a. _____

         b. _____

         c. _____

         d. _____

(312)   14.   The acronym RACE stands for:

         R _____

         A _____

         C _____

         E _____

(313)   15.   Bioterrorism is:

     _____

     _____

(313)   16.   Chemical terrorism can be delivered in the form of:

         a. _____

         b. _____

         c. _____

(312)   17.   The incubation period for Anthrax is 1 to _____ days.

(313)   18.   Sarin is a chemical agent that acts on the nerves and exposure may lead to
_____.

(314)   19.   Ways to protect yourself from radiation include _____
_____.

(314)   20.   The symptoms of acute radiation sickness (ARS) are:

     _____

     _____

     _____

(314)   21.   Using the principles of triage, place the following victims of a disaster in the priority order of treatment.

         a.   32-year-old male with fractured femur

         b.   3-year-old with a head injury and scalp laceration who is bleeding, but conscious

         c.   72-year-old with a broken arm and cuts to the hand and forearm; the bleeding is stopped

         d.   56-year-old who is unconscious with a serious head injury with part of the skull depressed, open abdominal wound, and burns over 80% of the body

      The priority order of treatment for these victims is: _____

(314) 22. The first step in handling victims of a biological or chemical terrorist attack as they arrive at the emergency room is _____ _____.

(314) 23. An important aspect of preventing poisoning in the home is to always keep poisonous substances in their _____.

(315) 24. Protective devices are to be used only as a(n) _____.

(315) 25. Measures that may help to decrease confusion in older adults when they enter a health care facility are:

_____

(315) 26. When applying a protective device, it is essential to be certain that the patient's movements or tugging will not impair _____ or _____.

(315) 27. To check the safe application of a protective device, see if you can insert your _____ between the patient and the device.

(319) 28. Ties for a protective device should be secured to _____ _____.

(315) 29. A protective device that immobilizes a body part should be removed every _____ and _____ performed to immobilized joints and muscles.

NCLEX-PN® EXAM REVIEW

*Directions: Choose the **best** answer(s) for each of the following questions.*

(311) 1. Safety precautions when serving meal trays include
1. opening all containers on the tray.
2. providing sufficient napkins.
3. cutting up meat before serving.
4. warning the patient about hot liquids.

(310) 2. Interventions by the nurse that help prevent patient falls are to (Select all that apply)
1. provide night lighting for trips to the bathroom.
2. allow the patient to walk only with assistance.
3. keep the pathway between the bed and bathroom clear.
4. allow minimal patient belongings in the room.

* 3. When planning for patient safety, consider the patient's (Select all that apply)
1. age.
2. sex.
3. educational level.
4. current condition.

(312-313) 4. Infection control guidelines for patient safety require that infectious waste such as soiled dressings be treated as biohazards and be
1. sterilized before disposal.
2. placed in impermeable, sealed bags.
3. burned as soon as possible.
4. placed in the utility room trash.

Student Name _____

(310)   5. In order to prevent falls by elderly patients, you should (Select all that apply)
1. encourage the use of nonskid mats in tub or shower.
2. insist on bright lighting at all times.
3. encourage use of firm, rubber-soled slippers.
4. keep side rails up when patient is in bed.

(319)   6. When securing the ties on a protective device it is essential that
1. the knot be easily undone in case of fire.
2. the knot be difficult to undo.
3. a double knot be used.
4. only a square knot be used.

(318)   7. When utilizing a safety belt for a patient in a wheelchair, you must
1. explain to the family exactly why it is being used.
2. document the specific reason the belt is needed.
3. fasten it to the chair loosely.
4. obtain the patient's permission for use.

(318)   8. When utilizing a limb immobilizer protective device, you must
1. massage the area proximal to its attachment frequently.
2. flex the joint before applying the device.
3. check the circulation and sensation distal to the device frequently.
4. exercise all joints at least twice per shift.

(310)   9. Medications may have side effects that contribute to the risk of falls, especially for the elderly. When evaluating a patient's drugs for side effects that may increase the risk of falling, look at those that affect the

_____

_____ system. (Fill in the blank)

(310)   10. A measure to promote patient safety after finishing a nursing procedure is to
1. explain the reason for the procedure.
2. elevate the head of the bed to semi-Fowler's position.
3. replace the bed in the lowest position.
4. tell the patient when you will return to the room.

(310)   11. Safety measures for the patient during ambulation include the use of (Select all that apply)
1. a gait belt any time the patient is unsteady.
2. two people at all times for ambulation.
3. a rolling IV pole for stability.
4. wearing of firm-soled shoes.

(310)   12. One measure to prevent nighttime wandering in the elderly is
1. administer sleeping medication at bedtime.
2. give a back rub and warm milk at bedtime.
3. place the patient in a room with another patient.
4. increase daytime stimulation to decrease napping.

(317)   13. The best choice for a protective device to assist a patient who cannot maintain an upright sitting posture in a wheelchair would be
1. a security vest.
2. a safety belt.
3. a protective jacket.
4. wrist immobilizing devices.

(318) 14. An important nursing action for the patient using wrist and ankle immobilizers is to
1. attach the ties properly to the side rails.
2. offer fluids at 4-hour intervals.
3. check on the patient every 2 hours while immobilized.
4. document their removal and exercises performed every 2 hours.

(312) 15. The first action to be taken in the event of a fire is to
1. activate the fire alarm.
2. rescue the patient.
3. contain the fire.
4. extinguish the flames.

CRITICAL THINKING ACTIVITIES

1. Your patient is a 78-year-old male with pneumonia who is quite confused. He is prone to falls. He has just been admitted and keeps trying to get out of bed. What measures should you use to keep him in bed without using a protective device?

2. In reviewing Table 20-4, what would you need to do in your home to make it safer from fire?

3. Check your home for poison safety. What do you need to do to protect people in your home from poisoning?

MEETING CLINICAL OBJECTIVES

Directions: The following suggested activities will help you meet the stated clinical practice objectives for the chapter. Review your school's clinical objectives for the week and outline a plan of activities that will help you meet them. If you are unsure how to meet them, consult with your instructor at the beginning of the clinical day.

1. Practice hospital bed-making at home until you can quickly and smoothly make the bed.

2. Locate the fire extinguishers, fire alarms, and escape routes for the unit to which you are assigned for clinical experience.

3. Review the procedures for the handling of biohazards in your clinical facility.

4. If protective devices are available in the skill lab, work with a peer in applying and securing the devices. Take turns being the patient to experience how it feels to have such a device in place.

5. Practice securing the ties of a protective device to the bed properly.

6. When assigned to a patient who is wearing a protective device, think of an alternate solution to the underlying problem.

Student Name _____

VOCABULARY BUILDING GLOSSARY

Term	Pronunciation	Definition
A. Individual Terms		
acronym	AC ro nym	a word made from the first letter of a related list of words (RACE)
altercations	al ter CA tions	arguments, disagreements
clutter	CLUT ter	lots of things around, messy
compromise	COM pro mise	to expose to danger by unwise action
diffused	dif FUSEd	spread around, scattered
frayed	FRAYed	worn at the edges, especially fabric with loose strings
glare	GLARE	a strong reflected light
hazard	HAZ ard	danger
miter	MI ter	joining two flat pieces together at an angle
noxious	NOX ious	harmful
predispose	pre di SPOSE	to make vulnerable, more likely to suffer from
prone	PRONE	likely to happen
slump	SLUMP	to slide or bend into a low position
solaria	so LAR i a	sun rooms (plural of solarium)
stifling	STI fling	preventing, or restricting from getting air
tact	TACT	to speak carefully about an uncomfortable subject so you will not offend
vigilance	VIG i lance	watching carefully over a period of time
warrant	WARR ant	to give sufficient reason or justification for some action
B. Phrases		
holistic patient care	ho LIST ic patient care	caring for the whole or total patient—the physical, mental, social, and spiritual parts of life
last resort	LAST re sort	something to do when nothing else works
neat and tidy	NEAT and TI dy	things picked up and organized in their proper places
refrain from	re FRAIN from	to hold back; not do something

COMPLETION

Directions: Fill in the blank(s) with the correct term(s) from the Vocabulary Building Glossary to complete each sentence.

1. Soft, _____ light prevents shadows in the room which can interfere with vision and predispose a patient to a fall.

2. Leaving used equipment in the room trash can lead to _____ odors.

3. A(n) _____ cord for the electric bed presents a fire hazard.

4. When correcting a nursing assistant's action, it is best to use _____.

5. Nursing instructors like patient rooms to be _____ without clutter lying about.

6. A patient who has a fever may find _____ from light uncomfortable.

7. Leaving a spill on the floor will _____ the safety of those working in the area.

8. The patient who has one-sided weakness is _____ to falls if allowed to ambulate unassisted initially.

9. One must be careful about intervening in _____ between angry family members.

10. It is necessary to _____ restricting a patient's movements unnecessarily.

VOCABULARY EXERCISES

English words may have many different meanings, as you have discovered. Sometimes these meanings are physical or tangible (meaning they can be touched or felt) and sometimes they are intangible (meaning they can not be touched—like an idea).

1. Below the table are Glossary words with two correct meanings. Some words have both tangible and intangible meanings. For those words, put the meanings in the correct place.

Word	Physical/Tangible	Emotional/Intangible
Example: frayed	*worn at the edges*	*irritated, annoyed*

Student Name_____

glare	(n) a strong reflected light/a look of anger or hatred, a harsh stare (v) to look hard at someone with anger or hatred
miter	making a corner with two pieces at an angle a tall pointed bishop's hat
prone	likely to happen lying face down
slump	to slide or bend into a low position to fall or sink down—financial market, sports record, etc.
stifle	preventing or restricting from getting air prevent someone from doing something

2. Opposites: Make sentences using these opposites from the Glossary.

   a. clutter/neat and tidy: _____

   _____

   b. glare/diffuse:_____

   _____

COMMUNICATION EXERCISES

Directions: Write what you would say in each of these situations:

1. to a patient before raising the bed rails? _____

   _____

2. to visitors talking and laughing loudly in the hall? _____

   _____

3. to a family whose elderly mother was put in restraints?_____

   _____

4. to a patient when serving morning tea? _____

   _____

GRAMMAR POINTS

The little word "as" has many important uses.

- Here it is used as a conjunction to hold two short clauses together. It means "because."
  "Floor or table fans are discouraged, as moving air currents spread microorganisms."
- Sometimes it is a preposition meaning "in the role of."
  "This medicine is used as a diuretic."
- Sometimes it is an adverb meaning "to the same amount."
  "Can you find something as effective as restraints?"
- "As" may mean "for example."
  "Immobility can cause such physical problems as muscle weakness, atrophy, contractures, constipation, and cognitive impairment."

Directions: What is the meaning of "as" in these sentences?

1. The physician's assistant can often act as a doctor.

_____

2. Restraints should be checked often as they can impair circulation.

_____

3. Patient rooms are often as nicely furnished as hotel rooms.

_____

4. Patients can be bothered by such loud noises as inconsiderate talking, noisy equipment, or blaring televisions.

_____

CULTURAL POINTS

In the United States environmental security and safety are important not only for the patient's comfort and safety, but because there are so many laws requiring it. Hospitals, institutions, agencies, and even individuals run great risks of legal action if they do not provide for the safety and security of the patients and staff. It is for this reason that the administrators and inspectors are so careful to see that the rules are enforced.

Review the chapter key points, answer the study questions, and complete the
critical thinking activities at the end of the chapter in the textbook.

CHAPTER 21

Measuring Vital Signs

Answer Key: Textbook page references are provided as a guide for answering selected questions. A complete answer key was provided for your instructor.

TERMINOLOGY

A. Matching

Directions: Match the terms in Column I with the definitions in Column II.

	Column I	Column II
(344)	1. _f_ apnea	a. State of having a fever
(338)	2. _b_ bradycardia	b. Pulse rate less than 60 bpm
(343)	3. _h_ bradypnea	c. Pulse rate greater than 100 bpm
(329)	4. _a_ febrile	d. Difference between the radial and apical pulse
(325)	5. _i_ hypoxia	e. Irregular heart rate
(340)	6. _e_ arrhythmia	f. Absence of breathing
(339)	7. _d_ pulse deficit	g. Rapid respiratory rate
(344)	8. _j_ stridor	h. Slow, shallow breathing
(338)	9. _c_ tachycardia	i. Decreased oxygen in the blood
(343)	10. _g_ tachypnea	j. High-pitched crowing sound on inspiration

B. Completion

Directions: Fill in the blank(s) with the correct word(s) from the terms list in the chapter in the textbook to complete the sentence.

(343) 1. The normal pattern of breathing is described as _____Eupnea_____.

(343) 2. The term used to describe difficult and labored breathing is
_____Dyspnea_____.

(327) 3. The _____ pressure is written below the line for BP.

(329) 4. When a fever begins to come down, the patient is in a state of
_____febrile_____.

(347) 5. If a silence is heard between sounds when auscultating blood pressure, it is termed a(n)
_____auscultatory gap_____.

(324) 6. The rate at which heat is produced when the body is at rest is the
_____.

(324)   7.   Heat production is a by-product of _Metabolism (cellular chemical reactions in the body._

(324)   8.   The _hypothalamus_ controls temperature by a(n) _feedback_ mechanism.

(325)   9.   The pulse rate multiplied by the stroke volume equals the _cardiac output._

REVIEW OF STRUCTURE AND FUNCTION

Directions: Write a brief answer for each question.

(324)   1.   Fever occurs when _____.

(324)   2.   Factors that affect the BMR are: _____

_____

(325)   3.   The mechanism of _____ attempts to cool the body by evaporation when a high fever occurs.

(325)   4.   The pulse is produced by _____.

(325)   5.   The pulse rate is normally dependent on the impulses emerging from the _____ in the heart.

(325)   6.   The character of the pulse is affected by the _____.

(325)   7.   Cardiac output is calculated by multiplying the _____ by the pulse _____.

(325)   8.   Ventilation is the _____ movement of air in and out of the lungs.

(325-326)   9.   Diffusion of oxygen and carbon dioxide occurs across the

_____.

(326)   10.   Structures directly involved in respiration are:

_____

_____

(326)   11.   A substance necessary in the alveoli to keep them open is

_____.

(326)   12.   The respiratory center is located in the _____ and _____ of the brain stem.

(326)   13.   The respiratory centers are signaled to alter rate or depth of respiration by the _____ in the carotid arteries and by the _____ receptors adjacent to the aortic arch.

(327)   14.   Systolic pressure is when there is:

_____

_____

Student Name_____

(327)   15.   Diastolic pressure occurs when:

_____

_____

(327)   16.   Blood pressure increases as _____ volume increases.

(327)   17.   Arterial blood pressure rises when there is an increase in _____
_____ resistance.

(327)   18.   If blood volume decreases, the blood pressure _____.

(327)   19.   When vascular wall elasticity decreases, the blood pressure will
_____.

(327)   20.   The lower-than-average temperature often found in the older adult may be a result of a decrease in _____ rate.

(327)   21.   The respiratory rate may be slightly _____ in the older
adult to compensate for a decrease in vital capacity and respiratory reserve.

SHORT ANSWER

Directions: Write a brief answer for each question.

(328-329)   1.   Name at least four factors that influence body temperature.

a.   _____

b.   _____

c.   _____

d.   _____

(327)   2.   What is the normal range for temperature in Fahrenheit and in Celsius?
_____ ° F   _____ ° C

(340)   3.   What is the normal pulse rate in the adult? _____

(340-341)   4.   In addition to the rate, what characteristics of the pulse should you note and be able to describe?

_____

(336)   5.   List the points on the body where the pulse can be palpated.

_____

_____

(338)   6.   When counting the apical pulse, the stethoscope is placed at the
_____ and counted for
_____.

(338)   7.   What are four pulse findings that should be reported?

a.   _____

b.   _____

c.   _____

d.   _____

(343)   8.   The normal range of respirations for a healthy adult is _____.

(343)   9.   The respiratory center of the brain is more sensitive to changes in the _____ levels.

(344)   10.   The average blood pressure of a healthy young adult is _____.

(347)   11.   Name at least five conditions/factors that are helpful in taking an accurate blood pressure reading.

a.   _____

b.   _____

c.   _____

d.   _____

e.   _____

(346)   12.   Low blood pressures are dangerous when they occur with symptoms of _____ or _____.

(346)   13.   One problem that the elderly may have related to blood pressure is _____ hypotension.

(339)   14.   To determine if the patient has a pulse deficit you would:

_____

_____

_____

APPLICATION OF THE NURSING PROCESS

Directions: Write a brief answer for each question.

1.   Jamie, age 14 months, has been ill with vomiting and diarrhea. He has been running an elevated temperature. His parents bring him to the clinic to see the nurse practitioner. Which type of thermometer would be best to use for Jamie and which route would you use to check his temperature?

_____

_____

2.   How would you take a pulse on a crying 4-year-old child?

_____

3.   If you check the radial pulse on your patient and find that it is irregular, what would you do next?

_____

Student Name_____

4. If your patient weighs 280 lbs., what type of equipment would you use to take the blood pressure?

_____

5. What is the best way to measure respirations on a clinic patient who has on a shirt and sweater?

_____

6. List one appropriate nursing diagnosis for each of the following situations:
   a. Patient with a temperature of 102.2° F (39.0° C) who is acutely ill:

   _____

   b. Patient with a respiratory rate of 28 who is quite short of breath:

   _____

   c. Adult patient with a heart rate of 128 who is dizzy:

   _____

   d. Adult patient whose blood pressure has been 168/98 on three readings on three different occasions:

   _____

7. Write one expected outcome for each of the above nursing diagnoses:
   a. _____
   b. _____
   c. _____
   d. _____

8. What evaluation data would you need to determine if each of the above expected outcomes was being met or was met?
   a. _____
   b. _____
   c. _____
   d. _____

9. What would you do if your ill, hospitalized patient's temperature registers 95.2° F (32.1° C) on the thermometer?

   _____

   _____

10. What would you do if when taking your patient's blood pressure, you hear the first sounds, they disappear, and then you hear them again?

   _____

   _____

NCLEX-PN® EXAM REVIEW

*Directions: Choose the **best** answer(s) for each of the following questions.*

(326) 1. Respiration is controlled by the
1. hypothalamus.
2. pons and medulla.
3. sinoatrial node.
4. lungs.

(327) 2. Systolic blood pressure is the pressure
1. exerted on the artery when the heart is at rest.
2. equal to that in the arteries at any given time.
3. in the arteries when intrathoracic pressure is greatest.
4. exerted on the artery during left ventricular contraction.

(327) 3. If overhydration occurs, the blood pressure will
1. increase.
2. decrease.
3. remain the same.
4. become muffled.

(327) 4. Which of the following are *true* regarding vital sign changes that occur with aging? (Select all that apply)
1. Normal temperature is higher than that of the average adult.
2. Heart rate remains normal, but rhythm may become slightly irregular.
3. Vital capacity increases as subcutaneous fat is lost.
4. Respiratory rate my rise as a decrease in vital capacity occurs.

(348) 5. When measuring a patient's blood pressure in the arm, the center of the bladder in the cuff should be placed
1. at the right outer edge of the arm.
2. over the antecubital space.
3. over the brachial artery.
4. at the inner edge of the arm.

(341) 6. When measuring respirations, the patient should NOT be (Select all that apply)
1. sitting up in bed.
2. talking to anyone.
3. resting quietly.
4. aware of the measuring.

(339) 7. An apical-radial pulse is taken to determine if there is
1. an arrhythmia.
2. skipped heartbeats.
3. an abnormal heart sound.
4. a pulse deficit.

(347) 8. A type of Korotkoff's sound that indicates the diastolic pressure in children and in some adults is
1. tapping.
2. knocking.
3. muffling.
4. silence.

(349) 9. When measuring blood pressure with an aneroid manometer, it is important to
1. deflate the cuff slowly while observing the dial.
2. support the arm below the level of the heart.
3. take a reading from both arms.
4. retake the pressure to verify the reading.

(344) 10. Biot's respirations occur in patients with increased intracranial pressure and are characterized by
1. increasing rapidity of breathing followed by slowing of the rate.
2. excessively slow, deep respirations followed by a period of apnea.
3. increase-decrease of rate and depth of respiration.
4. two or three shallow breaths followed by a period of apnea.

Student Name _____

(340) 11. As an infant grows, the heart rate slows. A heart rate within normal limits for a 6-month-old infant is _____ bpm. (Fill in the blank)

(340) 12. The respiratory rate varies from infancy to adulthood. A normal respiratory rate in the 7-year-old child will be _____ than an adult's. (Fill in the blank)

13. If a patient's blood pressure measures 146/92 on the left arm and 138/84 on the right arm, what would you do?
    1. retake the pressure on both arms.
    2. retake the pressure on the left arm.
    3. record both pressures on the chart.
    4. wait 30 minutes and take the pressures again.

14. When performing an assessment on a patient, you should
    1. check that all peripheral pulses are present.
    2. compare peripheral pulses from one side to the other.
    3. check peripheral pulses on the dominant side of the body.
    4. only check the radial and dorsalis pedis pulses.

15. Your patient's blood pressure measures 15 points higher than on her last visit. She has no history of hypertension. Which actions would be appropriate? (Select all that apply)
    1. Wait 15 minutes and take the pressure again.
    2. Tell her to return for a recheck in one week.
    3. Ask if something upsetting has happened.
    4. Inquire when the last meal was eaten.

(328) 16. Interference with accurate measurement of body temperature occurs if the patient
    1. has been chewing gum.
    2. just came in from the cold.
    3. rushed getting to the office.
    4. has been speaking before the temperature is measured.

CRITICAL THINKING ACTIVITIES

1. Take the respiratory rate of a healthy individual and a patient with a lower respiratory infection. List the possible physiological reasons for the difference in the respiratory rate.

2. Explain the mechanisms by which the body elevates temperature to combat a pyrogen.

3. Why do you think that taking a major class examination might raise your pulse rate?

MEETING CLINICAL OBJECTIVES

Directions: The following suggested activities will help you meet the stated clinical practice objectives for the chapter. Review your school's clinical objectives for the week and outline a plan of activities that will help you meet them. If you are unsure how to meet them, consult with your instructor at the beginning of the clinical day.

1. Practice taking the temperature by the various routes and with a glass thermometer and an electronic thermometer.

2. Practice taking blood pressure on as many patients as possible. Have an experienced nurse check your readings on a few people to be certain you are accurate.

3. Try to correlate each vital sign with what is happening in the patient's body to explain changes in vital signs.

4. Work with a classmate and check the respiratory rate on five people. You should both have the same results.

5. Practice taking the radial pulse on 10 different people. Have a classmate check the pulse by counting at the same time on at least three people to be certain that you are accurate.

6. Take an apical pulse on five different people. Have a classmate or instructor check your results. You should be within a couple of beats of each other.

STEPS TOWARD BETTER COMMUNICATION

VOCABULARY BUILDING GLOSSARY

Term	Pronunciation	Definition
A. Individual Terms		
abatement	a BATE ment	lessening, decreasing
alter	AL ter	to change
blunt	blunt	not sharp, with a flattened end
calibrated	CAL i BRAT ed	marked with measurements
clockwise	CLOCK wise	in the direction of the hands of the clock move
contraindicated	con tra IN di ca ted	shows treatment is not desirable
distract	dis TRACT	bring attention elsewhere
flared	flared	wide, opened
impaired	im PAIR ed	damaged
mode	mode	method
occlusive	oc CLU sive	closing off or obstructing
prone	prOne	likely; lying face down
peripheral	per IPH er al	outside the main area, to the edge
propelled	pro PELL ed	pushed with strong force
readily	READ i ly	quickly and easily
secrete	se CRETE	to manufacture and produce a substance

Student Name _____

simultaneously	si mul TAN e ous ly	occurring at the same time
superficial	su per FI cial	on the surface, shallow
unobtrusively	un ob TRU sive ly	quietly, without bringing attention to one's own action

B. Phrases

defining characteristics	de FIN ing char ac ter IS tics	signs or symptoms that explain an illness or nursing diagnosis
in conjunction with	in con JUNC tion with	together with, two or more things used together
jot down	JOT down	to make a written note
keep pace with	keep PACE with	to keep up with, to maintain equal position
owing to	OW ing to	because of, due to
restore the unit	re STORE the unit	put things in the room back in their original or correct places

COMPLETION

Directions: Fill in the blank(s) with the correct term(s) from the Vocabulary Building Glossary to complete the sentence.

1. The antibiotics were bringing about a(n) _____ of the patient's symptoms.

2. The wrong size blood pressure cuff will _____ the reading.

3. If the patient is allergic to the sulfonamides, those drugs are _____ for treatment of his upper respiratory infection.

4. Pushing the plunger on the syringe caused the medication to be _____ into the patient's body.

5. Because the patient was having difficulty breathing, his nostrils were
_____.

6. It is easy to measure the temperature and the pulse _____.

7. It is wise to _____ the patient when counting respirations.

8. To begin measuring blood pressure with an aneroid sphygmomanometer, you must turn the valve _____ to close it before beginning to squeeze the bulb.

9. A rectal temperature is measured with a thermometer that has a(n) _____ end.

10. When assessing circulation, besides measuring the radial pulse, you should also check the _____ pulses.

VOCABULARY EXERCISE

Blunt and *superficial* are not medical terms, but are used in the textbook for explanation of medical information. In the following sentences they are used to describe a person's conversation. Can you describe what the words mean in both cases? You may need to use a nonmedical dictionary.

His conversation is very blunt. If he thinks you are boring, he says so.

Her conversation is superficial. She never talks about anything important.

	Meaning in text	Meaning in conversation
blunt		
superficial		

WORD ATTACK SKILLS

Directions: Break these words into their parts and see if you can figure out the definition. Underline the accented syllable. Check your answer in the dictionary.

1. hemodynamics *(Skill 21-5)*

_____

2. antecubital space *(Skill 21-7)*

_____

PRONUNCIATION SKILLS

Directions: Underline the stressed syllable in these words, then practice saying them aloud to yourself or with a partner. The accent for the first word is underlined as an example.

<u>ap</u> ne a   bra dyp ne a   ta chyp ne a   eup ne a   dysp ne a

hy pox i a   ar rhyth mi a   tach y car di a   di as tol ic   a scul ta tory

feb rile   py rex i a   def er ves ence   di a phor e sis

sphyg mo man o me ter

COMMUNICATION EXERCISES

Directions: Read and practice the dialogue with a partner.

Sample Dialogue A

Nurse: "I'm going to take your vital signs and then I will look at your incision. Did you sleep well last night?"

Mr. S.: "I slept OK, except they woke me up twice to check me over."

Nurse: "I'm going to take your blood pressure first. Can you hold your pajama sleeve up for me?"

Mr. S.: "Sure. Like this?"

Nurse: "That's fine. This may be a little uncomfortable as I pump up the cuff. (Measures BP.). It's 142/86 this morning. That's better than it was yesterday."

Mr. S.: "I'm glad to hear that!"

Nurse: "Now let's take your temperature and count your pulse rate."

Student Name _____

Directions: Fill in the blanks in the conversation to complete the sentences for Sample B; read and practice this with a partner.

Sample Dialogue B

Nurse: "Slip this probe under _____ _____. The
          thermometer will 'beep' when it is done. Turn your _____ over for
          me, so I can feel your _____ more easily."

Mr. S.:   "OK."

Nurse: (Places fingers over artery.) "There it is. It is regular at 76 _____."

*Review the chapter key points, answer the study questions, and complete the
critical thinking activities at the end of the chapter in the textbook.*

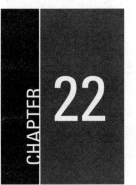

22 Assessing Health Status

CHAPTER

Answer Key: Textbook page references are provided as a guide for answering selected questions. A complete answer key was provided for your instructor.

TERMINOLOGY

A. Matching

Directions: Match the terms in Column I with the correct definitions in Column II.

		Column I		Column II
(359)	1.	_____ auscultation	a.	Tissue elasticity
(373)	2.	_____ cerumen	b.	Fluid in the interstitial spaces
(358)	3.	_____ edema	c.	Tissue damage or discontinuity of normal tissue
(362)	4.	_____ kyphosis		
(359)	5.	_____ lesion	d.	Involuntary fine movement of the body or limbs
(362)	6.	_____ lordosis		
(360)	7.	_____ olfaction	e.	Exaggerated lumbar curve
(358)	8.	_____ palpation	f.	Increased curve in the thoracic area of the spine
(358)	9.	_____ percussion	g.	Pronounced lateral curvature of the spine
(367)	10.	_____ quadrant	h.	Tapping on the body surface to produce sounds
(362)	11.	_____ scoliosis	i.	Ear wax
(358)	12.	_____ tremor	j.	One-quarter of an area
(358)	13.	_____ turgor	k.	Listening for sounds within the body with a stethoscope
			l.	Smelling for distinctive odors
			m.	Touch used to feel various parts of the body

B. Completion

Directions: Fill in the blank(s) with the correct word(s) from the terms list in the chapter in the textbook to complete the sentence.

(364) 1. Normal breath sounds heard over the central chest or back are called
_____; they are equal in length during inspiration and
expiration.

(365) 2. Soft, rustling sounds heard in the periphery of the lung fields are
_____ breath sounds.

(365) 3. The croaking sound of _____ indicates a partial obstruction of an upper air passage.

(365) 4. When auscultating the lungs, listen for any _____ sound by learning the normal breath sounds.

(365) 5. A musical, whistling, high-pitched sound produced by air being forced through a narrowed airway is termed a(n) _____.

(373) 6. The _____ hearing test compares bone and air conduction of sound and is performed with a tuning fork.

(373) 7. The _____ hearing test checks conduction of sound through bone.

(359) 8. An abnormal accumulation of serous fluid within the peritoneal cavity is called

_____.

(365) 9. Fluid is present in the lungs when _____ are auscultated.

(359) 10. The term _____ refers to paleness of the skin.

IDENTIFICATION

Directions: For each of the following problems, identify the correct form of assessment technique.

(358-359) 1. _____ excessive air in the abdominal area

(358-359) 2. _____ difficulty breathing

(359) 3. _____ hyperactive bowel sounds

(358) 4. _____ pain in the abdomen

(360) 5. _____ alcohol ingestion

(358) 6. _____ rash on the skin

(358, 360) 7. _____ presence of wound infection

(358) 8. _____ presence of muscle spasm

(358) 9. _____ laceration on forearm

(358) 10. _____ temperature elevation

a. Inspection
b. Palpation
c. Percussion
d. Auscultation
e. Olfaction

SHORT ANSWER

Directions: Write a brief answer for each question.

(369) 1. The physical examination generally includes the following major areas:

a. _____

b. _____

c. _____

d. _____

e. _____

f. _____

g. _____

Student Name _____

(371) 2. Give examples of examinations for which the following positions are used:

    a. lithotomy _____

    b. knee-chest_____

    c. Sims' _____

(375-376) 3. The areas and responses assessed during the neurological examination or "check" are:

    a. _____

    b. _____

    c. _____

    d. _____

(356) 4. Assessment information pertinent to daily care of the patient includes:

    a. _____

    b. _____

    c. _____

(368) 5. A nursing assessment of the areas of basic needs would include:

    a. _____

    b. _____

    c. _____

    d. _____

    e. _____

    f. _____

    g. _____

(370) 6. Topics for patient teaching regarding preventive health care are:

    a. _____

    b. _____

    c. _____

    d. _____

    e. _____

    f. _____

COMPLETION

Directions: Fill in the blank(s) with the correct word(s) to complete the sentence.

(360) 1. Olfaction may be used to detect a(n) _____ odor to the breath that may indicate diabetic acidosis.

(360) 2. When weighing an infant, you must keep _____ hovering to prevent a fall while adjusting the scale weights.

(362) 3. Blood pressure is never taken on an extremity containing a(n) _____ or on the side where a(n) _____ or lymph node dissection has occurred.

(360) 4. The heart valve sounds are heard best with the _____ of the stethoscope.

(365) 5. To check for dehydration in the elderly patient it is best to check the _____.

(366) 6. When checking peripheral pulses, they should be _____

(367) 7. When assessing for dependent edema, press the fingers into the tissue over the _____ just above the _____.

(367) 8. The planning phase of the nursing process requires that _____ be written for each nursing diagnosis.

(368) 9. One way to remember the areas to assess concerning basic needs is to recall the acronym _____.

(370) 10. Patients should be assessed from _____ at least once each shift.

(370) 11. When assessing patients, it is important to instruct the patient about the purpose of _____ that are ordered.

(371) 12. The purpose of properly draping the patient for the physician's examination is to prevent _____ during the exam.

(375) 13. The Glasgow coma scale is used to score the _____.

(377) 14. A patient who opens the eyes when spoken to, localizes pain, but is confused would have a Glasgow coma scale score of _____.

APPLICATION OF THE NURSING PROCESS

Directions: Write a brief answer for each question.

1. After gathering patient assessment data, what is the next step?

_____

_____

_____

(356) 2. The main purpose of assessing for cultural preferences and health beliefs is so that

_____.

(358) 3. The most important method for gathering data upon physical assessment is

_____.

Student Name_____

(367)   4.   How is the data obtained during assessment used to choose appropriate nursing diagnoses?

_____

_____

_____

(367)   5.   Although writing goals or expected outcomes occurs during the planning step of the nursing process, other planning tasks might include:

_____

_____

_____

(355)   6.   After the initial assessment, additional assessments should be made:

_____

_____

(375, 377)   7.   Evaluation of the assessment process is based on:

_____

_____

_____

NCLEX-PN® EXAM REVIEW

Directions: Choose the best answer(s) to each of the following questions. Some of these questions require synthesis of information with previously acquired knowledge and critical thinking.

1.   A 62-year-old male presents with abdominal pain, nausea, feelings of malaise, and fatigue. While collecting assessment data, an important question to ask him is
   1.   "What is your occupation?"
   2.   "Are you experiencing shortness of breath?"
   3.   "When did you have your last bowel movement?"
   4.   "Do you have a headache?"

(358)   2.   Various techniques are used to assess the abdomen, including inspection, auscultation, percussion and palpation. In order to determine the location of this patient's abdominal pain you would use _____. (Fill in the blank)

3.   While exploring the symptom of nausea, an appropriate question to ask is
   1.   "What did you eat prior to the onset of nausea?"
   2.   "How many hours are you sleeping each night?"
   3.   "Is your vision blurred?"
   4.   "Do you vomit easily?"

(359)   4.   A very pertinent part of the physical examination on this patient is
   1.   inspection of the extremities.
   2.   auscultation of bowel sounds.
   3.   auscultation of the lungs.
   4.   percussion of the flank areas of the back.

(371) 5. A 46-year-old female presents with menstrual difficulties, fatigue, and mood swings. A pelvic examination is ordered. You would place the patient in the lithotomy position with the feet in the stirrups and ask her to (Select all that apply)
1. move her buttocks to the edge of the table.
2. hold her breath during the exam.
3. let her knees fall apart.
4. tense her abdominal muscles.

6. When gathering a history from a patient with menstrual difficulties you would ask (Select all that apply)
1. "When was the first day of your last period?"
2. "How much water are you drinking daily?"
3. "When was your last bowel movement?"
4. "Is it possible you are pregnant?"

(375-376) 7. A 16-year-old male sustained a head injury while playing soccer. When performing a neurological check on him, you look at each pupil to determine
1. if the shape is regular.
2. if they have become smaller.
3. the state of consciousness.
4. whether one pupil is larger than the other.

(375-376) 8. When checking extraocular movements, you ask the patient to follow an object as it is moved into different positions and watch to see if
1. the pupils constrict when focusing on the object.
2. the pupils dilate when focusing on the object.
3. the eyes move in a normal coordinated manner.
4. there is blinking while trying to focus on the object.

(376) 9. To check extremity strength, you ask the patient to
1. touch his finger to his nose.
2. raise the left leg.
3. push the soles of the feet against your hands.
4. bend the right knee.

(376) 10. You check this patient's mental status by asking (Select all that apply)
1. where he is right now.
2. who the current president of the U.S. is.
3. what month it is.
4. where his parents are.

CRITICAL THINKING ACTIVITIES

1. Describe the steps in a focused cardiovascular assessment.

2. Teach a family member about the recommendations for periodic diagnostic testing. Points to cover:

3. From memory, list the equipment that would be needed for the physician to perform a physical examination on an adult male or female.

Student Name _____

MEETING CLINICAL OBJECTIVES

Directions: The following suggested activities will help you meet the stated clinical practice objectives for the chapter. Review your school's clinical objectives for the week and outline a plan of activities that will help you meet them. If you are unsure how to meet them, consult with your instructor at the beginning of the clinical day.

1. Practice performing an initial physical and psychosocial assessment on classmates and family members. Organize your approach so that it will be in a consistent order each time you perform such an assessment. Make up index cards to guide you; use an outline format. Use the cards when you are in the clinical setting.

2. Practice the neurological "check" on at least four people.

3. When assigned to the clinical setting where a proctosigmoidoscopy examination, a pelvic examination, and Pap smear may be done, review the procedure for setting up and assisting the physician with each exam.

4. Teach a female about self-breast examination and teach a male about self-testicular examination.

STEPS TOWARD BETTER COMMUNICATION

VOCABULARY BUILDING GLOSSARY

Term	Pronunciation	Definition
acronym	AC ro nym	a word made from initials of other words, (e.g., BP = blood pressure)
appraising	ap PRAI sing	evaluating
ascertaining	as cer TAIN ing	finding out information
astute	a STUTE	intelligent
holistic	ho LIS tic	relating to the total being (body, mind, and spirit)
opacity	o PAC i ty	not allowing light to pass through
patent	PA tent	open, unobstructed
patency	PA ten cy	amount of openness
sluggishly	SLUG gish ly	slowly
subsides	sub SIDES	goes down, becomes less strong

COMPLETION

Directions: Fill in the blank(s) with the correct word(s) from the Vocabulary Building Glossary to complete the sentence.

1. Performing a physical assessment is part of the process used when _____ the patient's condition.

2. A cataract causes a(n) _____ of the lens in the eye.

3. Nurses are taught to provide _____ care to patients, considering body, mind, and spirit.

4. While _____ information from the chart, the nurse discovered that the patient previously had a hip fracture.

5. A fever usually _____ when the patient is given acetaminophen.

6. PT is a(n) _____ for physical therapy.

7. Normal bowel sounds indicate that the bowel is _____.

8. When all assessment data have been gathered, a(n) _____ decision about the care needed for the patient can be made.

VOCABULARY EXERCISES

Directions: Complete the statement with one of the following words.

occluded   abnormal   sluggish   a word made from the initials of other words

1. *Adventitious* means _____.

2. An acronym is _____.

3. The opposite of patent is _____.

4. *Brisk* is the opposite of _____.

WORD ATTACK SKILLS

Pronunciation of Difficult Terms

A. *Directions: Practice pronouncing the following words. (The stressed syllable is written in capital letters, the "long mark" or macron (-) indicates that the sound of that letter is the same as the name of the letter.)*

A SCĪ tes	ech chy MŌ sis	er y THĒ ma
GUAĪ ac	LĒ sion	nys TAG mus
PĀ tent	pe TĒ che ae	RhŌN chus/RhŌN chi
RIN ne test	san GWIN e ous	STRĪ dor
tin NĪ tous	Weber (VĀ ber) test	

B. *Directions: Divide the following two words into syllables and put a line under the accented syllables; practice pronouncing the words with a partner.*

1. sphygmomanometer _____

2. ophthalmoscope _____

Abbreviations

Directions: Write the meaning for the following abbreviations.

1. PMI _____

2. PERRLA _____

Student Name_____

3. BSE _____

4. PCA_____

5. ADL _____

6. TSE _____

7. EOMS _____

8. GI _____

9. DRE _____

COMMUNICATION EXERCISE

Interviewing and communication skills include:

- Maintaining a relaxed, pleasant manner.
- Maintaining the correct degree of formality.
- Being respectful of the person and his or her privacy.
- Speaking carefully and distinctly where the patient can see your lips.
- Using correct pronunciation.
- Asking the person to repeat if you do not understand.
- Repeating the information received to make sure you understood it correctly.
- Saying so when you do not know something and then finding out the answer.

Here is a communication example for performing the beginning of a basic needs assessment *(Table 22-5)*:

Nurse:	"Good morning, Ms. T., I'm _____, your student nurse today. I need to gather some information about you and perform an examination. Is there anything you need before we begin?"
Ms. T.:	"I just need to turn and get out of this position first."
Nurse:	Let me help you to turn and sit up. Is that better?"
Ms. T.:	"Yes, I'm fine now."
Nurse:	(Visually assessing the patient) "Did you have any problems with mobility or muscle strength before this surgery?"
Ms. T.:	"I'm always stiff first thing in the morning, but after I'm up a while I can move around just fine. I'm not as strong as I used to be, but that is expected at 78 years old. I do have some arthritis in my hands and that makes it difficult to do some things, especially when it flares up."
Nurse:	"Does the arthritis prevent you from managing to bathe, groom, and dress?"
Ms. T.:	"No, I can do those things; it just takes me longer sometimes."
Nurse:	"What about cooking, eating, or cleaning up?"
Ms. T.:	"I can manage to cook OK with my electric can opener and large-handled knives and utensils. My daughter helps me clean really well once a month."
Nurse:	"How many hours a night do you usually sleep?"
Ms. T.:	"It varies; most of the time I'm in bed by 10:00, but sometimes I'll watch a movie that runs later. I usually wake up about 6:30. If I'm short on sleep, I'll nap after lunch."
Nurse:	"Do you awaken at night much?"

Ms. T.: "I have to get up once during the night to use the bathroom, but I only awaken more when I have been out to dinner and had more liquid than usual."

Nurse: "Does pain interfere with your usual activities or sleep?"

Ms. T.: "Well, right now it does, but then I just had the surgery yesterday. When my arthritis flares up I have to take a lot of ibuprofen and sometimes something stronger or I have trouble sleeping."

A. *Directions: Practice obtaining the rest of the information needed for the basic needs assessment with a partner. Ask the questions and have the partner supply the answer. Continue with the assessment depending on the answer given.*

B. *Directions: Fill in what you would say in the following dialogue regarding the psychosocial assessment of Ms. T.:*

Nurse: "Do you belong to a church or a spiritual group?"

Ms. T.: "Yes, I'm a member of the Presbyterian church. I go most Sundays."

Nurse: "What about your support system? Who can you count on when _____?"

Ms. T.: "My daughter is very helpful, but she lives an hour away. My friend, Betty, will help me and my neighbor, Jim, is available if I call him."

Nurse: "How would you describe your mental outlook? Are you ever _____? How do you handle upsetting events?"

Ms. T.: "I'm usually fairly happy, but I get lonely sometimes. I wouldn't really call it depressed, except when I was told I had to have this surgery. I'm glad that's over.

I talk with my friend Betty when I have a problem. If I feel down, I remind myself of how lucky I am to have so few health problems and to still be in my own place.

I find music will cheer me up too."

Nurse: "Will you be able to have someone care for you at home while you recover, or would you like to speak with the _____ to arrange your convalescence?"

Ms. T.: "My daughter is taking some time off of work and I will go to her house to recover."

Nurse: "Will you be able to obtain your _____ and _____ without a problem?"

Ms. T.: "Yes, my insurance will cover what I need. I have a supplemental policy from my years of employment."

Nurse: "What are your _____ at this point in time?"

Ms. T.: "My biggest fear is that this lump was malignant and I will have to undergo chemotherapy. I worry about who will take care of me if I get really sick. My daughter works full time and she has three small children."

Nurse: "Let's wait and see what the _____.

Now, considering your discharge tomorrow, let's see what you need to know. How will you _____ _____?"

Ms. T.: "How often should the dressing be changed? How do I clean the wound? Will it hurt?"

Student Name _____

C. *Directions: Write a short dialogue for a home health visit to a patient you have visited before. Include a quick assessment of general condition.*

CULTURAL POINTS

Think about what foods, practices, and beliefs from your culture might seem unusual to a nurse who grew up in a different culture. What suggestions can you make for how the nurse could deal with the differences? How will you deal with such differences when you have a patient from a culture different from your own? Do you think you will have an advantage in understanding how the patient might feel?

Review the chapter key points, answer the study questions, and complete the critical thinking activities at the end of the chapter in the textbook.

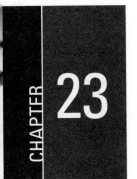

CHAPTER 23

Admitting, Transferring, and Discharging Patients

Answer Key: Textbook page references are provided as a guide for answering selected questions. A complete answer key was provided for your instructor.

TERMINOLOGY

A. Matching

Directions: Match the terms in Column I with the definitions in Column II.

Column I		Column II
(384)	1. _____ MSW	a. Health maintenance organization
(380)	2. _____ deductible	b. The amount the patient pays for each service before insurance pays
(386)	3. _____ autopsy	c. Examination of remains by a pathologist to determine cause of death
(380)	4. _____ HMO	
(386)	5. _____ coroner	d. County medical officer responsible for investigating unexplained deaths
(380)	6. _____ co-pay	e. Amount per calendar year a patient pays before insurance begins to pay for care
		f. Master's degree in social work

B. Completion

Directions: Fill in the blank(s) with the correct term(s) from the terms list in the chapter in the textbook to complete the sentence.

(384)   1. The _____ is the RN or social worker who coordinates home care after hospitalization when the patient needs it.

(379)   2. Prior authorization is not needed for a(n) _____, such as might occur after an automobile accident.

(380)   3. Most patients over 65 years of age are covered by _____, government health insurance for the elderly.

(380)   4. _____ is a state insurance program for the poor who cannot afford health insurance.

(379)   5. A(n) _____ admission would occur for a patient who was scheduled to have a hip replacement surgery.

(380)   6. _____ is a system of health care that was designed to lower the costs of health care.

SHORT ANSWER

Directions: Write a brief answer for each question.

(380)   1.   The role of the admitting department is to:

_____

_____

(380)   2.   You would cover the following points when orienting a patient to the patient unit:

    a. _____

    b. _____

    c. _____

    d. _____

    e. _____

    f. _____

    g. _____

(383)   3.   When a patient is transferred to another facility, the five types of information which must be sent with the patient are:

    a. _____

    b. _____

    c. _____

    d. _____

    e. _____

(384)   4.   Types of information to be included in the patient's discharge instructions when going home are:

    a. _____

    b. _____

    c. _____

    d. _____

    e. _____

    f. _____

(386)   5.   When it appears that a patient has died, the nurse must:

_____

_____

_____

_____

(381)   6.   If a patient brings valuables to the hospital, they should be

_____ or _____.

Student Name_____

(383)   7.   The nurse who notes that orders have been transcribed is legally responsible for their
_____.

(383)   8.   Orders are signed off by _____
_____.

(383)   9.   When a patient is transferred to another unit or facility it is important to also notify
_____.

(383)   10. Discharge planning begins at _____.

(384)   11. Discharge orders are written by _____.

(384)   12. The nurse is responsible for seeing that all _____ accompany the patient at discharge.

(384)   13. Home health services may include skilled nursing such as _____
_____.

(384)   14. Other home health services include:

_____

_____

(385)   15. If a patient decides to leave before he or she is discharged, the nurse must immediately
_____.

(384)   16. Responsibilities of the nurse when a patient wishes to leave against medical advice are:

_____

_____

_____

(385)   17. Patients who consider leaving against medical advice need to know that sometimes insurance
companies will _____.

(386)   18. List four ways you may be able to assist a significant other when a patient has died.

      a. _____

      b. _____

      c. _____

      d. _____

(386)   19. Three reasons an autopsy may have to be done are:

      a. _____

      b. _____

      c. _____

NCLEX-PN® EXAM REVIEW

*Directions: Choose the **best** answer(s) for each of the following questions.*

(380) 1. A priority during orientation to the patient unit is how to
1. work the TV.
2. call the nurse.
3. use the telephone.
4. obtain meals.

(381) 2. When a patient brings medications from home the nurse should
1. allow the family to administer them.
2. make a list of the medications and send them home with the family.
3. ask the physician to write an order for each medication so they can be administered to the patient.
4. place them in the bedside drawer and ask the patient to refrain from taking them.

(384) 3. Nursing duties at the time of discharge include (Select all that apply)
1. returning medications to the pharmacy.
2. arranging transportation home.
3. making certain the patient understands discharge instructions.
4. teaching regarding care at home.

(380) 4. Obtaining prior authorization for admission to the hospital is usually the responsibility of the
1. nurse assigned to the patient.
2. nursing unit to which the patient is assigned.
3. admitting office of the hospital.
4. the admitting physician's office.

(383) 5. When a patient is to be transferred to another facility, transportation by ambulance is arranged by the
1. nurse assigned to the patient.
2. hospital discharge planner.
3. attending physician.
4. patient's family.

(386) 6. An autopsy would most likely be necessary in which one of the following incidences?
1. A patient dies while recovering from a myocardial infarction (heart attack).
2. A 91-year-old patient who was being treated for congestive heart failure dies at home.
3. A patient with long-term diabetes dies while being treated for end-stage renal disease.
4. A patient dies while being treated for injuries sustained in an assault.

(380) 7. A male patient is admitted after sustaining a fall from a ladder at home. He has fractured his femur. He is assigned to you and you start his admission process. You appropriately say to him *first*
1. "So you fell off a ladder, sir?"
2. "Welcome to the unit. We'll take good care of you."
3. "My name is S.D., LPN/LVN. I will be your nurse for this shift."
4. "If you will put on the gown, I will be back in a bit."

(380) 8. The injured patient tells you "This is the first time I have ever been in a hospital as a patient." He appears apprehensive. Your best response would be
1. "We'll take good care of you here. Don't you worry."
2. "This must be very scary for you."
3. "Your wife, here, will watch out for you."
4. "I'll be happy to answer any questions or address your concerns."

Student Name_____

(384) 9. Your patient is ready for discharge. When preparing to send him home, it is most important to include on his discharge instruction sheet
   1. your name and home phone number.
   2. whether each medication should be taken with food.
   3. the social worker's name and phone number.
   4. a list of specific foods he is to eat.

(383) 10. A male patient is being transferred from your unit to the convalescent unit. It is important that you (Select all that apply)
   1. notify his family of the transfer before moving him.
   2. check all drawers, the closet, and bed linens for his personal possessions.
   3. transfer him by stretcher to the other unit.
   4. provide time for him to say goodbye to his roommate who has been there for several days.

(381) 11. A male patient has been transferred to your unit. The transferring nurse has given you a report on his condition and helped you settle him in bed. Your next priority would be to
   1. perform a head-to-toe assessment.
   2. read all the orders the physician has written.
   3. check his MAR to see what medications he is receiving.
   4. document the transfer in the chart.

(384) 12. There are no available beds on your unit. The ER has called wanting to transfer a patient and is inquiring if there is anyone who can be discharged. You know that a patient is ready to go home, but he has no discharge order. You know that
   1. the admitting office would have to call the physician.
   2. the unit secretary would need to contact the insurance company to verify the discharge.
   3. you would need to call the physician to see if he will order the patient discharged.
   4. you must check with the patient to see if he feels ready to go home.

CRITICAL THINKING ACTIVITIES

1. What information would be important for you to know when you enter a hospital as a patient?
2. How would you obtain needed information upon admission for a patient who is comatose?
3. What could you do to help an elderly patient who is worried about leaving his wife home alone when he is admitted to the hospital?

MEETING CLINICAL OBJECTIVES

Directions: The following suggested activities will help you meet the stated clinical practice objectives for the chapter. Review your school's clinical objectives for the week and outline a plan of activities that will help you meet them. If you are unsure how to meet them, consult with your instructor at the beginning of the clinical day.

1. Review the admission forms and then assist a staff nurse who is admitting a new patient. Orient the patient to the unit.

2. Help a nurse transfer a patient to another unit; listen carefully to the report given to the new nurse.

3. Collaborate with the social worker regarding discharge needs of an assigned patient. Describe the patient's home needs to the social worker.

4. Role play a situation in which a patient seeks to leave against medical advice.

5. Outline how you would interact with a family of one of your assigned patients should that patient suddenly expire.

STEPS TOWARD BETTER COMMUNICATION

VOCABULARY BUILDING GLOSSARY

Term	Pronunciation	Definition
alleviate	al LEV i ate	to make less difficult; relieve
bereaved	be REAVed	a person whose loved one has died
deterioration	de TER i or A tion	going into a worse condition
devastating	DEV as ta ting	overwhelming; causing great emotional stress
in general	in GEN er al	usually
lethargic	le THAR gic	showing little energy or interest, tired
protocols	PRO to cols	rules for action under certain conditions
significant other	sig NIF i cant OTH er	any close friend, partner, or family member who has as special relationship with the patient
synopsis	syn OP sis	summary
verified	VER i fIEd	checked to make sure it is correct

COMPLETION

Directions: Fill in the blank(s) with the correct word(s) from the Vocabulary Building Glossary to complete each sentence.

1. The patient's _____ was her male companion of 15 years.

2. Each nurse must follow the accepted _____ when allergies are identified during assessment.

3. The medication list of a confused patient should be _____ with the family.

4. When transferring a patient to another unit within the hospital, a(n) _____ is given of the patient's condition and current treatment.

5. Orienting the patient to the unit and hospital routine will _____ some anxiety.

6. Valuables must be treated with care as the loss of a prized piece of jewelry can be _____ to the patient.

Student Name_____

7. The patient was very _____ upon admission and wouldn't respond very well to questions.

8. _____, the patient is welcomed to the unit before beginning the assessment process.

VOCABULARY EXERCISE

Choose a family member, friend, or classmate, and write an assessment of the person from what you can perceive visually. If possible, take and record vital signs. Use the vocabulary in Table 23-1 in the textbook.

WORD ATTACK SKILLS

Directions: Write the opposite of the given term.

1. alert_____

2. lethargic _____

3. oral _____

4. labored _____

5. shallow _____

6. sighted _____

COMMUNICATION EXERCISE

Directions: Choose a partner and perform the following role plays. Switch roles between "patient" and "nurse."

- Role play introducing a patient to the unit.

- Now do the same role play in an unfriendly, impolite, or impatient manner. How does it feel when you are playing the role of the patient?

- Practice comforting or being available to listen to someone whose loved one has just died. What to say in case of death:

"I am sorry for the death of your loved one."
"I am sorry for your loss."
"I am sorry."
"I am so sorry."
"You have my sympathy."

CULTURAL POINTS

In some religions, such as Islam, it is often considered the duty of the nearest relative of the same sex to prepare the body for burial. This may be by washing it in a certain ritual way. When death is approaching for such a person, try to find out what would be usual for this culture to do so that you can accommodate the family after the death. If there is a conflict between family wishes and hospital rules, you will need to be very careful how you explain it to the family or ask the physician to talk to them.

Review the chapter key points, answer the study questions, and complete the critical thinking activities at the end of the chapter in the textbook.

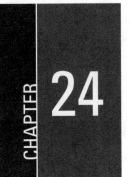

CHAPTER 24
Diagnostic Tests and Specimen Collection

Answer Key: Textbook page references are provided as a guide for answering selected questions. A complete answer key was provided for your instructor.

TERMINOLOGY

Directions: Fill in the blank(s) with the correct term(s) from the terms list in the chapter in the textbook to complete the sentence.

(400) 1. The technique of _____ is used to obtain a sample of bone marrow for diagnostic testing.

(400) 2. A breast _____ is often performed to determine whether a lump in the breast needs to be removed.

(408) 3. A(n) _____ is usually flexible, contains a fiberoptic light, and is used to view the interior of body structures.

(407) 4. Pressure must be placed over the site of insertion of the catheter used for an angiogram, or a(n) _____ may form.

(409) 5. One sign of liver disorders is _____ , with yellow skin and mucous membranes.

(392) 6. Blood chemistry tests are usually combined into a(n) _____ where many tests are performed sequentially at one time.

(408) 7. A colonoscopy is performed to detect _____ in the colon which might become malignant.

(412) 8. A Pap _____ consists of cells taken from the cervix and vagina for the detection of cervical cancer.

(401) 9. A(n) _____ is passed over the upper right quadrant of the abdomen to conduct an ultrasound study of the gallbladder.

(413) 10. When taking a throat culture, you would keep the swab sterile and only touch the _____ area and the back wall of the throat where it is inflamed.

MATCHING

Directions: Match the tests in Column I with the descriptions in Column II.

<table>
<tr><td></td><td></td><td>**Column I**</td><td></td><td>**Column II**</td></tr>
<tr><td>(390)</td><td>1.</td><td>_____ angiography</td><td>a.</td><td>Examination of the rectum and sigmoid colon with a proctoscope</td></tr>
<tr><td>(390)</td><td>2.</td><td>_____ MRI</td><td>b.</td><td>Computed tomography scan</td></tr>
<tr><td>(390)</td><td>3.</td><td>_____ culture</td><td>c.</td><td>Magnetic resonance imaging</td></tr>
<tr><td>(390)</td><td>4.</td><td>_____ CT scan</td><td>d.</td><td>Insertion of a needle into the subarachnoid space between the lumbar vertebrae to withdraw cerebrospinal fluid</td></tr>
<tr><td>(409)</td><td>5.</td><td>_____ cystoscopy</td><td></td><td></td></tr>
<tr><td>(412)</td><td>6.</td><td>_____ EEG</td><td>e.</td><td>Electrical recording of brain waves</td></tr>
<tr><td>(390)</td><td>7.</td><td>_____ IVP</td><td>f.</td><td>Radiography of an artery after injection with a contrast medium into the bloodstream</td></tr>
<tr><td>(390)</td><td>8.</td><td>_____ lumbar puncture</td><td></td><td></td></tr>
<tr><td>(390)</td><td>9.</td><td>_____ Pap smear</td><td>g.</td><td>Growing organisms in a laboratory culture medium</td></tr>
<tr><td>(390)</td><td>10.</td><td>_____ proctosigmoidoscopy</td><td>h.</td><td>Examination of the bladder through a cystoscope</td></tr>
<tr><td>(390)</td><td>11.</td><td>_____ thoracentesis</td><td>i.</td><td>Intravenous pyelogram</td></tr>
<tr><td>(392)</td><td>12.</td><td>_____ venipuncture</td><td>j.</td><td>Laboratory test to determine cervical (or other) cancer</td></tr>
<tr><td></td><td></td><td></td><td>k.</td><td>Insertion of a needle into a vein to withdraw blood</td></tr>
<tr><td></td><td></td><td></td><td>l.</td><td>Insertion of a needle into the pleural space to withdraw fluid or air or to instill medication</td></tr>
</table>

COMPLETION

Directions: Fill in the blank(s) with the correct word(s) from the textbook chapter to complete the sentence.

(389)   1.   Diagnostic tests are performed to aid in the _____ of disease.

(390)   2.   Magnetic resonance imaging is a(n) _____ method of visualizing parts within the body without the use of contrast media or ionizing radiation.

(400)   3.   Sonography uses _____ to outline structures.

(391)   4.   _____ is the study of blood and its _____.

(391)   5.   An increase in leukocytes is termed _____ and often indicates _____.

(391)   6.   The _____ test is used to monitor anticoagulant drugs such as sodium warfarin.

(392)   7.   Inflammatory conditions cause an increase in the erythrocyte _____ rate.

(392)   8.   Food and drink are withheld for _____ hours prior to some blood chemistry tests.

Student Name_____

(393) 9. Whenever obtaining blood for a diagnostic test, the nurse must
_____ to prevent contamination.

(392) 10. The blood of the diabetic patient is frequently tested using capillary blood and a(n)
_____.

(392) 11. Blood urea nitrogen (BUN) and creatinine levels are important indicators of
_____ function.

(398) 12. Because urine _____, specimens should be analyzed
soon after collection.

(400) 13. Tissues obtained by biopsy are examined by a(n) _____.

(403) 14. Fluoroscopy is used to examine _____ in the GI system.

(404) 15. Radionuclide studies are performed in the _____ department.

(390) 16. KUB stands for _____,
_____, _____.

(404) 17. When preparing the patient for an MRI, all _____
must be removed from the body.

(404-405) 18. The ECG represents the _____ of the cardiac cycle.

(406) 19. Cardiac catheterization determines the function of the
_____, _____,
and _____ circulation.

(408) 20. Pulmonary function tests provide information about
_____ function, lung
_____,and_____of
gases.

(404) 21. Common x-rays of the GI system include a(n) _____
and a(n) _____.

22. After any diagnostic test that utilizes a contrast medium or dye of some sort,
the patient is encouraged to _____ a lot of
_____.

(408) 23. A gastroscopy is usually performed in the _____ laboratory.

(409) 24. Colonoscopy examines the entire _____ for polyps,
areas of inflammation, and malignant lesions.

(409) 25. ERCP, _____, is used to identify a cause
of biliary obstruction such as _____,
_____, _____, or
tumor.

(401) 26. A stool specimen for ova and parasites must be sent to the laboratory
_____.

(416) 27. A thin prep Pap smear procedure differs from a regular Pap smear in that the specimen is
placed _____.

NCLEX-PN® EXAM REVIEW

*Directions: Choose the **best** answer(s) to each of the following questions.*

(391) 1. Teaching for the patient undergoing an upper GI in the morning would include
1. why a bowel prep is necessary.
2. the need for a liquid dinner.
3. the reason an IV line will be started.
4. not to take anything by mouth (NPO) after midnight.

(407) 2. Post-test nursing care specific to the patient who has had an arteriogram includes (Select all that apply)
1. taking vital signs frequently per the protocol schedule.
2. checking pulses distal to the catheter insertion site.
3. keeping the patient NPO for 4 hours.
4. ambulating the patient every 2 hours.

(392) 3. The patient's CBC revealed a Hgb of 11.8 gm/dL, a platelet count of 320,000/mm³, and a WBC of 7,500/µL. These results indicate
1. a low platelet count.
2. a high leukocyte count.
3. normal platelets and low WBCs.
4. normal WBCs and a low hemoglobin.

(410) 4. One of the nurse's main responsibilities in assisting with a lumbar puncture is to
1. hand the physician the instruments.
2. help the patient maintain the correct position.
3. sterilize the equipment after use.
4. maintain pressure on the puncture site afterward.

(416) 5. To prepare a Pap smear for the laboratory,
1. it must be "fixed" on the slide.
2. it has to be sent to the lab immediately.
3. a stain is applied to the slide.
4. the secretions must be kept moist.

(403) 6. Fluoroscopy is done during x-ray examination of the
1. liver.
2. extremities.
3. GI system.
4. lungs.

(409) 7. Pretest preparation for a colonoscopy that is not necessary for a barium enema includes
1. NPO after midnight.
2. colon prep.
3. increasing fluid intake.
4. pretest sedation.

(404) 8. One difference for the patient between an x-ray and an MRI study is that for the MRI the patient must
1. hold very still for an extended period.
2. remove normal clothing.
3. drink several glasses of water beforehand.
4. refrain from breathing for 2 minutes at a time.

(406, 409) 9. Which one of the following diagnostic procedures requires a signed consent? (Select all that apply)
1. colonoscopy
2. gallbladder sonogram
3. cardiac catheterization
4. pulmonary function test

(409)   10.   A part of the preparation for the
                 colonoscopy that differs from other
                 GI tests is that the patient must

           1.   take laxatives the day before
               the test.
           2.   be NPO for 12 hours before
               the test.
           3.   have an enema the morning of
               the test.
           4.   have a liquid diet for 2–3 days
               prior to the test.

APPLICATION OF THE NURSING PROCESS

Directions: Write a brief answer for each question.

1. Four assessment factors to be considered when a diagnostic test is to be performed on a patient are:

     a.   _____

     b.   _____

     c.   _____

     d.   _____

2. A nursing diagnosis that is appropriate for any patient who is not familiar with a diagnostic test to be performed is _____.

3. An expected outcome for the above nursing diagnosis might be _____ _____.

4. A very important part of nursing intervention prior to diagnostic tests is _____ _____.

5. An important part of nursing intervention after a diagnostic test has been performed is _____ _____ _____.

6. A part of the evaluation process when serial diagnostic tests are being performed is to _____ _____ _____.

CRITICAL THINKING ACTIVITIES

1. Make an outline of the teaching points you would cover for the patient undergoing a cardiac catheterization.

2. How would you prepare the patient who is to undergo an MRI of the brain?

3. If a patient asks how sonography works, what would you say?

MEETING CLINICAL OBJECTIVES

Directions: The following suggested activities will help you meet the stated clinical practice objectives for the chapter. Review your school's clinical objectives for the week and outline a plan of activities that will help you meet them. If you are unsure how to meet them, consult with your instructor at the beginning of the clinical day.

1. Outline pretest and post-test nursing care for patients undergoing three different diagnostic tests or procedures.

2. Interact with a patient who has fears regarding a diagnostic procedure. Plan ahead by reviewing therapeutic communication techniques.

3. While in clinical, tell the staff you would like opportunities to perform finger-stick blood glucose tests using a glucometer. Remember to wear gloves.

4. Seek opportunities to assist with a lumbar puncture, thoracentesis, paracentesis, bone marrow aspiration, or liver biopsy, or prepare to assist with these procedures. Outline your duties and the supplies you would need to gather. You might role play a simulated situation with a peer.

5. Prepare to calm and soothe a patient who is very anxious about having her first pelvic exam and Pap smear performed.

6. Teach a patient about an MRI diagnostic test. Place an outline on a card to help you review the points to cover.

STEPS TOWARD BETTER COMMUNICATION

VOCABULARY BUILDING GLOSSARY

Term	Pronunciation	Definition
ampule	am PULE	a small, sealed, glass or polyethylene container of a measured amount of medication
deteriorates	de TER i or ates	loses quality
diagnostic	di ag NOS tic	an analysis done to find the cause or source of a problem or illness
shunt (noun)	SHUNT	a passage between two natural channels, either a natural irregularity or man-made
shunt (verb)	SHUNT	to turn to one side; to bypass
titer	TI ter	the strength or concentration of one substance mixed with others
troubleshoot	TROU ble SHOOT	to look for a way to fix a problem

COMPLETION

Directions: Fill in the blank(s) with the correct term(s) from the Vocabulary Building Glossary to complete the sentence.

1. It was hoped that the _____ test would show what was wrong with the patient.

Student Name_____

2. The blood test showed a rise in the _____ of Rocky Mountain spotted fever antibodies.

3. Urine must be sent to the lab right away as it _____ when allowed to sit for any length of time.

4. When the machine would not turn on, the nurse had to _____ to find the problem.

WORD ATTACK SKILLS

Directions: In this chapter there are a number of suffixes (a word part at the end of the word) used to describe procedures. Look at the meanings of these suffixes. Find examples in the textbook and write them in the blanks.

1. -scope means an instrument to visually examine.

   _____

2. -scopy means a process of visual examination, using a -scope.

   _____

3. -graph means a recording instrument showing relationships by using a diagram.

   _____

4. -graphy means a process of recording.

   _____

PRONUNCIATION OF DIFFICULT TERMS

Directions: Divide the following words into syllables and put a line under the accented syllables. Practice pronouncing the words.

1. angiography _____
2. cholangiopancreatography _____
3. cystoscopy_____
4. electroencephalogram_____
5. gastroscopy _____
6. myocardial infarction _____
7. paracentesis_____
8. proctosigmoidoscopy _____
9. radiopaque _____
10. radioimmunoassays _____
11. thoracentesis_____

COMMUNICATION EXERCISE

Directions: Practice this dialogue with a partner.

A nurse explains to her patient, Mr. F., how to prepare for an exercise stress test, and what will happen.

Nurse: "Good morning, Mr. F. The doctor has ordered an exercise stress test for you."

Mr. F.: "Is that with a treadmill? Is that where I have to walk on one of those moving platforms?"

Nurse: "That's right. He wants to measure your heart performance and blood pressure while you exercise."

Mr. F.: "What will happen?"

Nurse: "The technician will attach wires to your skin with stick-on electrodes and place a blood pressure cuff on your arm. They will show the heart rate and pattern of electrical activity in your heart and your blood pressure while you exercise. The platform may move at a steady pace, or they may increase the speed or incline it gradually to see how exercise affects your heart."

Mr. F.: "I guess I can handle that OK."

Nurse: "I don't think it will be too difficult for you. You must not smoke or eat for at least 4 hours before the test."

Mr. F.: "Uh oh! Can I eat breakfast before the test?"

Nurse: "You can have a light breakfast as the test isn't scheduled until 1:00 P.M."

Mr. F.: "Well, that's good."

Nurse: "You can take your heart and blood pressure medications as usual."

Mr. F.: "OK."

Nurse: "I need you to sign this consent form, please."

Mr. F.: "OK, it doesn't sound too bad. Where do I sign?"

Nurse: "Here on this line. I hope the test shows your heart is OK."

Review the chapter key points, answer the study questions, and complete the critical thinking activities at the end of the chapter in the textbook.

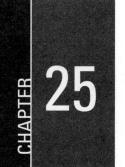

CHAPTER 25 Fluid, Electrolyte, and Acid-Base Balance

Answer Key: Textbook page references are provided as a guide for answering selected questions. A complete answer key was provided for your instructor.

TERMINOLOGY

A. Matching

Directions: Match the terms in Column I with the definitions in Column II.

<table>
<tr><th colspan="3">Column I</th><th colspan="2">Column II</th></tr>
<tr><td>(425)</td><td>1. _____</td><td>acidosis</td><td>a.</td><td>A mineral or salt dissolved in body fluid</td></tr>
<tr><td>(425)</td><td>2. _____</td><td>ascites</td><td>b.</td><td>Degree of elasticity of tissue</td></tr>
<tr><td>(428)</td><td>3. _____</td><td>alkalosis</td><td>c.</td><td>Abnormal accumulation of fluid within the</td></tr>
<tr><td>(421)</td><td>4. _____</td><td>dehydration</td><td></td><td>peritoneal cavity</td></tr>
<tr><td>(424)</td><td>5. _____</td><td>edema</td><td>d.</td><td>Decrease in pH</td></tr>
<tr><td>(420)</td><td>6. _____</td><td>electrolyte</td><td>e.</td><td>Condition of severe muscle cramps, carpal</td></tr>
<tr><td>(421)</td><td>7. _____</td><td>interstitial</td><td></td><td>pedal spasms, and laryngeal spasm</td></tr>
<tr><td>(421)</td><td>8. _____</td><td>intracellular</td><td>f.</td><td>Removal of water from a tissue</td></tr>
<tr><td>(432)</td><td>9. _____</td><td>stridor</td><td>g.</td><td>Increase in pH</td></tr>
<tr><td>(432)</td><td>10. _____</td><td>tetany</td><td>h.</td><td>Excessive accumulation of interstitial fluid</td></tr>
<tr><td>(421)</td><td>11. _____</td><td>transcellular fluid</td><td>i.</td><td>Shrill, harsh sound upon inspiration</td></tr>
<tr><td>(424)</td><td>12. _____</td><td>turgor</td><td>j.</td><td>Fluid in spaces surrounding the cells</td></tr>
<tr><td></td><td></td><td></td><td>k.</td><td>Fluid within the cells</td></tr>
<tr><td></td><td></td><td></td><td>l.</td><td>Gastrointestinal secretions</td></tr>
</table>

B. Completion

Directions: Fill in the blank(s) with the correct term(s) from the terms list in the textbook chapter to complete the sentence.

(421)   1. A young man involved in an auto accident sustained a severe cut to his leg and lost a lot of blood; he is suffering from _____.

(426)   2. A patient's lab work shows a low potassium value. This patient has

_____.

(428)   3. The electrolyte imbalance _____ can cause tetany.

(421)   4. The process by which substances move back and forth across the membrane until they are evenly distributed is called _____.

(422)   5.   _____ refers to the movement of pure solvent across a membrane.

(422)   6.   When solute and water are of equal concentration, a solution is

            _____.

(422)   7.   When a substance is introduced into the blood that makes the fluid in the vascular compartment _____, fluid will be drawn from the cells into the vascular compartment.

(422)   8.   If a patient is hydrated too quickly with isotonic solution, the vascular fluid becomes _____ and fluid will move into the tissues.

(422)   9.   The movement of fluid outward through a semipermeable membrane is termed

            _____.

(422)   10.   Substances, regardless of their electrical charge, may be moved from an area of lower concentration to an area of higher concentration by _____.

(425)   11.   A state of dehydration often causes the electrolyte imbalance

            _____.

(427)   12.   Burn patients often develop the electrolyte imbalance

            _____.

(428)   13.   The electrolyte imbalance, _____, usually only occurs in the presence of kidney failure.

(429)   14.   Respiratory acidosis occurs from an increase in _____.

(431)   15.   Metabolic acidosis often occurs in the _____ patient.

IDENTIFICATION

A. Directions: Indicate whether each of the following laboratory values is normal or if an electrolyte imbalance is present. If an imbalance is present, indicate what that imbalance is.

(425-426, 430)

1. K^+ 3.2 mEq/L _____

2. Na^+ 148 mEq/L _____

3. Ca^{++} 9.6 mg/dL _____

4. HCO_3^- 24 mEq/L _____

5. K^+ 4.9 mEq/L _____

6. Na^+ 132 mEq/L _____

B. Directions: For each of the following sets of blood gases, tell what type of problem exists: respiratory acidosis, metabolic acidosis, respiratory alkalosis, metabolic alkalosis.

(430)

1.   pH 7.32, pCO_2 47 mmHg, HCO_3^- 23 mEq/L _____

2.   pH 7.48, pCO_2 33 mmHg, HCO_3^- 26 mEq/L _____

3.   pH 7.30, pCO_2 38 mmHg, HCO_3^- 20 mEq/L _____

4.   pH 7.50, pCO_2 45 mmHg, HCO_3^- 28 mEq/L _____

Student Name_____

SHORT ANSWER

Directions: Write a brief answer for each question.

(419)   1. List the four main functions of water within the body:

        a. _____

        b. _____

        c. _____

        d. _____

(420)   2. List the primary location of these electrolytes:

        a. sodium _____

        b. potassium _____

(421)   3. Which two factors help to keep the fluid in the vascular compartment?

(432)   4. Intake and output records are evaluated to determine if there is _____

(432)   5. Another way to assess for alterations in fluid balance is to keep a record of _____

(424)   6. An early sign of decreased vascular volume from fluid volume deficit is _____

(432)   7. When imbalances in calcium or magnesium are suspected, assessment of _____ should be performed.

(432)   8. To assess for Chvostek's sign, you would _____

APPLICATION OF THE NURSING PROCESS

Directions: Write a brief answer for each question.

(426)   1. When assessing for signs of hypokalemia in the patient who is taking a digitalis preparation, you would ask about:

(433)   2. When assessing for fluid volume deficit in the elderly patient, you would assess:

(433)   3. The patient who is known to have a fluid volume deficit from loss of blood may also have the nursing diagnosis of:

(433) 4. Appropriate expected outcomes for the patient with the nursing diagnosis *Fluid volume deficit related to severe diarrhea* would be:

_____

_____

(433) 5. Actions to assist the patient who has severe diarrhea to regain and maintain fluid balance might be:

_____

_____

_____

_____

(432) 6. To evaluate the effectiveness of actions to combat fluid volume deficit, you would check:

_____

_____

_____

_____

NCLEX-PN® EXAM REVIEW

*Directions: Choose the **best** answer(s) for each of the following questions.*

(433) 1. A 76-year-old patient is admitted with vomiting and diarrhea of 3 days' duration. Besides assessing skin condition when looking for signs of dehydration, you would look for
1. dull eyes.
2. brittle nails.
3. dry mucous membranes.
4. dry hair.

(419) 2. Dehydration may occur more quickly for a 76-year-old than for a younger person because
1. there is less subcutaneous fat in the older adult.
2. the thirst mechanism is more active in the older adult.
3. there is a decrease in the urine-concentrating ability of the kidney in the older adult.
4. more antidiuretic hormone is produced in the older adult.

(424) 3. The patient is started on IV therapy. A sign that he is receiving too much or too rapid IV fluid, when compared with previous data, would be
1. full, bounding, pulse.
2. very rapid pulse rate.
3. decreasing urine output.
4. sudden vomiting.

(426) 4. When assessing a patient, you look for signs of electrolyte imbalance. A sign of hypokalemia would be
1. hypertension.
2. muscle weakness.
3. mental confusion.
4. oliguria.

(425) 5. Signs that the patient has developed hypernatremia would be (Select all that apply)
1. abdominal cramps.
2. low urine output.
3. intense thirst.
4. nausea and vomiting.

Student Name_____

(433) 6. The patient's condition improves and he is started on oral nourishment. The following amounts were entered on his I and O sheet: juice 120 mL, cereal 180 mL, tea 150 mL, urine 380 mL, IV fluid 1050 mL, emesis 50 mL. His oral intake was

_____.

(Fill in the blank)

(430) 7. A male, age 46, is admitted with decreased level of consciousness and symptoms of influenza. He is a diabetic. His blood gases are pH 7.32, CO_2 36, HCO_3^- 20. You would determine that his acid-base imbalance is
   1. respiratory acidosis.
   2. metabolic alkalosis.
   3. respiratory alkalosis.
   4. metabolic acidosis.

(430) 8. You would expect this patient's breathing to be
   1. deep and rapid.
   2. shallow and rapid.
   3. shallow and slow.
   4. regular rate and depth.

9. Because of the excess glucose in the patient's system, water is drawn from the cells into the vascular system and then excreted. An appropriate nursing diagnosis for him would be
   1. *Fluid volume overload.*
   2. *Ineffective tissue perfusion.*
   3. *Fluid volume deficit.*
   4. *Ineffective breathing pattern.*

(432) 10. One method of tracking fluid balance status in patients, in addition to recording I & O, is to
   1. determine acid-base status.
   2. encourage intake of oral liquids.
   3. check electrolyte laboratory values.
   4. compare weight from day to day.

(425) 11. A male patient has hyponatremia. Nursing interventions appropriate for him are (Select all that apply)
   1. discourage the intake of milk.
   2. restrict his fluid intake.
   3. give foods high in sodium.
   4. administer the ordered diuretic.

(421-422) 12. Osmosis differs from diffusion in that it refers to
   1. movement of solutes from the cells to the interstitial fluid.
   2. movement of solvent across a membrane.
   3. substances moved across a membrane with the use of energy.
   4. movement of fluid out of the vascular system.

(428) 13. Causes of calcium imbalance are (Select all that apply)
   1. diabetes mellitus.
   2. multiple myeloma
   3. arteriosclerosis.
   4. cancerous bone metastasis.

(426) 14. When teaching patients about calcium intake, you include that the absorption of dietary calcium is enhanced by
   1. vitamin B complex.
   2. vitamin C.
   3. vitamin D.
   4. iron.

(424) 15. A male patient is admitted with elevated blood pressure, rapid weight gain, edema, and restlessness. An appropriate nursing diagnosis for him would probably be
   1. *Fluid volume excess.*
   2. *Fluid volume deficit.*
   3. *Risk for fluid volume deficit.*
   4. *Impaired urinary elimination.*

CRITICAL THINKING ACTIVITIES

1. Prepare a teaching plan for the patient with kidney disease who needs to decrease his intake of potassium. What foods should be avoided?

2. Prepare a teaching plan for the Hispanic American patient who has hypertension. He will need to decrease the sodium in his diet. Outline the plan:

MEETING CLINICAL OBJECTIVES

Directions: The following suggested activities will help you meet the stated clinical practice objectives for the chapter. Review your school's clinical objectives for the week and outline a plan of activities that will help you meet them. If you are unsure how to meet them, consult with your instructor at the beginning of the clinical day.

1. Make a list of the food and drink containers used by the dietary department in your clinical facility and the amounts each holds.

2. Practice calculating intake for each patient assigned regardless of whether the patient is on intake and output recording.

3. Practice calculating the IV intake for each patient assigned who has an IV for the hours you are in clinical.

4. For each assigned patient, figure out what you would need to include in calculating output if it was to be recorded.

5. Assess each assigned patient for signs of hypokalemia, fluid volume deficit, or fluid volume excess.

6. Scan each assigned patient's laboratory values for abnormalities of electrolytes and acid-base balance.

STEPS TOWARD BETTER COMMUNICATION

VOCABULARY BUILDING GLOSSARY

Term	Pronunciation	Definition
buffer	BUF fer	a cushion; used to protect something from outside harm or irritation
compensatory	com PEN sa to ry	balancing a lack of one thing with more of another
considerable	con SID er a ble	large or lengthy
constituents	con STI tu ents	parts of a whole
deplete	de PLETE	use up or empty out
gradient	GRA di ent	a rate or degree of change
ingestion	in GES tion	the process of eating and drinking or taking something into the body orally
lethargic	le THAR gic	sleepy, tired, with little energy
obligatory	o BLIG a tory	necessary, required
pit	PIT	an indentation or small hollow
tented	TENT ed	coming to a point, like a tent
tracking	TRACK ing	keeping a record of; keeping track of
twitch	TWITCH	slight contraction or quiver

Student Name _____

COMPLETION

Directions: Fill in the blank(s) with the correct term(s) from the Vocabulary Building Glossary to complete the sentence.

1. It takes _____ time for the kidneys to adjust pH when the body becomes acidic.

2. The lungs blow off excess carbon dioxide as a(n) _____ mechanism when the body becomes too acidic.

3. Whenever the patient is receiving intravenous fluids, _____ intake and output is important.

4. When the body is in a state of alkalosis, muscles may _____ .

5. The patient experiencing ketoacidosis may become very _____ and may go into a coma.

6. Sodium bicarbonate is a(n) _____ and is given when acidosis needs to be corrected.

7. When the patient is taking a potassium-depleting diuretic, _____ of extra potassium is necessary.

VOCABULARY EXERCISES

Adjectives are often used to describe signs and symptoms.

irritable	scanty	weak	thready
moist	full	bounding	pale
dry	faint	sticky	
slow	elevated	rapid	

Directions: List the adjectives that might be used for signs and symptoms for the following:

1. lung sounds: _____

2. pulse: _____

3. blood pressure: _____

4. mucous membranes: _____

5. urine: _____

6. skin: _____

WORD ATTACK SKILLS

Directions: Opposites are often used when documenting assessment changes. Write the opposites for these words:

	Words		Opposites
1.	shallow	_____	active
2.	rapid	_____	decrease
3.	passive	_____	deep
4.	moist	_____	dry
5.	attraction	_____	excess
6.	gain	_____	repellent
7.	increase	_____	slow
8.	deficit	_____	loss

Prefixes and suffixes are word parts with specific meanings that are attached to words to change their meaning in some way. Recall that prefixes are added to the beginning of the word, suffixes to the end.

Negative prefixes meaning *no* or *not*: im-balance, dis-orientation, un-usual

Medical and scientific terms often use prefixes and suffixes.

Prefix	Meaning	Example	Meaning
hyper-	excessive, above	hypercalcemia	calcium excess/high calcium
hypo-	deficient, below	hypocalcemia	calcium deficiency/low calcium
ab-	away from	absorb	draw away from
ex-, extra-	out, outside	excrete	throw out/eliminate
		extracellular	outside of the cell
re-	again, behind	reabsorb	absorb again
intra-	within	intracellular	within/inside a cell
inter-	between	interstitial	between the parts of a tissue
trans-	across, through	transport	carry across
iso-	equal, same	isotonic	equal tension

Suffix	Meaning	Example	Meaning
-tonic	tension	hypertonic	greater tension/concentration
-emia	blood condition	hypercalcemia	excess calcium in the blood
-osis	abnormal condition	acidosis	abnormal amount of acid

PRONUNCIATION OF DIFFICULT TERMS

Directions: Practice pronouncing the following words.

interstitial = in ter STISH ial

turgor = TUR gor (compare with turgid = TUR gid)

Student Name_____

COMMUNICATION EXERCISE

With a partner, write and practice a dialogue explaining to a patient why you will be measuring intake and output and what the patient will need to do (use the call light, remember what he or she eats and drinks, etc.).

Review the chapter key points, answer the study questions, and complete the critical thinking activities at the end of the chapter in the textbook.

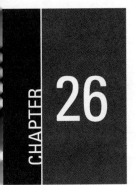

CHAPTER 26

Concepts of Basic Nutrition and Cultural Considerations

Answer Key: Textbook page references are provided as a guide for answering selected questions. A complete answer key was provided for your instructor.

TERMINOLOGY

A. Matching

Directions: Match the terms in Column I with the definitions in Column II.

Column I			Column II
(444)	1.	_____ amino acid	a. Processes of taking in nutrients and absorbing and using them
(449)	2.	_____ cholesterol	b. Process of converting food into substances that can be absorbed and utilized
(446)	3.	_____ carbohydrate	c. Essential substance for the building of cells
(442)	4.	_____ digestion	d. Body's main source of energy
(448)	5.	_____ fat	e. Metabolized form of sugar in the body
(446)	6.	_____ fiber	f. Table sugar
(446)	7.	_____ fructose	g. Sugar found in fruit
(446)	8.	_____ glucose	h. Sugar found in milk
(446)	9.	_____ lactose	i. Carbohydrate that is not broken down by digestion
(452)	10.	_____ mineral	j. Substance that supplies nine calories per gram consumed
(440)	11.	_____ nutrition	k. A component of fat
(457)	12.	_____ obesity	l. Essential nutrients taken in through food or supplements
(443)	13.	_____ protein	m. Inorganic substances contained in animals and plants
(446)	14.	_____ sucrose	n. Excessive accumulation of body fat
(449)	15.	_____ vitamin	o. Building blocks of protein

B. Completion

Directions: Fill in the blank(s) with the correct term(s) from the terms list in the chapter in the textbook to complete the sentence.

(444)   1.   A(n) _____ contains all nine essential amino acids and are of animal source.

(444)   2.   Plant sources of protein are _____ because they do not contain all essential amino acids.

(446)   3.   Proteins from plant sources that are combined in the diet to achieve complete protein intake are called _____.

(444)   4.   Nine amino acids are considered _____ because they must be consumed through food sources.

(444)   5.   The liver can manufacture 11 _____ amino acids.

(445)   6.   A disorder of malnutrition that results from severe starvation is _____.

(445)   7.   A condition of severe protein deficiency that occurs in infants after weaning from breast milk in countries where food is scarce is _____.

(445)   8.   The _____ diet excludes all sources of animal food.

(449)   9.   Most _____ are unsaturated fat, with the exception of coconut oil and palm oil.

(449)   10.   Animal food sources provide the most _____ fats.

(449)   11.   When the fat-soluble vitamins A, D, E, and K are ingested in excessive quantities they can cause _____.

(454)   12.   Foods prepared in the _____ manner are prepared for use according to Jewish law.

REVIEW OF STRUCTURE AND FUNCTION

Directions: Match the structures in Column I with the functions in Column II.

	Column I		Column II
(441) 1.	_____ tongue	a.	Absorbs nutrients
(441) 2.	_____ salivary glands	b.	Assists in changing food to a semiliquid state
(442) 3.	_____ stomach	c.	Absorbs fluid and electrolytes
(442) 4.	_____ small intestine	d.	Secrete saliva containing enzymes
(442) 5.	_____ liver	e.	Secretes bile for the digestion of fats
(442) 6.	_____ gallbladder	f.	Secretes digestive enzymes and insulin
(442) 7.	_____ large intestine	g.	Stores and concentrates bile
(442) 8.	_____ pancreas	h.	Manipulates food, mixing it with saliva

SHORT ANSWER

Directions: Write a brief answer for each question.

(448-449)   1.   Fat's main function in the body is to _____.

Four other functions of fat are:

a.   _____

b.   _____

Student Name _____

        c. _____

        d. _____

(449)   2. The three essential fatty acids important to good nutrition are _____
_____.

(449)   3. The recommended daily allowance of fat is _____% of total calories.

(443)   4. Protein is essential for rebuilding _____ and
_____.

       Other functions of protein are:

       _____

       _____

       _____

(444)   5. Protein intake should be _____% of the total daily calories.

(446)   6. Carbohydrates should make up about _____% of the daily diet. Each gram of carbohydrate supplies _____ calories.

(446)   7. Functions of carbohydrates include:

        a. _____

        b. _____

        c. _____

        d. _____

        e. _____

(452)   8. Minerals are necessary for proper _____ and
_____ function and act as catalysts for many cellular functions.

(452)   9. Other functions of minerals include:

        a. _____

        b. _____

        c. _____

(452) 10. A general rule regarding water requirements is that the patient needs to take in an amount equal to the recorded fluid output plus _____.

(452, 454) 11. Give one example of how each of the following factors might influence nutrition.

        a. Age:_____

        b. Illness:_____

        c. Emotional status: _____

        d. Economic status:_____

        e. Religion: _____

        f. Culture:_____

(455)   12.   By _____ months of age, the birth weight of the infant should _____. By the end of the first year the birth weight should _____.

(457)   13.   It is often difficult to get _____ to eat much.

(457)   14.   School-age children often desire _____ more than other foods and parents must set a good example of proper nutrition.

(457)   15.   Adolescents tend to consume many _____ and may not eat a balanced diet.

(457)   16.   Often, adults only eat the _____ meal at home and this often leads to inadequate nutrition and _____.

(458)   17.   The group most at risk for inadequate nutrition is _____.

(449)   18.   A cup of 2% milk contains _____ grams of fat whereas a cup of 1% milk contains _____ grams of fat.

(449)   19.   A Whopper with cheese hamburger contains _____ grams of fat.

(443)   20.   The American Heart Association Eating Plan for Healthy Americans suggests you choose fats with _____ grams or less of saturated fat per serving.

(461)   21.   A BMI over _____ indicates the person is overweight.

IDENTIFICATION

A.   Directions: Indicate the vitamin responsible for each function.

(450-451)
1. _____ Maintenance of epithelial cells and mucous membranes
2. _____ Promotes bone and teeth mineralization
3. _____ Needed for carbohydrate metabolism
4. _____ Helps regulate energy metabolism
5. _____ Necessary for blood clotting
6. _____ Metabolism of amino acids
7. _____ Formation of red blood cells
8. _____ Helps maintain normal cell membranes
9. _____ Essential for certain enzyme systems
10. _____ Aids in hemoglobin synthesis

B.   Directions: List a primary function in the body of each of the following minerals and one consequence of deficiency.

(453-454)

1.   Calcium _____

Deficiency causes: _____

2.   Chloride _____

Deficiency causes: _____

3. Magnesium _____

   Deficiency causes: _____

4. Phosphorus_____

   Deficiency causes: _____

5. Potassium _____

   Deficiency causes: _____

6. Sodium _____

   Deficiency causes: _____

7. Chromium _____

   Deficiency causes: _____

8. Fluorine _____

   Deficiency causes: _____

9. Iodine _____

   Deficiency causes: _____

10. Iron _____

    Deficiency causes: _____

11. Zinc_____

    Deficiency causes: _____

APPLICATION OF THE NURSING PROCESS

Directions: Write a short answer for each question.

(459) 1. While assessing E.O., you find she weighs 142 lbs. and is 64" tall. What is her BMI?

           _____

(461) 2. E.O. has just been diagnosed with colon cancer and is preparing to undergo surgery and then chemotherapy. What is a probable nursing diagnosis for this patient related to her nutritional needs?

           _____

(461-462) 3. Write two expected outcomes for the above nursing diagnosis.

           a. _____

           b. _____

(462) 4. Indicate two nursing interventions to assist E.O. to meet each of the expected outcomes.

           a. _____

           b. _____

           c. _____

           d. _____

(462) 5. Indicate an evaluation statement for each of the above expected outcomes that would indicate that they are being met.

a. _____

b. _____

(459, 461) 6. What type of data found on assessment might indicate that these outcomes are not being met?

_____

7. If the outcomes are not being met, what would you do?

_____

_____

NCLEX-PN® EXAM REVIEW

*Directions: Choose the **best** answer(s) for each of the following questions.*

(461) 1. Your female patient is 76 years old and has arthritis in her hands. When performing a nutritional assessment for her you would particularly want to know
   1. if her family eats with her often.
   2. if she can easily prepare her own food.
   3. if she eats only one hot meal a day.
   4. whether she has any food dislikes.

(461) 2. A 46-year-old male is 5'8" tall and weighs 158 lbs. He has the intestinal flu and is suffering from severe nausea, vomiting, and diarrhea. Appropriate nursing diagnoses for this patient might be (Select all that apply)
   1. *Nutrition, imbalanced: less than body requirements*
   2. *Nutrition, imbalanced: more than body requirements*
   3. *Fluid volume excess*
   4. *Fluid volume deficit*

(462) 3. A 64-year-old female who is recovering from hip surgery has little appetite. In order to encourage her to eat you would (Select all that apply)
   1. remind her that protein is essential to healing.
   2. create an attractive and pleasant environment.
   3. offer to feed her some extra bites after she is finished.
   4. encourage family to sit with her while she eats.

(462) 4. From the following evaluation statements, which statement would indicate that the expected outcome of "Patient will gain 1 lb. per week" is being met?
   1. Made appropriate food choices from a 2500 calorie menu.
   2. Consumed 60% of food and fluids at dinner.
   3. Gained 0.5 lb. since day before yesterday.
   4. Lost 3 lbs. during chemotherapy treatment.

Student Name _____

(458)   5. Your patient is 30 lbs. overweight. You are discussing a weight loss plan with him. You explain that the only way to realistically lose weight is to cut calories or
1. revise the amount of fat consumed.
2. eat only high-protein foods.
3. revise the amount of carbohydrates eaten.
4. increase the daily activity level.

(442)   6. You use the Food Guide Pyramid to help the patient construct an appropriate balanced diet. You explain that the greatest number of servings of food per day should come from the
1. grain group.
2. meat group.
3. fruit group.
4. vegetable group.

(443)   7. Because the patient also has a high cholesterol level, you recommend that he reduce red meat to one to two times a week and obtain adequate protein in the diet by eating
1. fish or poultry several times a week.
2. two eggs each morning for breakfast.
3. protein fortified cereal for two meals a day.
4. pasta with tomato sauce several times a week.

(458)   8. You explain to the patient that the most effective way to lose weight—other than cutting calories—and keep it off is to
1. eat more fruits and vegetables.
2. drink 6–8 glasses of water a day.
3. exercise for at least 30 minutes five times a week.
4. totally abstain from alcoholic beverages.

(443)   9. The patient eats a lot of Mexican dishes. In trying to cut down on his fat intake, he should
1. refrain from eating any Mexican dishes.
2. eat soft tacos rather than fried tacos.
3. ask for meat enchiladas rather than cheese enchiladas.
4. use extra hot peppers on food to "cut the fat."

(461)   10. Your patient is an 82-year-old widow who lives alone and lives on a very limited income. Her arthritis makes it difficult for her to shop and prepare her meals. In order to improve her nutritional intake, you might suggest she try
1. taking her noon meal at the corner senior daycare center.
2. asking a neighbor to shop for fresh foods for her twice a week.
3. buy a microwave oven and cookware and learn to use it.
4. buy a freezer so her daughter can prepare meals for her on the weekends for the rest of the week.

(447)   11. The patient checks a frozen dinner her daughter put in her freezer. She sees it contains 9 grams of fat and 396 calories. She understands that this means that
1. 36 calories come from fat.
2. 27 calories come from fat.
3. 9% of the meal is fat.
4. 81 calories come from fat.

(445)   12. A lacto-vegetarian will eat
1. any food except for eggs.
2. plant foods only.
3. plant and dairy foods.
4. poultry and plant foods.

(449) 13. Vitamin supplements should be taken only as recommended because if taken in large quantities fat-soluble vitamins can cause
1. gastric irritation.
2. diarrhea.
3. weight gain.
4. toxicity.

(444) 14. A mainstay of the Asian diet that is a good source of protein is
1. mushrooms.
2. rice.
3. soybeans.
4. bamboo shoots.

(455) 15. If a baby weighed 8 lbs. at birth, at one year of age he should weigh
1. 24 lbs.
2. 32 lbs.
3. 16 lbs.
4. 20 lbs.

(457) 16. When solid foods are introduced into the baby's diet, they should (Select all that apply)
1. begin with puréed meat dishes.
2. start with cooked fruits.
3. be sweetened with honey.
4. be introduced gradually, one food at a time.

(457) 17. A guideline that is helpful in getting a toddler to eat more is to (Select all that apply)
1. eat with him or her.
2. keep foods from touching each other on the plate.
3. serve only one food at a time.
4. feed "finger foods."

(457) 18. A good snack for a school-age child is
1. peanut butter on apple slices.
2. buttered popcorn.
3. cookies and milk.
4. chocolate-covered ice cream bar.

(458) 19. When considering the nutritional needs of the elderly adult, you know that
1. nutrient requirements do not change with age.
2. more calories are needed for tissue repair.
3. the taste for sweets decreases with age.
4. preferences for foods often change.

(454) 20. Minerals are essential for various functions in the body. Iodine is necessary in the diet for the function of the _____ _____. (Fill in the blank)

CRITICAL THINKING ACTIVITIES

1. Your friend wants to go on a high-protein diet, cutting out carbohydrates in the form of grain products and sweets. If a multivitamin tablet is not taken daily, what possible disorders might this friend develop from vitamin B-group deficiencies?

2. J.L., a 16-year-old neighbor, leads a very active teen life. She rarely eats meals at home. She is concerned about weight gain. How could you counsel her about managing her diet while eating at fast-food restaurants?

3. A.R., age 2, will not eat much of anything but Cheerios and milk. What teaching could you do for her mother to assist her to improve A.R.'s diet?

4. Analyze your own diet. Is the calorie intake appropriate to maintain a normal weight? Is the diet well-balanced? What changes should be made?

MEETING CLINICAL OBJECTIVES

Directions: The following suggested activities will help you meet the stated clinical practice objectives for the chapter. Review your school's clinical objectives for the week and outline a plan of activities that will help you meet them. If you are unsure how to meet them, consult with your instructor at the beginning of the clinical day.

1. Find and look through the diet manual for the clinical facility to which you are assigned.
2. Perform a nutritional assessment on a patient from a different culture. Work with the patient to plan an appropriate balanced diet that contains sufficient protein, but is low fat.
3. Teach a patient about foods needed to increase potassium intake when the patient is on furosemide (Lasix), a potent diuretic.

STEPS TOWARD BETTER COMMUNICATION

VOCABULARY BUILDING GLOSSARY

Term	Pronunciation	Definition
child rearing	CHILD REARing	caring for and educating children
comprise	com PRISE	include, form
compromised	COM pro MISEd	endangered
consume	con SUME	eat
finicky	FIN ick y	very particular, with definite likes and dislikes
Meals on Wheels	MEALS on WHEELS	a program where a meal is prepared and delivered to an elderly person's home by volunteers
peer	PEER	a person of similar age, ability, social status
sparingly	SPAR ing ly	in small amounts

VOCABULARY EXERCISES

Directions: Underline the Vocabulary Building Glossary words used in the sentences below.

1. Child rearing comprises feeding, clothing, nourishing, training, loving, and educating a child.
2. Finicky eaters consume some foods sparingly.
3. The lack of green vegetables in his diet compromised his health.
4. Many volunteers for the Meals on Wheels program are retired and enjoy helping their peers.

COMMUNICATION EXERCISE

Often in English speech, especially informal conversation, words are left out and certain sounds are omitted between words, within a word, or even changed, depending on the sounds that follow. English learners need to understand these omissions when they hear them. They may even choose to use some of them in order to sound more like a native speaker.

Directions: In the following conversation, see where the omissions occur. Draw a line under them and write the words as they would be spoken and written in formal speech.

Nurse: "Morning, Ms. A. How're you today?"

Ms. A.: "I'm OK, but I wish they'd gimme a better breakfast!"

Nurse:	"Whaddaya mean? What'd you have?"
Ms. A.:	"Just some lukewarm watery tea, an' cold oatmeal 'n' milk—with no salt. An' the toast was dry 'n' cold."
Nurse:	"Doesn't sound very appetizing. I'll speak to dietary. Didya call the nurse 'n' ask fer hot tea?"
Ms. A.:	"Naw. 't wasn' worth it. I'm goin' home today anyway."
Nurse:	"That's good news. But ya' know you're on a low-sodium diet. That means your not 'sposed to have salt added to your food."
Ms. A.:	"Not even a little in cooking?"
Nurse:	"Not if ya want to follow doctor's orders and keep your blood pressure down. We don't want to see you back in here again."
Ms. A.:	"No offense, but I don' wanna BE back here again. I'll jus' hafta try ta get usta it, I guess."
Nurse:	"That's the spirit. Now let me take your vital signs."

Words that should be used:

1. _____
2. _____
3. _____
4. _____
5. _____
6. _____
7. _____
8. _____
9. _____
10. _____
11. _____
12. _____

CULTURAL POINTS

1. When planning a diet for any patient, it is good to find out what they like to eat and suggest a diet that includes as many of their preferred foods as is healthy and look at ways to modify those foods so they can be kept in the diet. However, if a person really loves salty French fries, they might prefer mashed potatoes to baked fries with no salt.

2. With patients from other cultures, you may want to ask about their usual diet and see if there are ways it can be modified to meet their current dietary needs. Another consideration is that the ethnic group may have special types of foods it believes will aid in healing, such as hot and cold (temperature or character). Vietnamese women may fear losing heat during labor and delivery and prefer a special diet of salty, hot foods. North Americans usually look at soups, especially chicken soup, hot drinks like tea, and puddings as comforting and healing foods when they are sick.

Review the chapter key points, answer the study questions, and complete the critical thinking activities at the end of the chapter in the textbook.

CHAPTER 27

Diet Therapy and Assisted Feeding

Answer Key: Textbook page references are provided as a guide for answering selected questions. A complete answer key was provided for your instructor.

TERMINOLOGY

A. Completion

Directions: Fill in the blank(s) with the correct term(s) from the terms list in the chapter in the textbook to complete the sentence.

(472)   1.   Eating a high-fat diet increases the risk of _____ and narrowing of the arteries.

(472)   2.   It is recommended that people who have _____ decrease their sodium intake to decrease edema.

(472)   3.   Excessive blood glucose is a problem in people who have

_____.

(469)   4.   More young women than young men develop _____, a disorder in which as few calories as possible are eaten in an effort to remain very thin.

(470)   5.   The diagnosis of _____ requires that a person have an excessive accumulation of fat tissue as determined by the body mass index (BMI) rating.

(470)   6.   The disorder in which a person induces vomiting to control weight gain is called

_____.

(472)   7.   Diet and exercise are recommended to control the high blood pressure that occurs with the disorder _____.

8.   To be diagnosed with _____, a patient must have a blood pressure above 140/90 on at least three occasions.

(476)   9.   A(n) _____ tube is inserted percutaneously with the aid of an endoscope inserted into the stomach.

(486)   10.   Most feeding solutions have _____ when compared to water or saline because of the concentration of solutes.

(476)   11.   A(n) _____ tube is used for either evacuation of stomach contents or the instillation of feedings.

IDENTIFICATION

Directions: Identify foods that are allowed on a clear-liquid and full-liquid diet. Mark the foods allowed on a clear liquid diet with a "C." Mark the foods only allowed on a full-liquid diet with an "F" and foods that are allowed on both diets with a "B." Mark foods not included in either diet with an "N" for not allowed.

(469)

1. _____ orange juice
2. _____ tea
3. _____ vegetable beef soup
4. _____ egg nog
5. _____ Cream of Wheat cereal
6. _____ mashed potatoes

7. _____ Jell-O
8. _____ popsicles
9. _____ custard
10. _____ margarine
11. _____ milk
12. _____ ice cream

SHORT ANSWER

Directions: Write a brief answer for each question.

(466)   1. The nurse's role in promoting the goals of diet therapy is to:

a. _____

b. _____

c. _____

(469)   2. Postoperative patients progress from being NPO to _____
_____.

(469-470)   3. For the disorders of anorexia nervosa and bulimia, both
_____ and _____
counseling are necessary.

(471)   4. Appropriate weight gain during pregnancy is _____ lbs. during the first trimester
and _____ per week during the second and third trimesters.

(471)   5. Alcoholism often causes a _____ deficiency.

(470)   6. Obesity is thought to contribute to the risk of:

_____

_____

(472)   7. Diet therapy for cardiovascular disease focuses on the reduction of
_____ and _____.

(472)   8. In order to help patients with cardiovascular disease plan an appropriate diet, you teach
them that one teaspoon of salt contains _____ of sodium.

(472)   9. The difference between type 1 diabetes and type 2 diabetes is that in type 2 diabetes, insulin
is _____.

247

Student Name_____

(472-473) 10. Patients with diabetes are at higher risk for:

    a. _____

    b. _____

    c. _____

    d. _____

    e. _____

(472) 11. The goal of diabetes treatment is to keep the blood glucose between _____ mg/dL.

(475) 12. Dietary considerations for the HIV/AIDS patient include:

    a. _____

    b. _____

    c. _____

    d. _____

    e. _____

    f. _____

(477) 13. Feeding tubes are often used to increase nutrition in patients at risk of malnutrition from the effects of:

    a. _____

    b. _____

    c. _____

    d. _____

(477) 14. When a patient has a nasogastric or small-bore feeding tube in place it is essential to check tube placement when _____ .

(480) 15. Advantages of the PEG tube over the nasogastric or small-bore feeding tube are:

_____

_____

(480-481) 16. To check the placement of the PEG tube—which must be done before each feeding or the administration of medication—you would:

_____

_____

(482) 17. The normal amount of formula given at one feeding is _____ ounces.

(482) 18. Tube feeding solutions should be administered slowly to prevent _____ and _____ .

19. What might happen if feeding tube placement is not checked before administering a feeding?

_____

_____

_____

(486)   20.   Four principles to follow when administering a tube feeding are:

a. _____

b. _____

c. _____

d. _____

APPLICATION OF THE NURSING PROCESS

Directions: Write a short answer for each question.

(487)   1.   J.K. is suffering from malnutrition due to inflammatory bowel disease. She is started on TPN. Four assessments you must make regarding her nutritional status and safety with this treatment are:

a. _____

b. _____

c. _____

d. _____

(475)   2.   T.P. has AIDS. He has sores in his mouth that make eating painful. He has frequent diarrhea and is rapidly losing weight. He is depressed about his diagnosis and has little appetite. He is started on tube feedings. In planning care for him you determine that appropriate nursing diagnoses related to nutrition problems are:

_____

_____

_____

_____

(475)   3.   Appropriate expected outcomes for these nursing diagnoses might be:

_____

_____

_____

_____

(486)   4.   Four actions to be implemented to decrease the risk of injury to the patient receiving a tube feeding are:

a. _____

b. _____

c. _____

d. _____

Student Name _____

(483)   5. Indicate the correct order for actions in administering a feeding via feeding tube.
- a. _____ Unclamp the tube.
- b. _____ Flush the tube with water.
- c. _____ Check the placement of the tube.
- d. _____ Elevate the patient's head and upper body.
- e. _____ Prepare the feeding bag.
- f. _____ Check for residual feeding in the stomach.
- g. _____ Start the feeding.
- h. _____ Reclamp tube.

6. Three evaluation statements that would indicate that tube feeding is a successful intervention for the nursing diagnosis of *Nutrition, imbalanced: less than body requirements* for the above patient would be:

a. _____

b. _____

c. _____

NCLEX-PN® EXAM REVIEW

*Directions: Choose the **best** answer(s) to each of the following questions.*

1. A patient, like several of her co-workers, is gaining weight. As a way to reduce calories, besides reducing fat in the diet, she (like most Americans) should reduce the intake of _____ _____. (Fill in the blank.)

2. A patient condition that greatly increases caloric need and causes a need for nutritional creativity is
   1. healing joint replacement.
   2. severe burns.
   3. infection with fever.
   4. inflammatory bowel disease.

(484)   3. Your patient is receiving tube feedings. If he has a stomach residual of 85 mL at the time the next tube feeding is due, you should
   1. hold the feeding and notify the physician.
   2. go ahead and give the next feeding.
   3. check the patient for constipation.
   4. mix the next feeding at 2x strength ordered.

(484)   4. After giving the patient's intermittent tube feeding, you would
   1. immediately clamp the tube.
   2. leave the tube open for 10 minutes.
   3. flush the tube with a small amount of water.
   4. instill 30 mL of air to clear the tube.

(484-485)   5. Your patient has a percutaneous endoscopic gastrostomy (PEG) feeding tube in place. Care for him related to this tube would include (Select all that apply)
   1. cleansing the abdomen around the insertion site each shift.
   2. auscultating for bowel sounds each shift.
   3. checking tube placement every shift and prior to feeding.
   4. cleansing the nare with a moist cotton-tipped swab every shift.

(484)   6. The rationale for leaving the patient in an elevated position after each feeding is
1. to prevent nausea.
2. to prevent reflux.
3. to decrease the chance of diarrhea.
4. for gravity flow into the intestine.

(472)   7. Your patient, age 18, has type I diabetes. She is trying to adjust her diet and exercise to maintain her blood glucose within normal limits. Her blood glucose is 142 mg/dL at 4 P.M. This reading is
1. within normal limits.
2. high.
3. low.
4. not important.

(472)   8. The purpose of trying to maintain the patient's blood glucose within normal limits is to
1. prevent complications of diabetes.
2. help her to feel better.
3. assist with the maintenance of a normal diet.
4. prevent further weight loss.

9. The patient is placed on a 2000 calorie diabetic diet. If she eats 64 grams of carbohydrates, 4 grams of fat, and 8 grams of protein for breakfast, she has already consumed how many calories of the day's allotment?
1. 624
2. 324
3. 364
4. 304

(469)   10. The patient becomes nauseated and starts vomiting. You recommend that she stick to a clear-liquid diet and take plenty of fluids. Foods that she could have on this diet are (Select all that apply)
1. milkshakes.
2. chicken noodle soup.
3. apple juice.
4. beef broth.

CRITICAL THINKING ACTIVITIES

1. Make out a diet plan for a patient with hypertension that is balanced and contains no more than 2000 calories a day. Include snacks.

2. Outline ways to assist a home care cancer patient to increase calorie and protein intake.

3. Plan ways to assist an African American patient with hypertension and atherosclerosis to adapt his diet to low-fat based on cultural eating patterns and food preferences.

MEETING CLINICAL OBJECTIVES

Directions: The following suggested activities will help you meet the stated clinical practice objectives for the chapter. Review your school's clinical objectives for the week and outline a plan of activities that will help you meet them. If you are unsure how to meet them, consult with your instructor at the beginning of the clinical day.

1. Seek assignment to a patient who is receiving tube feedings; outline the assessment and care needed for this patient.

2. Seek assignment to a patient who is receiving TPN. List the signs and symptoms of complications that you must watch for in this patient.

Student Name_____

3. Develop a diet teaching plan for a new diabetic patient.

4. Review laboratory results on each assigned patient checking nutritional parameters.

STEPS TOWARD BETTER COMMUNICATION

VOCABULARY BUILDING GLOSSARY

Term	Pronunciation	Definition
binge	BINGE	extreme activity, to excess
bland	BLAND	mild, having little taste or seasoning
collaboration	co LAB o RA tion	working together
differentiate	dif fer EN ti ate	explain how several things are different from each other
discrepancies	dis CREP an cies	disagreements in facts or figures (in a chart or record)
exacerbation	ex A cer BA tion	increase; worsening
instilled	in STILLed	put into
malabsorption	mal ab sorp tion	not properly absorbing food from the intestines
nares	NAR es	nostrils, the two openings in the nose
prevalent	PREV a lent	commonly found
prior to	PRI or to	before
purging	PURG ing (purj ing)	causing bowel evacuation
rationale	ra tion Ale	the reason why something is done
resection	RE sec tion	cutting out a piece of an organ (such as the bowel)
trimester	TRI mes ter	three months

COMPLETION

Directions: Fill in the blank(s) with the correct term(s) from the Vocabulary Building Glossary to complete the sentence.

1. There were some _____ when what the patient said he usually ate and what the family indicated he ate that would explain his weight gain.

2. A low-sodium diet is very _____ but can be improved with the use of other herbs when cooking.

3. Colon cancer often requires _____ of the bowel.

4. The person with bulimia often tends to be a(n) _____ eater.

5. The nurse often works in _____ with the dietitian when trying to change a person's dietary habits.

6. The first _____ of pregnancy is a time of very rapid fetal growth.

7. Eating hot, spicy food or caffeine often causes a(n) _____ of gastritis.

8. After giving a tube feeding, water must be _____ into the tube to clear the formula so that clumping and clogging does not take place.

PRONUNCIATION EXERCISE

Directions: The sound "L" is difficult for some people to pronounce. Compare how the sounds "N," "L," and "R" are made.

First make the sound "N" by placing the tongue against the roof of the mouth, touching the teeth all around with the sides of the tongue. Use your voice, and the sound "N" will come through your nose.

Practice: nice   no   never   nutrition   nurse   anorexia   nares

To make the sound "L," keep the tip of the tongue against the roof of the mouth, but narrow and lower the tongue so the sides of the tongue are not touching the teeth. Use your voice to say "L." The sound and the air goes over the sides of your tongue and out of your mouth.

Practice: glucose   cell   "tolerate oral fluid"

Practice alternating the sounds: no/low   night/light   knife/life   knock/lock   need/lead

ten/tell   nab/lab   nook/look   snow/slow   connect/collect   never/lever

To make the sound "R," drop the tip of the tongue so it does not touch the roof of the mouth. The sides of your tongue should touch your back teeth. The air flows out over the tip of the tongue through the middle of the mouth.

Practice: radiation   rationale   prior   rapid   residual

To Review:

"N"—The tongue touches the roof of the mouth and the teeth on all sides. Sound goes out the nose.

"L"—The tip of the tongue touches the roof of the mouth and the air flows out the sides

"R"—The tip of the tongue does not touch the roof of the mouth and the air flows out the middle.

Practice: lay/ray   long/wrong   gleam/green   glass/grass   laser/razor   illustrate/irrigate

flee/free   tell/tear

Now practice the words with "L," "R," and "N" in the Vocabulary Building Glossary and the terms list.

PRONUNCIATION OF DIFFICULT TERMS

Directions: Practice pronouncing the following words with a peer.

anorexia nervosa	an o REX i a ner VO sa
atherosclerosis	ATH er o scler O sis
diabetes mellitus	DI a be tis mel LI tis
esophageal	e soph a GE al (ee sof ah jee al)
hyperosmolality	HY per os mo lal i ty
lipoprotein	li po PRO tein
percutaneous	per cu TAN e ous

Student Name _____

endoscopic	EN do SCOP ic
gastrostomy	gas TROS to my
triglycerides	tri GLI cer ides (tri gliss er ides)

COMMUNICATION EXERCISES

1. Here is an example of a therapeutic communication with a patient who needs to alter his diet.

   Mr. H. has hypertension. Although he has been started on medication, his blood pressure has not come down as much as desired. It is necessary to find out if he is following diet and exercise guidelines that were given to him a few weeks ago.

   Nurse: "Mr. H., your blood pressure is not coming down as much as we would like. You are still in the hypertensive range. Have you looked at the diet and exercise guidelines we gave you?"

   Mr. H.: "Yes, I read them over. I'm taking a walk as often as I can. I'm not adding any salt at the table anymore either."

   Nurse: "Let's look more closely at the foods you are eating and the way they are prepared. What did you have for breakfast today?"

   Mr. H.: "I had bacon and eggs with an English muffin and orange juice for breakfast. Oh, and coffee, of course."

   Nurse: "How often do you eat that type of breakfast?"

   Mr. H.: "About three or four times a week, I guess."

   Nurse: "Bacon in particular has a lot of sodium in it. Would it be possible to leave off the bacon all but one or two of those days?"

   Mr. H.: "I guess I could try that."

   Nurse: "Now, tell me about yesterday's lunch and dinner."

   Mr. H.: "For lunch we went to the deli and I had a pastrami sandwich and a dill pickle, cole slaw, and iced tea. For dinner, we had ham and sweet potatoes, peas, cottage cheese and fruit salad, and iced tea. For dessert there was ice cream."

   Nurse: "OK, let's see, the pastrami and dill pickle are loaded with sodium. A green salad with oil and vinegar dressing is usually lower in sodium than cole slaw because of the type of dressing that is on that. Ham is preserved and is very high in sodium. Peas and cottage cheese also have some sodium in them as do all milk products like ice cream. From the reading of the guidelines you did do you recall other things that might be substituted for these foods?"

   Mr. H.: "I think that fresh fish seemed lower in sodium than ham or pastrami. An apple might have less sodium than a dill pickle. A sorbet bar might have less sodium than ice cream and still satisfy my sweet tooth. I don't recall much else."

   Nurse: "Why don't you and your wife go over the guidelines again and we will talk about it when you come in to have your blood pressure checked again next week?"

   Mr. H.: "I guess we could do that. I'll try to think more about what I am eating."

2. Practice this conversation using "L" with a partner.

   Nurse: "Hello, Mr. M. How are you feeling?"

   Mr. M.: "Less good than last night. My left leg is a little sore."

   Nurse: "Let's look at it."

Mr. M.:	"I can't lift it even a little."
Nurse:	"Dr. Lincoln should look at it. I'll leave a call for her to drop by on her rounds."
Mr. M.:	"Can I have my lunch now? I'm awfully hungry."
Nurse:	"It's a little early. It's only eleven o'clock. Would you like me to order you some lemonade and a light snack?"
Mr. M.:	"Only a little lemon and a lot of sugar. That's the way I like it."
Nurse:	"I'll leave your request with the kitchen help. See you later."

Review the chapter key points, answer the study questions, and complete the critical thinking activities at the end of the chapter in the textbook.

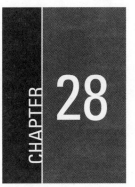

CHAPTER 28

Assisting with Respiration and Oxygen Delivery

Answer Key: Textbook page references are provided as a guide for answering selected questions. A complete answer key was provided for your instructor.

TERMINOLOGY

A. Matching

Directions: Match the terms in Column I with the definitions in Column II.

<table>
<tr><td colspan="3">**Column I**</td><td>**Column II**</td></tr>
<tr><td>(491)</td><td>1.</td><td>_____ anoxia</td><td>a. Adhesive, sticky</td></tr>
<tr><td>(512)</td><td>2.</td><td>_____ apnea</td><td>b. Machine that measures oxygen saturation of the blood</td></tr>
<tr><td>(505)</td><td>3.</td><td>_____ cannula</td><td></td></tr>
<tr><td>(491)</td><td>4.</td><td>_____ dyspnea</td><td>c. Device supplying moisture to air or oxygen</td></tr>
<tr><td>(494)</td><td>5.</td><td>_____ cyanosis</td><td>d. Above-normal level of carbon dioxide in the blood</td></tr>
<tr><td>(504)</td><td>6.</td><td>_____ expectorate</td><td></td></tr>
<tr><td>(506)</td><td>7.</td><td>_____ humidifier</td><td>e. Tube for insertion into a cavity or vessel</td></tr>
<tr><td>(491)</td><td>8.</td><td>_____ hypercapnia</td><td>f. Device that dispenses liquid in a fine spray</td></tr>
<tr><td>(491)</td><td>9.</td><td>_____ hypoxia</td><td>g. Difficulty breathing</td></tr>
<tr><td>(504)</td><td>10.</td><td>_____ nebulizer</td><td>h. Absence of breathing</td></tr>
<tr><td>(495)</td><td>11.</td><td>_____ oximeter</td><td>i. Bluish color around lips and of mucous membranes from lack of oxygen</td></tr>
<tr><td>(494)</td><td>12.</td><td>_____ retraction</td><td></td></tr>
<tr><td>(494)</td><td>13.</td><td>_____ stridor</td><td>j. Cough up and spit out secretions</td></tr>
<tr><td>(494)</td><td>14.</td><td>_____ tachypnea</td><td>k. Low level of oxygen in the blood</td></tr>
<tr><td>(508)</td><td>15.</td><td>_____ tenacious</td><td>l. Muscles move inward upon inspiration</td></tr>
<tr><td></td><td></td><td></td><td>m. Condition of being without oxygen</td></tr>
<tr><td></td><td></td><td></td><td>n. Shrill, harsh sound made when breathing is obstructed</td></tr>
<tr><td></td><td></td><td></td><td>o. Rapid breathing</td></tr>
</table>

B. Completion

Directions: Fill in the blank(s) with the correct term(s) from the terms in the chapter in the textbook to complete the sentence.

(512)   1.   In the emergency or short-term situation, a(n) _____ tube is often used to maintain a patent airway.

(512)   2.   For longer-term assisted ventilation, a(n) _____ is performed.

(517) 3. A(n) _____ is needed to insert a tracheostomy tube.

(492) 4. The process of_____ uses the respiratory muscles and diaphragm to draw air into the lungs.

(492) 5. The passive relaxation of the respiratory muscles causes _____ and air flows out of the lungs.

(491) 6. When there is a lower level of oxygen in the blood than normal, the patient has

_____.

7. The exchange of air between the lungs and the atmosphere is called

_____.

8. _____ is the exchange of oxygen and carbon dioxide between the atmosphere and the body cells.

REVIEW OF STRUCTURE AND FUNCTION OF THE RESPIRATORY SYSTEM

Directions: Identify the correct structure to match the function performed by the respiratory system.

chemoreceptors   central nervous system (CNS)
mucous membranes   alveolar membrane
bronchi   upper airway passages
alveolar macrophages   blood

(493) 1. _____ controls respiration.

(493) 2. _____ channel air to and from the lungs.

(493) 3. _____ phagocytize inhaled bacteria and foreign particles.

(493) 4. _____ sense changes in oxygen or carbon dioxide and signal the brain stem.

(493) 5. _____ secrete mucus to assist cilia to cleanse respiratory tract of foreign particles.

(493) 6. _____ allows diffusion of oxygen and carbon dioxide from alveoli into the bloodstream.

(493) 7. _____ transports oxygen to the cells and carbon dioxide to the lungs.

(492) 8. _____ warm and humidify air on its way to the lungs.

SHORT ANSWER

Directions: Write a brief answer for each question.

(493) 1. Three causes of hypoxemia are:

a. _____

b. _____

c. _____

Student Name_____

(508)   2. List one advantage of each of these oxygen delivery methods.

    a. Nasal cannula _____

    b. Simple mask _____

    c. Partial rebreathing mask_____

    d. Non-rebreathing mask _____

    e. Venturi mask _____

    f. Tracheostomy collar _____

    g. T-bar_____

(505-506) 3. List four safety precautions to be observed when patients are receiving oxygen therapy.

    a. _____

    b. _____

    c. _____

    d. _____

(494)   4. Five symptoms that indicate the patient should be assessed for possible hypoxia are:

    a. _____

    b. _____

    c. _____

    d. _____

    e. _____

(495-496) 5. Nursing responsibilities for the patient undergoing pulse oximetry are:

(509)   6. List four reasons an artificial airway may be used.

    a. _____

    b. _____

    c. _____

    d. _____

SEQUENCING

Directions: Place the following actions in correct sequential order (1, 2, 3, etc.) for the following situation: You are waiting in line at the grocery store when the person in front of you collapses.

(502)

_____ Check the carotid pulse (which is absent).

_____ Call for help.

_____ Shake and shout name or "Are you OK?" (No response.)

_____ Give two breaths.

_____ Position hands for chest compressions.

_____ Give two quick, short breaths.

_____ Give 15 chest compressions.

_____ Tilt head and open airway.

_____ Form seal around nose and mouth with your mouth.

_____ Check for presence of respiration (none).

_____ Continue CPR sequence.

APPLICATION OF THE NURSING PROCESS

Directions: Write a brief answer for each question.

(514) 1. G.C. is 1 day post-op from gallbladder surgery. She says she "doesn't feel right" and seems a bit short of breath after being up for her bath. What would you do to assess her respiratory status?

_____

_____

_____

_____

_____

(513-514) 2. You find that G.C. has diminished breath sounds in the right lower lobe, a respiratory rate of 24, pulse of 92, and some shortness of breath upon exertion. What would be the appropriate nursing diagnosis for her, relevant to her respiratory status?

_____

(514) 3. Write an expected outcome for the chosen nursing diagnosis.

_____

(514) 4. What nursing actions would assist G.C. in meeting the expected outcome?

_____

_____

_____

_____

Student Name _____

(523-524) 5. How would you determine if the nursing interventions are effective in helping G.C. meet the expected outcome?

_____

_____

_____

_____

NCLEX-PN® EXAM REVIEW

*Directions: Choose the **best** answer(s) for each of the following questions.*

(506) 1. Your patient, age 72, has developed hypostatic pneumonia while recovering from extensive trauma from a motor vehicle accident. He is started on oxygen via nasal cannula. He has no preexisting respiratory disease. You know that a normal rate of oxygen flow for him would be _____ L/min. (Fill in the blank)

(503) 2. Your patient is beginning to show signs of restlessness and irritability. A nursing action that might help is to have him
1. turn, cough, and deep-breathe.
2. take a good nap.
3. submit to a back rub.
4. take some pain medication.

(505-506) 3. Important nursing actions for the patient while undergoing oxygen therapy are to (Select all that apply)
1. safety check electrical equipment.
2. cleanse nares frequently.
3. increase calorie intake.
4. place the head of the bed at 30 degrees.

(503) 4. The physician has ordered postural drainage your patient. The best time to perform this procedure is
1. mid-morning.
2. after breakfast.
3. mid-afternoon.
4. before meals.

(503) 5. Other nursing actions to assist patients with pneumonia to obtain better oxygenation are to (Select all that apply)
1. have them up in a chair as much as possible.
2. ambulate them three times per day.
3. insist they stay as quiet as possible.
4. encourage deep-breathing and coughing.

(506) 6. A factor in keeping the patient's secretions thinned so they can be coughed up—other than using a humidifier—is to
1. use chest percussion treatments.
2. encourage a sitting position while awake.
3. increase his fluid intake.
4. suction him once every 2 hours.

(509) 7. A patient, age 64, has an endotracheal tube in place. She suffered a head injury 6 days ago in a fall and is comatose. The endotracheal tube should be replaced by a tracheostomy tube, if an airway is still needed, after _____.
(Fill in the blank)

(509) 8. F.P. remains comatose and in need of ventilation. A tracheostomy tube is inserted. When suctioning the tracheostomy, the suction pressure should be set between _____ mm Hg. (Fill in the blank)

(518-520) 9. For proper technique in suctioning the patient's tracheostomy, you would
1. rotate and use intermittent suction while introducing the catheter into the bronchus.
2. suction for 20 seconds at a time.
3. rotate the catheter and use suction while pulling the catheter out of the bronchus.
4. suction for 5 seconds at a time.

(512) 10. The patient is receiving positive-pressure ventilation. This means that her cuffed tube must be
1. inflated for ventilation to be most effective.
2. deflated for suctioning procedure.
3. replaced every 3 days.
4. repositioned each shift to prevent ulceration.

CRITICAL THINKING ACTIVITIES

1. How could you help the patient who has sustained fractured ribs and is having difficulty deep-breathing and coughing perform these needed exercises?

2. What would you say to the patient who has a chest tube about what to expect when the tube is taken out?

3. Outline a teaching plan to explain to a patient about the purpose of pulse oximetry and how it works.

MEETING CLINICAL OBJECTIVES

Directions: The following suggested activities will help you meet the stated clinical practice objectives for the chapter. Review your school's clinical objectives for the week and outline a plan of activities that will help you meet them. If you are unsure how to meet them, consult with your instructor at the beginning of the clinical day.

1. Find a preoperative patient to whom you can teach the techniques for proper deep-breathing and coughing.

2. Assist a patient to correctly use an incentive spirometer.

3. Help a patient assume positions for postural drainage of the lungs. If a patient is not available, practice the positioning with a family member.

4. Ask to be assigned to a patient who is receiving oxygen. Practice adjusting the flow rate and correctly applying the delivery device.

5. Go with another nurse to perform tracheostomy care, then ask to be assigned to a tracheostomy patient so that you can perform the needed care.

6. Practice tracheostomy suctioning in the skill lab if possible with a peer observing your technique.

7. Review chest tube care and then ask to be assigned to a patient with a chest tube.

Student Name_____

| **STEPS TOWARD BETTER COMMUNICATION** |

VOCABULARY BUILDING GLOSSARY

Term	Pronunciation	Definition
ambient	AM bi ent	surrounding; "ambient light" means the light that is around, available
brink	BRINK	edge, almost occurring
combustion	com BUS tion	the process of burning; "supports combustion" means it enables the process of burning
copious	COP i ous	a very large amount, abundant
intertwined	in ter TWINed	twisted together, connected

COMPLETION

Directions: Fill in the blank(s) with the correct word(s) from the Vocabulary Building Glossary to complete the sentence.

1. The patient was coughing and producing _____ sputum.

2. The patient's respiratory illness was worsening and he was on the _____ of respiratory failure.

3. Oxygen administration was discontinued and the patient was observed for a while on _____ oxygen in the room air.

4. It is dangerous to cause a spark in a room where oxygen is being used because oxygen will support _____.

WORD ATTACK SKILLS

Directions: Note the use of these prefixes and suffix.

-pnea = breathing
a- = not
dys- = difficult, poor
tachy- = rapid
brady- = slow

Even though the following words have the same root, the prefixes change the accent and therefore the pronunciation:

AP ne a
bra dy NE a (the p is silent)
dysp NE a
ta chyp NE a

(Note: hypercapnia is spelled with an i; it has a different meaning than pnea. -capnia refers to carbon dioxide.)

PRONUNCIATION OF DIFFICULT TERMS

Directions: Practice pronouncing the following words.

alveolar macrophages	AL ve O lar MAC ro PHAG es
atelectasis	AT e LEC ta sis
chemoreceptors	CHE mo re CEP tors
endotracheal	en do TRACH e al
hypercapnia	hy per CAP ni a
obturator	ob tu RA tor
oximeter	ox IM e ter
tracheostomy	trach e OS to my

GRAMMAR POINTS

Usually, the verb tense called the "present continuous" or "present progressive" is used when an action is happening right now: You are reading these words and you are answering the questions. It is used to answer the question "What are you doing?" "I am taking vital signs." It is formed by using the simple present form of be + verb + -ing.

This same verb tense may be used to describe activities that stop and start during a longer period that includes the present time. You can use this form when you interview patients to learn about symptoms they are having:

Are you coughing? (Not this minute, but today, or over the past few days continuing until now.)

Are you wheezing?

Are you experiencing shortness of breath?

How are you feeling? (This can mean "now," or in general over recent days.)

How much are you smoking?

Are you drinking a lot of water?

Are you getting any exercise?

COMMUNICATION EXERCISES

1. With a partner, write a dialogue describing to a patient who has a chest tube what to expect when the tube is taken out (Critical Thinking Activity #2 above). Practice the dialogue with your partner.

2. With a partner, practice the guidelines for interviewing the patient with a respiratory problem. See Table 28-5.

Review the chapter key points, answer the study questions, and complete the critical thinking activities at the end of the chapter in the textbook.

CHAPTER

29 Promoting Urinary Elimination

Answer Key: Textbook page references are provided as a guide for answering selected questions. A complete answer key was provided for your instructor.

TERMINOLOGY

A. Matching

Directions: Match the terms in Column I with the definitions in Column II.

Column I			Column II
(529)	1. _____	anuria	a. Needing to urinate at night during sleep hours
(530)	2. _____	cystitis	b. Pus in the urine
(558)	3. _____	dysuria	c. Narrowing, usually of a tube or opening
(531)	4. _____	hematuria	d. To urinate
(529)	5. _____	nocturia	e. Absence of urine
(530)	6. _____	oliguria	f. Inflammation of the bladder
(530)	7. _____	polyuria	g. Decreased urine output
(531)	8. _____	pyuria	h. Blood in the urine
(539)	9. _____	stricture	i. Painful urination
(527)	10. _____	void	j. Excessive urination

B. Completion

Directions: Fill in the blank(s) with the correct term(s) from the terms list in the chapter in the textbook to complete the sentence.

(534) 1. When it is too tiring for a patient to walk to the bathroom, toileting may be done with the _____ chair.

(529) 2. Sometimes running water in the sink will help a patient initiate _____.

(529) 3. Urine left in the bladder after urination is called _____.

(534) 4. Various medications cause urine _____ as a side effect, particularly in the male.

(529) 5. When the patient is unable to control the bladder sphincter, urinary _____ occurs.

(557) 6. A(n) _____ is an artificially created opening on the abdomen for the discharge of urine.

(539)   7. Urinary _____ is performed when the patient is unable to eliminate urine from the bladder.

(540)   8. A(n) _____ is only suitable for use on the male patient.

REVIEW OF STRUCTURE AND FUNCTION OF THE URINARY SYSTEM

Directions: Match the structures in Column I with the functions in Column II.

Column I	Column II
(528) 1. _____ kidney	a. Carries urine from the bladder to the outside of the body
(528) 2. _____ bladder	
(528) 3. _____ ureter	b. Extracts metabolic waste
(528) 4. _____ nephron	c. Manufactures urine
(528) 5. _____ urethra	d. Carries urine from the kidney to the bladder
(529) 6. _____ sphincter	e. Controls the release of urine from the bladder
	f. Holds 1000–1800 mL of urine

IDENTIFICATION

Directions: Mark the items from a urinalysis report with an "X" if they are abnormal. (Answer requires synthesis and application of knowledge.)

(531)

1. _____ Color: dark amber
2. _____ Character: slightly cloudy
3. _____ Specific gravity: 1.025
4. _____ pH: 6.0
5. _____ Glucose: 1+
6. _____ Protein: 0
7. _____ Ketones: 0
8. _____ Leukocytes: moderate
9. _____ Erythrocytes: 0
10. _____ Bilirubin: slight
11. _____ Pyuria: trace

SHORT ANSWER

Directions: Write a brief answer for each question.

(538-539)   1. Describe three nursing measures to assist patient to urinate normally.

   a. _____

   b. _____

   c. _____

(539)   2. List four reasons urinary catheterization may be ordered.

   a. _____

   b. _____

     c. _____

     d. _____

(540) 3. When catheterizing a patient you accidentally contaminate the catheter. You must:

_____

(551) 4. Intermittent catheterization is used for patients who:

_____

(552-553) 5. Three reasons bladder irrigation may be ordered are to:

     a. _____

     b. _____

     c. _____

(556) 6. An important principle to be applied when irrigating the bladder is:

_____

(556-557) 7. Urinary incontinence can be managed by:

_____

_____

_____

(530) 8. Symptoms of cystitis are:

_____

COMPLETION

Directions: Fill in the blank(s) with the correct word(s) to complete the sentence.

(527) 1. The average adult voids from _____ times a day.

(529) 2. Foul-smelling urine may indicate _____.

(530) 3. Each patient should void at least every _____ hours.

(531) 4. Urine specimens should be tested immediately, because after _____ of standing, the urine changes characteristics.

(532) 5. When instructing the patient on how to collect a 24-hour urine specimen you would tell him or her to void and _____ the specimen at the beginning of the test.

(532) 6. Urine is strained when it is suspected that the patient has a urinary _____.

(534) 7. A fracture pan is used when the patient is unable to _____ on a regular bedpan.

(529) 8. Men generally have an easier time voiding when in the _____ position.

(540) 9. A(n) _____ catheter is curved and is easier to insert into the male when the prostate is enlarged.

(552) 10. A bladder _____ may be used to soothe irritated bladder tissues and promote healing.

(529) 11. The lighter the shade of urine, the more _____ it is.

(534) 12. When placing a fracture pan, the wide lip goes _____.

(550) 13. When catheterizing a female, it is wise to identify the location of the _____ and the _____ before opening the catheter kit.

(551) 14. Suprapubic catheters are often used after gynecologic surgery so that _____ can be reestablished before the catheter is removed.

(553-555) 15. When performing a bladder irrigation, you must be careful not to exert _____ which might damage the bladder and cause pain.

APPLICATION OF THE NURSING PROCESS

Directions: Write a brief answer for each question.

(530) 1. If V.O., age 72, states that he has been experiencing a very frequent need to urinate, what questions would you ask to further assess the situation?

_____
_____
_____
_____

(532-533) 2. If the assessment data indicate V.O. seems to be having trouble with an enlarged prostate, what would be three possible nursing diagnoses for him? Place a "*" next to the most appropriate one.

_____
_____
_____
_____

3. Write two expected outcomes for the starred nursing diagnosis.

a. _____

b. _____

4. A tendency for a man who is experiencing frequent urination is to decrease fluid intake. What would you tell V.O. about his fluid intake?

_____
_____
_____

Student Name_____

(558)   5.   Treatment for V.O.'s problem takes time to be effective. How would you evaluate progress toward meeting the expected outcomes?

_____

_____

_____

NCLEX-PN® EXAM REVIEW

*Directions: Choose the **best** answer(s) for each of the following questions.*

(529)   1.   Your male patient, age 56, has been having urinary problems with urine retention and is to undergo diagnostic testing and treatment. He is to having tests to determine the status of his kidney function. One test used to see if the kidney is concentrating urine correctly is a
1.   urine culture.
2.   specific gravity.
3.   24-hour urine test.
4.   microscopic exam of urine.

(529)   2.   Continued urine retention can eventually damage the kidneys. If that happens, the kidneys will not be able to remove waste materials from the body or
1.   regulate fluid balance.
2.   absorb nutrients for cellular growth.
3.   help regulate body temperature.
4.   secrete hormones needed for growth.

(531)   3.   You obtain a urine specimen for urinalysis from the patient. Which characteristics of the specimen are abnormal? (Select all that apply)
1.   aromatic odor
2.   1+ protein
3.   cloudy appearance
4.   straw color

(532)   4.   A 24-hour urine collection must be done precisely. When collecting a 24-hour urine specimen, it is important to (Select all that apply)
1.   limit fluids to less than 1000 mL per day.
2.   start the test with an empty bladder.
3.   add the voiding at the end of the test to the container.
4.   force fluids to at least 3000 mL per day.

5.   Data that would indicate that the patient was experiencing retention of urine would be
1.   voiding 15 times a day.
2.   cloudy urine.
3.   low specific gravity of urine.
4.   palpation reveals a distended bladder.

(547-549)   6.   A Foley catheter is ordered for the patient to relieve his symptoms until treatment can correct the situation. When a urinary catheter is left in place for more than a couple of days in a male, it should be
1.   taped to the leg.
2.   taped to the abdomen.
3.   looped on the upper thigh.
4.   replaced every 3 days.

(547-549) 7. There are several actions that help insure success when catheterizing the male patient. When inserting the catheter into the penis, if resistance is felt, an appropriate action is to (Select all that apply)
   1. have him bear down and apply pressure to the catheter.
   2. remove the catheter and try a smaller one.
   3. tell him to take a deep breath and twist the catheter while inserting it.
   4. hold the penis at a 90 degree angle to the body.

(550) 8. Your 68-year-old female patient had surgery yesterday. She had experienced episodes of incontinence prior to surgery. She is recovering from a hip fracture and pinning. She has a Foley catheter in place. You know that it is **most** important to
   1. encourage fluid intake of 3000 mL a day.
   2. be certain the catheter and drainage tubing are free from kinks.
   3. empty the Foley bag when it is 3/4 full.
   4. assess the output every 2 hours.

(557) 9. The first step in beginning a urine continence training program is to
   1. toilet the patient every 2 hours.
   2. increase fluid intake to dilute the urine.
   3. collaborate with other health care workers.
   4. assess when voidings are occurring.

(557) 10. Besides scheduled toileting, one action that may assist the patient to regain bladder control is to
   1. teach her Kegel exercises.
   2. ambulate her regularly.
   3. use absorbent panty liners to prevent wetness.
   4. restrict fluids to 1000 mL per day.

CRITICAL THINKING ACTIVITIES

1. Write an outline for a specific teaching plan for a multiple sclerosis patient who has lost nerve control over the bladder and needs to learn to self-catheterize.

2. Write a specific teaching plan for a newly married woman who is having recurrent cystitis.

3. Explain to an older male family member why symptoms of prostate enlargement and urinary retention should be treated as soon as possible. Outline the points you would cover:

MEETING CLINICAL OBJECTIVES

Directions: The following suggested activities will help you meet the stated clinical practice objectives for the chapter. Review your school's clinical objectives for the week and outline a plan of activities that will help you meet them. If you are unsure how to meet them, consult with your instructor at the beginning of the clinical day.

1. With a peer, practice comfortably placing a bedpan under a patient. Use water to partially fill the pan and practice removing it without spilling.

Student Name _____

2. Practice catheterization procedure until you can do it efficiently and aseptically five times in the skill lab or simulated at home. Have a peer check your technique as you do the procedure.

3. Ask to observe catheterization procedures on your assigned unit before attempting to perform one.

4. Seek opportunity to obtain a sterile specimen from a Foley catheter.

5. Teach a patient how to obtain a midstream urine specimen.

6. Seek opportunity to remove a Foley catheter.

STEPS TOWARD BETTER COMMUNICATION

VOCABULARY BUILDING GLOSSARY

Term	Pronunciation	Definition
bulbous	BUL bous	shaped like a lightbulb, with a larger rounded end
dependent	de PEN dent	1) relying on someone or something else; 2) hanging down
deficit	DEF i cit	below the normal or desired level
diversion	di VER sion	an alternative way, going a different way
distal	dis tal	away from the center of the body or point of attachment
hypertrophy	hy PER tro phy	increase in volume of a tissue or organ, caused by enlargement of existing cells
impede	im PEDE	get in the way of, block, slow down
instillation	in STIL LA tion	addition, putting into
invalid	in VAL id	not correct, not able to be used
invalid	IN val id	a person who is ill, or weakened by ill health or injury
patency	PA tent cy	having a clear passage
prone	PRONE	1) likely to do or have something; 2) lying face down
pucker	PUCK er	to draw together in small wrinkles, tighten in a circle
stasis	STA sis	a slowing or stopping of the normal flow of a bodily fluid

COMPLETION

Directions: Fill in the blank(s) with the correct term(s) from the Vocabulary Building Glossary to complete the sentence.

1. Some people have a very _____ nose.

2. A stone can _____ urine flow from the kidney if it lodges in a ureter.

3. Older adults often develop _____ of urine in the bladder because they do not empty it completely.

4. One treatment for bladder cancer may be a(n) _____ of chemotherapy agents into the bladder.

5. Many women are very _____ to bladder infections induced by bacteria entering the urethra during intercourse.

6. The urinary meatus will _____ if it is touched with a swab when preparing to catheterize the female patient.

7. A urinary catheter must remain _____ or urine will back up into the kidney and may cause tissue damage.

VOCABULARY EXERCISES

Directions: Make six sentences using the different meanings of the three words dependent, invalid, *and* prone *(two sentences for each word).*

1. _____

2. _____

3. _____

4. _____

5. _____

6. _____

PRONUNCIATION OF DIFFICULT TERMS

Directions: Practice pronouncing the following words.

catheterization   CATH e ter i ZA tion
erythrocytes   e RY thro cytes
hypertrophy   hy PER tro phy
leukocytes   leu ko cytes
micturition   mic tu ri tion
reagent   re AG ent
urostomy   ur OS to my

COMMUNICATION EXERCISE

With a peer, practice your pronunciation by role playing the "Communication Cue" in the chapter in the textbook.

Review the chapter key points, answer the study questions, and complete the
critical thinking activities at the end of the chapter in the textbook.

CHAPTER 30 Promoting Bowel Elimination

Answer Key: Textbook page references are provided as a guide for answering selected questions. A complete answer key was provided for your instructor.

TERMINOLOGY

A. Matching

Directions: Match the terms in Column I with the definitions in Column II.

Column I		Column II
(576)	1. _____ ostomy appliance	a. Waste eliminated from the colon
(563)	2. _____ constipation	b. Opening from the abdomen into the intestine
(565)	3. _____ diarrhea	c. Expel feces
(562)	4. _____ defecate	d. Entrance of ostomy
(567)	5. _____ excoriation	e. Passage of hard, dry feces
(563)	6. _____ flatus	f. Enlarged veins inside or outside the rectum
(563)	7. _____ hemorrhoids	g. Partially digested blood in the stool
(563)	8. _____ melena	h. Stool having high fat content
(575)	9. _____ ostomy	i. Gas
(563)	10. _____ steatorrhea	j. Abrasion of the skin
(561)	11. _____ stool	k. Device to gather and contain ostomy output
(575)	12. _____ stoma	l. Frequent, watery stools

B. Completion

Directions: Fill in the blank(s) with the correct term(s) from the terms list in the chapter in the textbook to complete the sentence.

(572) 1. When an elderly person is on bed rest and is receiving narcotic pain medications, _____ may occur as constipation worsens.

(561) 2. Another term for stool is _____.

(565) 3. Bowel _____ is extremely upsetting to patients and not much fun for nurses either.

(563) 4. When there is a small amount of bleeding in the intestine it often appears as _____ blood in the stool.

(572)   5. A(n) _____ occurring when an impaction is being removed can cause cardiac dysrhythmia and an alteration in blood pressure.

(562)   6. Intra-abdominal pressure is created by performing the _____ and is used to initiate defecation.

(576)   7. A(n) _____ may be performed when the bowel has been invaded by cancerous tumor.

(562)   8. The intestinal villi _____ with aging and nutrient absorption may decrease in some elderly patients.

(575)   9. A(n) _____ is an opening into the small intestine for the diversion of intestinal contents.

(577) 10. Whenever the patient has an ostomy, meticulous _____ care is needed to keep the skin around the stoma in good condition.

(576) 11. The material discharged by an intestinal ostomy is called _____.

REVIEW OF STRUCTURE AND FUNCTION OF THE INTESTINAL SYSTEM

Directions: Match the structures in Column I with the functions in Column II.
(562)

Column I

1. _____ small intestine
2. _____ large intestine
3. _____ sigmoid colon
4. _____ rectum
5. _____ rectal sphincter
6. _____ vermiform appendix
7. _____ intestinal muscle layers
8. _____ villi
9. _____ anus
10. _____ ileocecal valve

Column II

a. Reabsorbs water, sodium, and chloride
b. Absorb food substances
c. Attaches transverse colon to rectum
d. No known digestive function
e. Controls movement of substances into the large intestine
f. Allows passage of feces to outside of body
g. Processes chyme into a more liquid state
h. Controls release of feces
i. Expand and contract to move chyme and feces
j. Stores feces for expulsion

SHORT ANSWER

Directions: Write a brief answer for each question.

(566)   1. Four factors that can interfere with normal bowel elimination are:

a. _____
b. _____
c. _____
d. _____

Student Name _____

(563)   2. Give the possible cause for each of the following abnormal stool characteristics:

    a.   Melena: _____

    b.   Occult blood: _____

    c.   Pale-colored stool: _____

    d.   Mucus: _____

    e.   Foul-smelling stool that floats in water: _____

    f.   Liquid stool: _____

    g.   Hard, dry stool:_____

(576)   3. Preoperative assessment of the patient who is to undergo an ostomy may reveal fear of:

    a.   _____

    b.   _____

    c.   _____

    d.   _____

(576)   4. One intervention that can be helpful to the patient who is to have an ostomy is:

    _____

    _____

(574)   5. Three types of intestinal diversions are:

    a.   _____

    b.   _____

    c.   _____

(568)   6. Four ways to prevent constipation are:

    a.   _____

    b.   _____

    c.   _____

    d.   _____

(568)   7. Rectal suppositories work to promote bowel movements by:

    a.   _____

    b.   _____

    c.   _____

(576)   8. Conditions that may require a bowel ostomy are:

    a.   _____

    b.   _____

    c.   _____

    d.   _____

APPLICATION OF THE NURSING PROCESS

Directions: Write a brief answer for each question.

(566)   1.   When assessing for normal bowel function you would:

_____

_____

_____

(565-566)   2.   R.M., age 56, is hospitalized due to trauma from a fall off of a ladder. He is receiving narcotic pain medication. He is normally a very active man. From this data, you know that he should have which nursing diagnosis related to bowel function?

_____

(566)   3.   Write an expected outcome for the above nursing diagnosis.

_____

(568)   4.   Interventions to prevent bowel problems for R.M. would be:

_____

_____

(568)   5.   To evaluate whether the expected outcome is being met, you would evaluate:

_____

_____

NCLEX-PN® EXAM REVIEW

*Directions: Choose the **best** answer(s) for each of the following questions.*

(656)   1.   Your male patient, age 45, is recovering from abdominal surgery and has developed constipation. His bowel pattern at home is once every day. He has not had a bowel movement in 3 days. The physician orders a rectal suppository to stimulate defecation. When inserting a rectal suppository, you should place it _____ inches above the outer sphincter. (Fill in the blank)

(569)   2.   The suppository does not work and an enema is ordered. When giving an enema to a patient in bed, the best patient position for instilling the solution is the _____ _____. (Fill in the blank)

(570)   3.   When administering the enema to the patient, you would position the solution container no higher above his buttocks than _____ inches. (Fill in the blank)

(570)   4.   Restricting the height of the solution container prevents
1.   bubbling and flatus from occurring in the bowel.
2.   the solution from running much too slowly.
3.   the solution from going too high in the colon.
4.   the solution from entering at too high a pressure.

Student Name _____

(570) 5. The amount of solution you would use for an average patient's enema is
1. 300–500 mL.
2. 1500–2000 mL.
3. 400–800 mL.
4. 500–1000 mL.

(569) 6. The amount of soap you would add to the water for a soapsuds enema for the patient is
1. 30 mL per 1000 mL.
2. 10 mL per 500 mL.
3. 5 mL per 1000 mL.
4. 2 mL per 500 mL.

(568) 7. The patient needs diet counseling to prevent further constipation. You would explain that he should (Select all that apply)
1. increase the amount of fluid taken daily.
2. eat cold cereal every morning.
3. consume more milk products.
4. increase vegetable and whole grain intake.

8. Your male patient, age 82, has a new colostomy because of colon cancer. Sometimes an elderly patient cannot manage self-care due to preexisting problems with
1. fragile skin.
2. arthritis.
3. back problems.
4. transient dizziness.

(577) 9. He is very concerned about odor from his colostomy. You might teach him that one way to prevent excessive unpleasant odor is to
1. eat lots of fresh fruit.
2. avoid gas-forming foods.
3. eat only cooked vegetables.
4. avoid too much fresh fruit.

(576) 10. When planning for teaching about his colostomy care, you explain that he should report to the doctor if the
1. effluent is always formed.
2. effluent is very soft.
3. stoma is pale in color.
4. appliance needs emptying several times a day.

CRITICAL THINKING ACTIVITIES

1. E.D. is a 36-year-old executive who eats on the run for most meals. She is having difficulty with increasing constipation. Outline a teaching plan for her to combat this problem. Consider her lifestyle.

2. Prepare to instruct a clinic patient how to collect a stool specimen at home for testing for occult blood. Outline your points of instruction:

3. Prepare a teaching plan for a patient who needs to learn to self-catheterize a continent diversion. Plan outline:

MEETING CLINICAL OBJECTIVES

Directions: The following suggested activities will help you meet the stated clinical practice objectives for the chapter. Review your school's clinical objectives for the week and outline a plan of activities that will help you meet them. If you are unsure how to meet them, consult with your instructor at the beginning of the clinical day.

1. If a skill lab is available, practice giving an enema to a mannequin with a peer to observe technique. Practice until you are comfortable with the equipment and the procedure.

2. Work on a bowel training program with a patient or relative who has a long-standing problem with constipation.

3. Ask for an opportunity to obtain and test a stool specimen for occult blood.

4. Seek clinical opportunities to give various types of enemas.

5. Contact the agency enterostomal therapist and ask to go along on patient visits and teaching sessions.

6. Attend the local ostomy society meeting.

7. Obtain a copy of the literature available for ostomy patients from the local chapter of the American Cancer Society.

8. In the clinical setting, seek opportunity to assist with colostomy, ileostomy, and urostomy care.

STEPS TOWARD BETTER COMMUNICATION

VOCABULARY BUILDING GLOSSARY

Term	Pronunciation	Definition
commode	com MODE	a toilet seat
compromised	COM pro mised	affected by exposing to danger or problems
distension	dis TEN sion	swelling, or pushing out because of internal pressure
heed	HEED	pay attention to
induced	in DUCEd	caused; brought on by
longitudinal	lon gi tud in al	lengthwise; along the long part of something
oblique	o blique (o BLEEK)	slanting; not straight across, but at a sharp angle
scanty	SCAN ty	a slight or small amount
tepid	TEP id	slightly warm
triggering	TRIG ger ing	starting a reaction
wafer	WA fer	a thin, flat, round disc

COMPLETION

Directions: Fill in the blank(s) with the correct term(s) from the Vocabulary Building Glossary to complete the sentence.

1. Patients who are prone to constipation need to learn to _____ the urge for defecation.

2. Constipation often causes abdominal _____, making the patient quite uncomfortable.

3. A tap water enema distends the bowel, _____ defecation.

4. A karaya _____ is often used on the skin to protect it when an ostomy appliance is applied to the stoma.

5. The appliance plate had to be trimmed to a(n) _____ angle in order to fit properly on the abdomen.

Student Name _____

6. A portable _____ is often used for bed rest patients and is placed beside the bed.

7. When a patient has an impaction, _____ amounts of liquid stool may be passed intermittently.

WORD ATTACK SKILLS

Directions: If an ostomy is an opening into the intestine, where specifically are the following located?

1. colostomy _____

2. ileostomy _____

3. urostomy _____

PRONUNCIATION OF DIFFICULT TERMS

Directions: Practice pronouncing the following words.

chyme   CHYME (kime)

ileocecal   il e o CE cal

longitudinal   lon gi TUD in al

oblique   o BLIQUE (o BLEEK)

sphincter   SPHINC ter (sfink ter)

steatorrhea   STE a tor rhe a

villi   VIL li (VIL eye)

COMMUNICATION EXERCISES

1. Read and practice the following dialogue.

    Nurse: "Good morning, Mr. H. How are you feeling today?"

    Mr. H.: "Oh, not so good."

    Nurse: "Why? What's the matter?"

    Mr. H.: "I'm having my surgery today."

    Nurse: "That does make you nervous, I know. Is there anything in particular you are worried about?"

    Mr. H.: "I suppose they think I will pull through the surgery or they wouldn't do it."

    Nurse: "Of course they do. Did the doctor talk to you about the risks?"

    Mr. H.: "Yeah, and I guess that is OK. I'll pull through. It is just that they are going to put in an os-something."

    Nurse: "An ostomy. They will make a small hole in your abdominal wall that connects to your intestine."

    Mr. H.: "And then they will put on that bag thing. I won't even be able to go to the bathroom and I'll have a bulge under my clothes."

    Nurse: "It can be adjusted so it hardly shows. We'll show you how."

Mr. H.:   "But it's full of crap and I'll smell and nobody will want to be around me—especially my girlfriend!"

Nurse: "Why don't I schedule you for a visit with someone from the Ostomy Association. They can help you with your questions and your feelings. It helps to talk to someone who has been through it."

Mr. H.:   "OK. I think I am going to need all the help I can get!"

2A. Here is a dialogue concerning assessment of bowel function.

Ms. D., age 56, has begun having considerable abdominal bloating and some hard, dry stools. She has come to see the doctor because of this problem.

Nurse: "Ms. D., I need to ask you some questions about your bowel function."

Ms. D.:   "OK."

Nurse: "When did you first notice this abdominal bloating?"

Ms. D.:   "It started about 8 months ago, but has become progressively worse."

Nurse: "Have you noticed any particular relationship between the bloating and what you eat?"

Ms. D.:   "I would say there is, but I can't pin down what foods seem to make it worse. I suspect wheat, tomato, sugar, wine, and who knows what else. Spicy food affects me too."

Nurse: "So, you have more bloating when you eat any of these foods?"

Ms. D.:   "It seems that way, but then now I seem to bloat up if I eat anything."

Nurse: "Tell me about your usual diet and fluid intake. Do you eat enough fiber?"

Ms. D.:   "I have cereal and fruit juice for breakfast during the week. For lunch I eat yogurt, an apple, and some crackers. I have a couple of low-fat, fruit-filled cookies for dessert. For dinner we eat salad every night as well as some fresh fruit as an appetizer. I fix a casserole with pasta or we have chicken or stir fry. We eat a piece of meat on the weekends. Once in a while we will have a grilled pork chop during the week. We have bread with dinner. Our portions are very moderate. I have a piece of hard candy for dessert later in the evening and light ice cream or frozen yogurt once or twice a week. I drink decaf for breakfast and mid-morning, lots of water during the day, and a diet coke mid-afternoon. We eat some peanuts or pretzels at cocktail time and I drink tonic with lime—once in a while with a capful of gin in it. I have wine with dinner about three times a week. No more than one or two glasses though."

Nurse: "It seems like you are eating pretty well. You could use more vegetables though."

Ms. D.:   "Oh, I use raw vegetables in the salad every night. My husband doesn't like cooked vegetables other than potatoes very much. We do eat potato several times a week and I eat the skin."

Nurse: "That sounds pretty good. What about your bowel movements?"

Ms. D.:   "I have small, harder stools, sometimes three or four a day, sometimes every other day. The pattern isn't consistent."

Nurse: "Do you ever have alternating constipation and diarrhea?"

Ms. D.:   "Not really. I'll have a loose stool sometimes if I eat really spicy food or drink a lot of wine."

Nurse: "What about pencil-thin stool?"

Ms. D.:   "Occasionally after a severe episode of bloating, I will have soft, pencil-like stool. It quickly returns to normal."

Nurse: "Have you ever noticed blood in your stool?"

Ms. D.:	"No, I have only ever had blood if I had a hemorrhoid flare-up. I developed one hemorrhoid during the last week of pregnancy."
Nurse:	"What about abdominal cramping?"
Ms. D.:	"I do have intermittent cramping, especially in the middle of the night. It is diffuse but seems to start somewhere around my belly button."
Nurse:	"About how often does this happen?"
Ms. D.:	"It varies; it may occur several nights in one week and then not again for two or three weeks."
Nurse:	"OK, Ms. D. The doctor will examine you and then will probably order some tests. We can probably find some medication that can help you with this problem."

2B. Using the example above, write a dialogue evaluating an elderly patient who lives alone and has been experiencing constipation. Make dietary recommendations.

3. Write out a dialogue for contacting the enterostomal therapist as suggested for a clinical activity. Explain who you are, why you want to go on patient visits, and make arrangements for the time and place to meet. Practice the dialogue, then make the contact. (If possible, have a peer whose first language is English critique your dialogue and help you practice the pronunciation.)

Review the chapter key points, answer the study questions, and complete the critical thinking activities at the end of the chapter in the textbook.

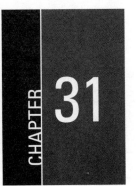

CHAPTER 31

Pain, Comfort, and Sleep

Answer Key: Textbook page references are provided as a guide for answering selected questions. A complete answer key was provided for your instructor.

TERMINOLOGY

A. Matching

Directions: Match the terms in Column I with the definitions in Column II.

Column I	Column II
(594) 1. _____ acupressure	a. Feeling of distress or suffering
(594) 2. _____ acupuncture	b. Naturally occurring, opiate-like peptides
(594) 3. _____ analgesic	c. Manipulation of the joints and adjacent tissues of the body
(595) 4. _____ bolus	
(594) 5. _____ chiropractic	d. Insertion of fine sterile needles into various points on the body
(585) 6. _____ endorphins	
(600) 7. _____ insomnia	e. Line or passageway of energy that passes through the body
(594) 8. _____ meridian	
(601) 9. _____ narcolepsy	f. Pressure applied to various points on the body
(594) 10. _____ nonsteroidal anti-inflammatory drugs (NSAIDs)	g. Nonopioid pain medications that have no steroidal effect
	h. Drug that relieves pain
(583) 11. _____ pain	i. Difficulty in getting to sleep or staying asleep
(600) 12. _____ sleep apnea	j. Periods when breathing stops during sleep
	k. Uncontrollable falling asleep during usual waking hours
	l. Concentrated dose given in a short period

SHORT ANSWER

Directions: Write a brief description of each of the following methods used to relieve pain and promote comfort.

(592)   1. Biofeedback technique: _____

_____

_____

(592)   2. Distraction technique: _____

_____

_____

(597-598)   3.   Epidural analgesia: _____

_____

(592)   4.   Guided imagery: _____

_____

_____

(593)   5.   Hypnosis: _____

_____

_____

(592)   6.   Meditation technique:_____

_____

_____

(595, 597)   7.   Patient-controlled analgesia:_____

_____

_____

(592)   8.   Relaxation technique: _____

_____

_____

(589-590)   9.   TENS: _____

_____

_____

(584)   10.   The gate control theory is one view of pain transmission and ways to interrupt it. According to this theory, massage and vibration work to relieve pain by:

_____

(586-587)   11.   Nociceptive pain treatment can be directed at any one of the four phases of that type of pain. Give one way pain can be interrupted or decreased for each phase:

    a.   Transduction: _____

    b.   Transmission: _____

    c.   Perception: _____

    d.   Modulation: _____

(592)   12.   Engaging in interesting activity reduces pain perception by:

_____

_____

(584)   13.   Anxiety increases pain perception causing _____

_____.

Student Name_____

(594)   14. The three basic categories of medications for pain relief are:

    a. _____

    b. _____

    c. _____

(595, 597) 15. PCA can be used via _____ or _____.

(587)   16. The reason that objective assessment of pain is very difficult is because pain is _____ _____.

(598)   17. Sleep and rest affect pain. A person who is rested shows both increased pain _____ and a greater response to _____.

(600)   18. Sleep may be interrupted due to:

    a. _____

    b. _____

    c. _____

    d. _____

(598)   19. Lack of sleep can cause _____ and _____.

(598)   20. The body receives the most rest during which phase of sleep? _____

(598-599) 21. Describe the stages of the sleep cycle.

    a. Stage 1: _____

    b. Stage 2: _____

    c. Stage 3: _____

    d. Stage 4: _____

    e. REM sleep: _____

(600)   22. Lifestyle factors that affect sleep are:

    a. _____

    b. _____

    c. _____

    d. _____

    e. _____

(600)   23.   Environmental factors that affect sleep are:

a. _____

b. _____

c. _____

(600)   24.   Obstructive sleep apnea can be successfully treated by:

_____

(600)   25.   Snoring may be caused by:

a. _____

b. _____

(590)   26.   Heat for the relief of pain and swelling can be applied by:

a. _____

b. _____

c. _____

d. _____

e. _____

f. _____

(601)   27.   Narcolepsy is characterized by:

_____

(601)   28.   A diagnosis of narcolepsy is achieved by:

_____

(590)   29.   Three uses of cold for pain or discomfort are:

a. _____

b. _____

c. _____

(590, 592) 30.   Precautions when using ice packs are:

a. _____

b. _____

APPLICATION OF THE NURSING PROCESS

Directions: Write a brief answer for each question.

(587)   1.   Your patient, L.F., age 36, was seriously injured in a motorcycle accident. He has multiple fractures and is intubated and on a ventilator. How would you assess his need for pain medication?

_____

_____

_____

_____

Student Name _____

(588)   2. Besides the obvious nursing diagnosis of *Pain*, what other nursing diagnoses might be appropriate based on the above information?

_____

_____

_____

_____

      3. Write one expected outcome for each of the above nursing diagnoses.

_____

_____

_____

_____

      4. List four nursing actions that might be helpful in decreasing L.F.'s pain, based on the above information.

    a. _____

    b. _____

    c. _____

    d. _____

      5. List one evaluation statement for each action above that indicates progress toward the expected outcomes.

    a. _____

    b. _____

    c. _____

    d. _____

NCLEX-PN® EXAM REVIEW

*Directions: Choose the **best** answer(s) for each of the following questions.*

(595)   1. Your female patient has fallen and injured her elbow. It is not fractured, but there is considerable swelling and pain. She asks which over-the-counter analgesic would be best to take for the discomfort. You tell her that one with NSAID properties would be best. Which of the following would it be best to take?
    1. acetaminophen
    2. aspirin
    3. ibuprofen
    4. oxymorphone

(590)   2. The patient asks what else she can do for the elbow pain. You suggest the use of cold on the elbow because it will
    1. directly reduce swelling which will reduce pain.
    2. distract from the pain.
    3. relax the muscles, reducing pain.
    4. focus attention to the area, stimulating healing.

(590, 592) 3. In instructing the patient how to apply ice packs, you would tell her that it is best to
1. apply the ice directly to the skin.
2. use the ice pack for 15 minutes several times a day.
3. alternate the ice pack with a heat pack.
4. apply the ice pack for an hour at a time.

(590, 592) 4. Ice cubes, ice water compresses, commercial cold packs, and frozen vegetables are often used to ice an area. You would tell her to use

_____

_____ as her ice for the elbow as it will conform best to the area. (Fill in the blank)

(592) 5. The patient tells you she is supposed to finish a work project this afternoon, but she probably cannot now. You tell her to go ahead and work because
1. her elbow will heal anyway.
2. the elbow is already swollen.
3. using the arm will decrease the swelling.
4. the distraction of work will decrease the pain.

(611) 6. A female patient comes to the clinic complaining of insomnia. She has had difficulty sleeping for the past 2 months, is tired all the time, and her work is suffering. In assessing the problem, you would ask her about (Select all that apply)
1. pattern of caffeine intake.
2. what medications she takes and when.
3. how she uses her leisure time.
4. stresses and problems in her life.

(600) 7. The patient having difficulty sleeping lives right off the freeway in an apartment complex where many young people live. You wonder if her problem might be due to
1. socializing.
2. too much noise.
3. loneliness.
4. too little exercise.

(601) 8. One thing you would ask the patient to do to try to locate the reason for her insomnia is to
1. discuss the problem with her friends.
2. review times in her life when she had no insomnia.
3. keep a diary related to sleep and problems encountered.
4. take a warm bath each time she cannot go back to sleep.

(601) 9. You would advise the patient with insomnia to (Select all that apply)
1. get up at the same time each day and avoid naps.
2. to take a warm bath or shower before retiring.
3. to eat a large snack before going to bed.
4. to eliminate alcohol and nicotine for at least 2 hours before bedtime.

(601) 10. You suggest that she include a warm dairy product in her bedtime snack to promote sleep through (Select all that apply)
1. warmth it provides to the body.
2. filling the stomach and preventing hunger.
3. analgesic effect of the protein in it.
4. its L-tryptophan content.

Student Name_____

CRITICAL THINKING ACTIVITIES

1. Write an imaging scenario to induce relaxation and reduce pain for a patient.

2. Look up the medications listed in Table 31-3 and list the potential side effects of each medication.

3. Write out and record a relaxation exercise that you can use for your own relaxation.

MEETING CLINICAL OBJECTIVES

Directions: The following suggested activities will help you meet the stated clinical practice objectives for the chapter. Review your school's clinical objectives for the week and outline a plan of activities that will help you meet them. If you are unsure how to meet them, consult with your instructor at the beginning of the clinical day.

1. Observe a nurse setting up a PCA pump and go with him or her to instruct the patient in its use.

2. Practice the use of alternative pain control techniques for a family member or friend for relief from a bad headache, muscle spasm, or other pain.

3. Use your own guided imagery "script" with patients to reduce pain.

4. Perform a sleep assessment on a patient. Assist the patient with methods that can be used to enhance sleep within the hospital environment.

STEPS TOWARD BETTER COMMUNICATION

VOCABULARY BUILDING GLOSSARY

Term	Pronunciation	Definition
A. Individual Terms		
adjuvant	ad ju vant	auxiliary; assisting
complementary	com ple MEN ta ry	a useful addition that makes something complete
divert	di VERT	move from one place to another
distraction	dis TRAC tion	focusing attention away from one thing to another
enhanced	en HANCed	made better
grimacing	GRIM a cing	twisting the facial muscles
induce	in DUCE	to gently cause; to make happen by gentle persuasion
jet lag	jet lag	a tired feeling caused by long distance travel into different time zones
pantomime	PAN to mime	to use hand, body, and facial movement without words to help someone understand what you are trying to say
perception	per CEP tion	the way a person sees or feels something
phantom	phan tom	a ghost; something unseen that comes and goes
stoic	STO ic	not showing feelings, especially pain
stressors	STRESS ors	things that cause stress

transient	TRAN si ent	temporary
verify	ver i fy	to prove something is true; to confirm

B. Phrases

a fair degree	a FAIR de GREE	quite a bit; a lot
during the course of the night	dur ing the course of the night	over the whole time of the night
over-the-counter medications	O ver the COUN ter med i CA tions	medication available without a prescription
on occasion	on oc CAS ion	sometimes
shift work	SHIFT work	when work is continuous over 24 hours and some people work in the day, some in the evening and some at night; each of these periods is a *shift*
to suffer from	to SUF fer from	to be ill with something or have a problem over a long period

COMPLETION

A. Directions: Fill in the blank(s) with the correct term(s) from the Vocabulary Building Glossary to complete the sentence.

1. An antidepressant is sometimes added along with analgesic medication as a(n) _____ medication.

2. The person with serious _____ occurring in his or her life will often experience more pain from an injury.

3. Playing card games is one form of _____ used to reduce the sensation of pain.

4. When working with a person whose language you do not speak, you may need to use _____ to help them understand what you are trying to say.

5. Computer games can help _____ a patient's attention away from pain.

6. The effects of pain medication may be _____ by giving a soothing back massage.

7. Each patient's _____ of pain is different.

8. Men, in general, are more _____ regarding pain and do not show their feelings.

9. Chiropractic adjustment may be a(n) _____ treatment to physical therapy for back pain.

10. The patient who has had an amputation may experience _____ pain seeming to be in the missing part.

Student Name _____

B. Directions: Make sentences using the phrases above in the Vocabulary Building Glossary. Try to use at least two of the phrases in each sentence. Example:

<u>On occasion</u> I <u>suffer from</u> headaches.

1. _____
2. _____
3. _____
4. _____
5. _____
6. _____

VOCABULARY EXERCISES

Directions: Exercise I—Use Table 31-1, "Descriptive Terms for Pain," in the textbook in the following exercises. Work in pairs or small groups with a native English speaker and an English learner.

1. To express degree of pain, draw a line which goes from no pain to the worst degree of pain, and write the descriptive words on it in the order of the degree of the pain. Now pantomime (using gestures without speaking) that degree of pain for each word so that someone who does not understand English would know what you mean, and could indicate his or her own degree of pain.

2. Pantomime the meanings for the terms for quality of pain. Make sure the English learner understands the meaning of the word correctly, and that the partner can correctly identify the term being pantomimed.

COMMUNICATION EXERCISES

1. After practicing describing pain in the Vocabulary Exercise above, take turns with a partner describing pain nonverbally, and documenting it for the chart.

2. With a partner, role play questioning a patient about pain and writing the results on the chart. This time, ask and answer orally. Charting:

_____

_____

_____

_____

PRONUNCIATION OF DIFFICULT TERMS

Directions: Practice pronouncing the following words with a partner.

acupressure	AC u pres sure
acupuncture	AC u punc ture
analgesic	an al GE sic
anti-inflammatory	an ti in FLAM a tor y
biofeedback	bi o FEED back

endorphins	en DOR phins
epidural	ep i DUR al
meridian	me RID i an
myocardial infarction	my o CARD i al in FARC tion
narcolepsy	NAR co lep sy

CULTURAL POINTS

What is the attitude toward pain in your native culture? Is it OK for some people to show pain (like women and children) but not others (like men and older people)? How are children treated when they cry? What are they told? How do you think this affects them when they are grown up? How could such cultural views affect their medical treatment? Talk about this with one of your peers.

Review the chapter key points, answer the study questions, and complete the critical thinking activities at the end of the chapter in the textbook.

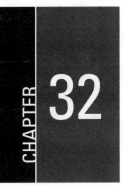

32 Complementary and Alternative Therapies

Answer Key: Textbook page references are provided as a guide for answering selected questions. A complete answer key was provided for your instructor.

TERMINOLOGY

Directions: Fill in the blank(s) with the correct term(s) from the terms list in the textbook chapter to complete the sentence.

(609) 1. _____ techniques apply pressure to certain points on the body to relieve pain or other symptoms.

(609) 2. Oils from plants are used in _____ to promote pleasurable feelings.

(609-610) 3. People with back pain often find relief with _____ treatment.

(604) 4. Therapies that augment mainstream medical treatment are called _____ therapies.

(605) 5. _____ or *curanderismo*, is a holistic approach to illness.

SHORT ANSWER

Directions: Write a brief answer for each question.

1. Two ways in which complementary and alternative therapies might be used in integrative medicine are:

   _____

   _____

   _____

(606-607) 2. Four body-mind therapies are:

   a. _____

   b. _____

   c. _____

   d. _____

(607, 609) 3. If asked by a patient about the advisability of using an herbal preparation, you should:

_____

_____

_____

COMPLETION

Directions: Fill in the blanks.

(604) 1. _____ therapy may be used along with pain medication to increase a patient's comfort.

(604) 2. The _____ has been established to provide evidence-based research regarding the efficacy of various complementary and alternative therapies.

(604-606) 3. _____, _____, _____, and _____ are examples of alternative medical systems.

(605) 4. Naturopathic medicine is a(n) _____ directed at prevention of disease and healing of the body.

(605) 5. _____, a branch of Chinese medicine, has been found by the National Institute of Health studies to be an effective method to treat pain.

NCLEX-PN® EXAM REVIEW

*Directions: Choose the **best** answer(s) to the following questions. Choose all answers that apply.*

(605) 1. Qi Gong exercise emphasizes
   1. muscle strengthening.
   2. breathing and coordination.
   3. increased circulation.
   4. relaxation.

(605) 2. Acupuncture needles are placed
   1. in the area of pain.
   2. along meridians of the body.
   3. to stimulate or disperse the flow of energy.
   4. only on the extremities.

(606) 3. American Indian medicine is based on the belief that
   1. spirit, mind, and emotions all interact with the environment.
   2. spirits of those departed are needed to heal the living.
   3. disease is caused by a disharmony in the patient's connection to nature.
   4. a depletion of energy is what causes illness.

(606) 4. Biofeedback therapy trains the patient to
   1. use the mind to control the flow of energy in the body.
   2. gain control over "involuntary" processes.
   3. balance "male" and "female" parts of the person.
   4. control particular internal physiologic processes.

(607) 5. Humor has proven to be helpful as a complementary therapy and can often
   1. quickly cure the patient's problem.
   2. speed the course of healing.
   3. decrease pain sensations.
   4. help create a positive outlook.

Student Name _____

CRITICAL THINKING ACTIVITIES

1. Use the computer to find information on the herb saw palmetto, often used to aid the patient with prostatic hypertrophy (prostate enlargement).

2. Explore further the practice of chiropractic medicine and the disorders it is used to treat.

MEETING CLINICAL OBJECTIVES

1. Assess the use of herbal medications and dietary supplements by each assigned patient. Determine if any of the substances used interfere with prescribed medications.

2. Explore the Internet for other sites that provide reliable information on alternative and complementary therapies.

3. Devise a short relaxation exercise that you can easily use with any patient. Develop an imagery exercise for a specific patient after assessing what type of images might work best for that patient.

STEPS TOWARD BETTER COMMUNICATION

VOCABULARY BUILDING GLOSSARY

Term	Pronunciation	Definition
comprise	com PRISE	to include, to be made up of
efficacy	EFF i ca cy	usefulness, giving the desired result
proactive	PRO ac tive	taking positive action for oneself
integrative	in te GRA tive	including several different aspects or ideas
inherent	in HER ent	inborn, or naturally existing in something
polarities	po LAR i ties	opposites, like the North and South poles
meridians	me RID i ans	lines between specific points (on the globe, lines that run between the North and South poles)
purgatives	PURG a tives	strong laxatives, causing bowel evacuation
wafted	WAF ted	moved gently through the air
enhancing	en HAN cing	making stronger or better
medium	MED i um	a method or means by which something is done ("artistic method")
circumspect	CIR cum SPECT	cautious, careful in actions
intercessory	in ter CESS o ry	asking for help or assistance as a go-between
alignment	a LIGN ment	straightening (into a line)
conduit	CON du it	a pipe, channel or method for transmitting something
augment	AUG ment	to supplement, add something

COMPLETION SENTENCES

Directions: Fill in the blank(s) with the correct word(s) from the Vocabulary Building Glossary above.

1. The child seems to be _____ good natured.

2. He took the car in for _____ of the wheels.

3. The smell of the jasmine _____ in through the open window.

4. Reading, writing, spelling, and pronunciation _____ the lessons in the English class.

5. The school newspaper was the _____ / _____ for making registration announcements. (*Two words can be used here.*)

VOCABULARY EXERCISES

1. Explain the difference between *alternative* and *complementary*.

2. What is the difference between *complementary* and *complimentary*? If you are not sure, ask a native speaker or check your dictionary.

3. Can you give examples for two meanings of the word *medium*?

WORD ATTACK SKILLS

When you find long words that look difficult or impossible to pronounce, look for root words that you recognize and break the word into parts you know, and then put the word back together again.

EXAMPLE: bioelectromagnetic-based

Find and pronounce the words *electro* and *magnet*. Add the pieces to them: bio electro, magnet ic. Practice saying the two new words, *bioelectric* and *magnetic*. Now put those two words together and practice them, then add the word *based*. Now practice the whole word and read it in the sentence: "Bioelectromagnetic-based theories are based on the use of electromagnetic fields." Note: In English, sometimes the stress will change in the new word. Underline the stressed syllable.

Bioelectromagnetic-based *(610)** Bio/electro/magnet/ic-based   BI o e LEC tro mag *NET* ic-BASE d

Contraindications *(607)*

Polarities *(605)*

_____

*Numbers within parentheses indicate page within the text chapter where the word is used.

Student Name_____

PRONUNCIATION OF DIFFICULT TERMS

Directions: Practice pronouncing the following words:

bioelectromagnetic   BI o e LEC tro mag *NET* ic

necessity   ne CESS i ty

efficacy   EFF i cacy

IDIOMATIC USAGE

*(604)**   mainstream—the most commonly accepted opinion or style

                Bilingual education was becoming mainstream for a while.

(604)   well versed—thoroughly understanding

                The nurse was well versed in the use of the stethoscope.

(605)   "Like cures like." Use a substance to cure a problem caused by that substance. For example, some people take a drink of whiskey in the morning to make them feel better after drinking too much whiskey the night before. (This is also sometimes known as using "the hair of the dog that bit them.")

(605)   root cause—the original reason causing something to happen. A systemic infection may be the root cause of recurrent fevers. A love of money is the root cause of many evils.

(605)   "journeys to other planes of existence"—goes into a trance or psychological state where they feel they are talking to other people or are in another place.

(606)   sweat lodge—a small building built by American Indians and used like a steam bath or sauna to cleanse themselves in both body and spirit. Water spilled on hot rocks in the sweat lodge creates steam.

(609)   hot flashes—a sudden sensation of extreme warmth accompanied by perspiration and reddening of the face. Women during menopause often experience hot flashes.

_____

*Numbers within parentheses indicate page within the text chapter where the word is used.

COMMUNICATION EXERCISE

With a partner, practice a dialogue between a nurse and patient cautioning the patient to be sure to inform her doctor that she is using or thinking about using alternative or complementary therapies. Be sure she also knows that she should tell her doctor or pharmacist of any herbal medications she is using, so that they will not conflict with prescribed medications.

CULTURAL POINTS

Ask other classmates what alternative therapies are commonly used in their countries or families. Share any experiences that may have come from those therapies.

Review the chapter key points, answer the study questions, and complete the
critical thinking activities at the end of the chapter in the textbook.

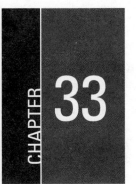

Student Name _____

CHAPTER 33
Pharmacology and Preparation for Drug Administration

Answer Key: Textbook page references are provided as a guide for answering selected questions. A complete answer key was provided for your instructor.

TERMINOLOGY

A. Matching

Directions: Match the terms in Column I with the definitions in Column II.

<table>
<tr><th></th><th></th><th>Column I</th><th></th><th>Column II</th></tr>
<tr><td>(617)</td><td>1.</td><td>_____ anaphylaxis</td><td>a.</td><td>Drug name not protected by trademark</td></tr>
<tr><td>(624)</td><td>2.</td><td>_____ contraindications</td><td>b.</td><td>How drugs enter the body, are metabolized,</td></tr>
<tr><td>(616)</td><td>3.</td><td>_____ degrade</td><td></td><td>reach the site of action, and are excreted</td></tr>
<tr><td>(613)</td><td>4.</td><td>_____ generic</td><td>c.</td><td>Break down</td></tr>
<tr><td>(622)</td><td>5.</td><td>_____ noncompliance</td><td>d.</td><td>Drug's effect on cellular physiology, biology,</td></tr>
<tr><td>(616)</td><td>6.</td><td>_____ pharmacodynamics</td><td></td><td>and its mechanism of action</td></tr>
<tr><td>(615)</td><td>7.</td><td>_____ pharmacokinetics</td><td>e.</td><td>Results of drug action not related to intended</td></tr>
<tr><td>(616)</td><td>8.</td><td>_____ side effects</td><td></td><td>action</td></tr>
<tr><td>(613)</td><td>9.</td><td>_____ trade name</td><td>f.</td><td>Severe allergic reaction</td></tr>
<tr><td>(622)</td><td>10.</td><td>_____ unit dose</td><td>g.</td><td>Not taking drugs as prescribed</td></tr>
<tr><td></td><td></td><td></td><td>h.</td><td>Name protected by trademark</td></tr>
<tr><td></td><td></td><td></td><td>i.</td><td>Reasons not to administer</td></tr>
<tr><td></td><td></td><td></td><td>j.</td><td>Single dose</td></tr>
</table>

B. Completion

Directions: Fill in the blank(s) with the correct term(s) from the terms list in the chapter in the textbook to complete the sentence.

(616) 1. A drug such as an antibiotic is called a(n) _____ because it produces a response.

(616) 2. A drug such as an antihistamine is called a(n) _____ because it blocks a response.

(617) 3. A(n) _____ occurs when one drug interferes with the way the other drug acts when taken alone.

(624) 4. Every drug administered in the agency is entered on the
_____ after it is given.

(613)   5. Knowing the side effects of a drug and how it works helps nurses figure out the _____ of the drug.

(617)   6. Alcohol causes a(n) _____ when consumed while taking a drug that depresses the central nervous system.

(617)   7. Some drugs have a very narrow _____ and if a patient takes an extra pill, toxicity may develop.

(617)   8. Impaired hearing is a(n) _____ of several drugs, including furosemide, a diuretic.

SHORT ANSWER

Directions: Write a brief answer for each question.

(613)   1. Drugs are generally classified by:

   a. _____

   b. _____

   c. _____

(615)   2. General action of drugs in the body is to:

   _____

(622)   3. Patients are often noncompliant in taking their drugs because:

   _____

   _____

(620)   4. Factors that affect how a drug works in a child's body are:

   _____

(620-622)   5. List five things that should be considered when giving medications to an elderly patient:

   a. _____

   b. _____

   c. _____

   d. _____

   e. _____

(622)   6. When medications are prescribed for the home care patient, the nurse should:

   _____

   _____

   _____

(613)   7. In the hospital the responsibility for the security of controlled drugs is _____.

Student Name_____

(614)   8.   For a drug to receive approval by the FDA it must meet standards in these five areas:

     a. _____

     b. _____

     c. _____

     d. _____

     e. _____

(625)   9.   The five rights of drug administration are:

     a. _____

     b. _____

     c. _____

     d. _____

     e. _____

(625)   10.   Information the patient should be taught about each drug includes:

     a. _____

     b. _____

     c. _____

     d. _____

     e. _____

     f. _____

(619)   11.   According to the new medication safety guidelines, the abbreviation "qhs" should not be used and the term _____ should be used instead.

(620)   12.   If an ordered drug dosage seems odd, or the drug ordered does not seem appropriate for the patient, you should:

     _____

(629)   13.   Drugs whose dosages should be checked by another nurse when you prepare them are:

     _____

IDENTIFICATION

Directions: Identify the meaning of each of the following abbreviations and symbols. Write the correct letter in the blank provided for each one.

(Table 33-5)

1.	_____	ac	a.	Intradermal
2.	_____	gtt	b.	Before meals
3.	_____	ID	c.	After meals
4.	_____	OS	d.	Left eye
5.	_____	pc	e.	Without

6.	_____ qs	f.	Drop
7.	_____ s	g.	Immediately
8.	_____ STAT	h.	Three times a day
9.	_____ tid	i.	Quantity sufficient

DRUG KNOWLEDGE

Directions: Using a drug handbook or a pharmacology textbook, look up the drug furosemide and fill in the information requested.

1. Classification: _____

2. Usual PO adult dosage:_____

3. Routes of administration: _____

4. One contraindication:_____

5. When it should be taken: _____

DRUG CALCULATIONS AND CONVERSIONS

Directions: Correctly convert or calculate the answer for each question.

1. 8 g = _____ gr

2. 180 gr = _____ g

3. 5 gr = _____ mg

4. 4.5 gr = _____ g

5. 180 mg = _____ gr

6. You are to give 10 cc of Robitussin. How many teaspoons would this be? _____

7. The patient weighs 54 lbs. You are to administer 70 mg of drug per kg of body weight. How many capsules will you give if each capsule contains 425 mg? _____

8. The order reads: 15 mEq KCl. You have available 30 mL of KCl with 2 mEq/mL. How many mL will you put in the patient's orange juice? _____

9. Vitamin E 400 U is ordered. You have on hand capsules with 200 U each. How many will you give? _____

10. You are to give 10 mg of morphine IM. The vial reads 15 mg/1 mL. How much will you give? _____

APPLICATION OF THE NURSING PROCESS

Directions: Write a brief answer for each question.

(623, 625) 1. C.T. is admitted to your home care agency after her stay in the rehabilitation institute is finished. She has suffered a stroke and has hemiparesis. She has a history of heart disease with

Student Name_____

atrial fibrillation (arrhythmia) and congestive heart failure. She also has osteoarthritis of the knees and hands. What questions would you ask to establish a medication history and find out what medications she is currently taking?

_____

_____

_____

_____

_____

_____

_____

2. What other information would you need in order to manage C.T.'s medication regimen?

_____

_____

_____

_____

_____

_____

3. The physicians believe that C.T. suffered the stroke because she was not taking her medications regularly. What would be the appropriate nursing diagnosis for C.T. regarding her use of medications?

_____

4. Write an expected outcome for this nursing diagnosis.

5. What interventions might you use to assist C.T. in meeting the expected outcome?

_____

_____

_____

_____

6. How would you evaluate whether the expected outcome is being met? Write evaluation statements that would indicate the outcome is being met:

_____

_____

_____

_____

NCLEX-PN® EXAM REVIEW

*Directions: Choose the **best** answer(s) for each of the following questions.*

(623)   1.   Which one of the following orders means to give the medication three times a day after meals?
1.   Ferrous sulfate 10 mg PO tid ac.
2.   Ferrous sulfate 10 mg PO bid pc.
3.   Ferrous sulfate 10 mg PO tid pc.
4.   Ferrous sulfate 10 mg PO bid ac.

2.   Which one of the following forms of a drug will be absorbed the quickest?
1.   capsule
2.   tablet
3.   suspension
4.   ointment

3.   A drug is only totally safe for a pregnant woman to take if it does not (Select all that apply)
1.   enter the mother's bloodstream.
2.   cross the placental barrier.
3.   enter the fetal brain.
4.   have any adverse effect on the mother.

(615)   4.   Drugs are metabolized in different ways in the body. Most drugs are mainly metabolized by the _____

_____.
(Fill in the blank)

(616)   5.   Sufficient fluid intake to eliminate drugs properly is at least
1.   1000 mL/day.
2.   1500 mL/day.
3.   30 mL/kg/day.
4.   50 mL/kg/day.

(616)   6.   The "duration of action" of a drug is the time the drug
1.   takes to be metabolized.
2.   exerts a pharmacological effect.
3.   takes to be excreted.
4.   is OK to take before it is no longer effective.

(617)   7.   Toxic effects of a drug are reached when
1.   the blood level reaches the therapeutic range.
2.   adverse effects occur.
3.   side effects appear.
4.   the blood level rises above the therapeutic range.

(623, 625)   8.   Although the physician orders the drug, before administering the drug the nurse is responsible for determining (Select all that apply)
1.   whether the patient has experienced side effects from the drug.
2.   contraindications for taking the drug.
3.   the reason the drug is prescribed.
4.   whether the dose is within safe limits.

(620-622)   9.   Elderly patients who have arthritis and are taking anti-inflammatory drugs must be monitored for
1.   gastrointestinal bleeding.
2.   orthostatic hypotension.
3.   rapid, irregular pulse.
4.   dehydration.

(629)   10.   Unit dose drugs should be opened for administration
1.   at the bedside.
2.   after the second check of the medication.
3.   in the medication room.
4.   at the medication cart at the patient's door.

Student Name _____

CRITICAL THINKING ACTIVITIES

1. Prepare to teach a patient about taking the drug digoxin. Outline points to cover:

2. Explain to a family member why it is illegal to share prescription tranquilizers with another family member. Outline the points you would make:

3. List the points of assessment that should be completed before a drug is administered to a patient:

MEETING CLINICAL OBJECTIVES

Directions: The following suggested activities will help you meet the stated clinical practice objectives for the chapter. Review your school's clinical objectives for the week and outline a plan of activities that will help you meet them. If you are unsure how to meet them, consult with your instructor at the beginning of the clinical day.

1. Look up three drugs that your assigned patient is taking; pay particular attention to the nursing implications for each drug.

2. Accompany a nurse who is using the unit dose system to administer drugs.

3. Have a staff nurse show you how to correctly obtain and record a controlled substance drug.

4. Teach a patient about a new drug that has been prescribed.

STEPS TOWARD BETTER COMMUNICATION

VOCABULARY BUILDING GLOSSARY

Term	Pronunciation	Definition
categorize	CAT e gor ize	to put into categories, or similar groups
compliant	com PLI ant	willing to do as instructed
decree	de CREE	to make a rule
erroneously	er RON e ous ly	incorrectly, in error
incompatible	in com PAT i ble	do not work well together
readily	READ i ly	quickly and easily
susceptible	sus CEP ti ble	easily affected
tactful	TACT ful	polite, careful, indirect
to be knowledgeable about	to be KNOW ledge able (NAW lej a ble) a BOUT	to know about

COMPLETION

Directions: Fill in the blank(s) with the correct term(s) from the Vocabulary Building Glossary to complete the sentence.

1. Some drugs are _____, especially in the intravenous form, and may not be given together.

2. If a patient is not _____ with the medication schedule at home, you must be _____ when working with her on correcting the problem.

3. A liquid form of a drug is more _____ absorbed by the body.

4. If you do not perform the five rights and check the drug three times before administering it, you may give it _____.

5. If you can _____ an unfamiliar drug and know the action of that drug category, you will know most of the possible side effects of the unfamiliar drug.

WORD ATTACK SKILLS

Directions: Word Families—Look at the meanings of different forms of the words within a word family.

de VISE (dee vīze)	(verb) To think of or figure out a new method or system for doing something
de VICE (dee vïs)	(noun) Something such as a piece of equipment designed for a special purpose
com PLY (verb)	To do as instructed
com PLI ance (noun)	Doing as instructed
com PLI ant (adjective)	One who is doing as instructed
NON com PLI ance (noun)	Not doing what is instructed, not following rules or instructions

Kinetics means movement; therefore, **pharmacokinetics** means movement of drugs through the body.

Dynamics means actions and interactions; therefore, **pharmacodynamics** means the action and interaction of the drug in the body.

PRONUNCIATION OF DIFFICULT TERMS

Directions: Practice pronouncing the following words.

agonist	AG on ist
anaphylaxis	AN a phy LAX is (AN a pha LAX is)
antagonist	an TAG on ist
contraindications	CON tra in di CA tions
efficacy	ef FI ca cy
gastrointestinal	gas tro in TES tin al
noncompliance	NON com PLI ance
pharmacodynamics	PHAR ma co dy NAM ics
pharmacokinetics	PHAR ma co ki NET ics
synergistic	SYN er GIS tic

Student Name_____

GRAMMAR POINTS

Various verb tenses: did you take/have you taken/are you taking

When you are communicating with a patient, it is often very important to know **when** something happens—when the pain or symptom occurs or when the medication was taken. To do this, both you and the patient must understand the time that you are talking about. If you are not sure, clarify by using time words such as yesterday, now, this morning, last night, three o'clock, etc.

Verb Tense or Time	Question	Answer
Simple Present (action is ongoing)	Do you take any medicine? Do you feel any pain?	I take ibuprofen every morning. My knee feels achy.
Present Progressive (action is happening now)	What over-the-counter medicines are you taking?	I am taking ibuprofen for my arthritis.
Simple Past (action completed)	What medicine did you take today?	I took my ibuprofen this morning.
Present Perfect (action has happened before this present time)	Have you taken your medicine this morning? Have you had any pain today?	Yes, I've already taken it. *or* Yes, I took it before breakfast. (Answer may be in the past) No, I haven't had any pain since yesterday.
Present Perfect Progressive (happening from the past up to this present time) Used for telling "how long a time."	How long have you been using ibuprofen? How long has your knee been hurting?	I've been using it for a couple of years now. It has been hurting for about a month.

COMMUNICATION EXERCISES

1. With a partner, prepare to assess an older adult's medication history. Use points for assessment in "Application of the Nursing Process" in this chapter to create a scenario dialogue about assessing what drugs and over-the-counter medicines this older, sometimes forgetful, person is taking. Practice the dialogue together.

2. Develop a script to assess what your patient knows about the drugs he or she is taking (why, when, how many, etc.) and any side effects he or she may be experiencing. Practice with a partner. Use three different common drugs for this exercise.

3. Develop a script that teaches the patient about furosemide.

CULTURAL POINTS

Think about your native culture's attitude toward drugs and medications and try to analyze it. Are the people afraid of medications, or do they expect the doctor to give them something every time they visit? Do they prefer herbal medicine, prescription pills, or injections? How does that compare with what you learned in this chapter?

In the U.S., there is a great reliance on prescription drugs, and belief—sometimes to an adverse degree—that they can cure anything. However, more people are turning to herbal remedies found in health food stores and pharmacies. Popular magazines and newspapers often have articles on the use of herbal medicine, as well as news about drugs being developed. One reason for this increased interest may be the very high cost of drugs in the U.S. as well as movement toward more natural and holistic methods. It should be remembered that herbal remedies may become toxic in high doses or interact with each other and with prescription medications. A drug history must include all types of herbs and medications the patient is taking.

Review the chapter key points, answer the study questions, and complete the
critical thinking activities at the end of the chapter in the textbook.

CHAPTER 34

Administering Oral, Topical, and Inhalant Medications

Answer Key: Textbook page references are provided as a guide for answering selected questions. A complete answer key was provided for your instructor.

TERMINOLOGY

A. Matching

Directions: Match the terms in Column I with the definitions in Column II.

Column I

(649) 1. _____ buccal
(652) 2. _____ cerumen
(654) 3. _____ douche
(654) 4. _____ fornices
(646) 5. _____ meniscus
(649) 6. _____ ophthalmic
(652) 7. _____ otic
(649) 8. _____ sublingual
(637) 9. _____ topical
(654) 10. _____ transdermal

Column II

a. The base of the curvature of liquid medication in a container
b. Under the tongue
c. Through the skin
d. Eye
e. Inner cheek
f. Ear
g. Vaginal irrigation
h. Archlike structures
i. Applied to the skin or mucous membrane
j. Ear wax

B. Abbreviations

Directions: Fill in the correct abbreviation or symbol for the indicated word in the following paragraph.

(Table 33-5)

V.S. is being treated for asthma. Her medications are not adequately controlling her symptoms. The doctor orders a nebulizer treatment for her immediately (_____) to relieve her bronchospasm. He tells her to discontinue the antihistamine she has been taking as it does not seem to be helping. He prescribes oral (_____) montelukast sodium (Singulair) to be taken with water in the evening. He puts her on another metered dose inhaler (_____), triamcinolone acetonide (Azmacort), and tells her to use the new inhaler tid.

SHORT ANSWER

Directions: Write a brief answer for each question.

1. List the possible patient identifiers that may be used for identification purposes when administering medications:

_____

_____

_____

_____

(633)   2. When administering medications, nurses are legally responsible for knowing:

a. _____

b. _____

c. _____

d. _____

e. _____

f. _____

(636)   3. When considering a written drug order's legality, you would check to see that it includes:

a. _____

b. _____

c. _____

d. _____

e. _____

f. _____

g. _____

(635-636)   4. List the correct drug classification for each of the following drug actions:

a. inhibit clotting of blood _____

b. reduce congestion and allergic reactions _____

c. relieve anxiety and promote sleep _____

d. relieve cough_____

e. inhibit the growth of or kill microorganisms_____

f. relieve depression _____

g. increase mental alertness and function _____

h. reduce inflammation and pain _____

(640)   5. The reason the unit-dose medication administration system is considered safer than the prescription system of delivery is that _____

_____.

Student Name_____

(658)   6. Medications that should not be crushed for administration via an enteral feeding tube are:

      a. _____

      b. _____

      c. _____

(645, 661) 7. Three special considerations for administering oral and topical medications to an elderly patient are:

      a. _____

      b. _____

      c. _____

(633)   8. Describe the legal and professional responsibilities of the LPN/LVN related to medication administration.

      _____

      _____

      _____

(649)   9. One method that seems to help an elderly person who has difficulty swallowing to take a pill is to instruct the person to:

      _____

      _____

COMPLETION

Directions: Fill in the blank(s) with the correct word(s) to complete the sentence.

(633)   1. Any medication order that is unclear, incomplete, or ambiguous must be
      _____.

(636)   2. The primary system of measuring medication dosage in the United States is the
      _____ system.

(636-637) 3. It is good practice to check any conversions and calculations for a divided dose with
      _____.

(638)   4. Topical medications are those applied to the _____ or
      _____.

(639)   5. When stat medication orders are written, the medication must be administered
      _____.

(639)   6. Medication orders are automatically canceled whenever a patient undergoes
      _____ or _____.

(639)   7. Medication orders written by the physician are transcribed onto the
      _____ which is used for the actual administration of
each medication.

(639)   8. Medication cards are usually used only with a fixed system of medication administration such as when medications are dispensed from a(n) _____
      or _____.

(641)   9.   Automated controlled dispensing systems are used to monitor and control _____.

(642)   10.   Ointments are used to keep the medication in _____ contact with the skin.

(642)   11.   The difference between a lotion and a liniment is that while a liniment is rubbed into the skin a lotion is _____ the skin.

(642-643) 12.   The most common type of medicinal irrigation is the _____ irrigation.

(642)   13.   Suppositories are a semisolid, cylinder-shaped medication inserted into the _____, _____, or _____, or ostomy _____ on the abdomen.

(645, 647) 14.   When pouring a liquid medication, always read the amount poured at the _____ of the fluid.

(649)   15.   If a sublingual medication is swallowed rather than dissolved under the tongue, the medication becomes totally _____.

APPLICATION OF THE NURSING PROCESS

Directions: Write a brief answer for each question.

(643)   1.   When administering medications, three assessments you should make in addition to following the five rights of medication administration are:

     a.   _____

     b.   _____

     c.   _____

     2.   The patient who is suffering from extended nausea and vomiting would probably be given the nursing diagnosis _____.

(643, 645) 3.   The five goals of medication administration are:

     a.   _____

     b.   _____

     c.   _____

     d.   _____

     e.   _____

(645)   4.   When implementing medication administration, it is best to follow the five rights of medication administration and to check each medication label _____.

(658, 661) 5.   An evaluation statement indicating that antibiotic therapy for a wound infection has been effective might be:

     _____

     _____

Student Name_____

NCLEX-PN® EXAM REVIEW

*Directions: Choose the **best** answer(s) to each of the following questions.*

(646-649) 1. You are assigned to give medications to five patients during your shift. Each patient has more than one medication ordered. When checking each medication while using the unit dose system, you would
1. verify the medication name and dosage and set the dose pack to one side.
2. verify the date, time, medication name, dosage, and route.
3. compare the medication administration sheet with the physician's order sheet before pulling out the medications.
4. verify the medication name and dosage, open the package and place the pill in a medication cup.

(646-649) 2. When performing the necessary medication checks for your patients using the unit dose system, the third check is performed
1. before returning the patient's medication bin or drawer to its place.
2. just before going to the patient's bedside.
3. after identifying the patient and before opening the package.
4. before throwing away the package the pill came in.

(643) 3. Each time you administer medications to one of your patients, in addition to properly identifying the patient by comparing the name and number of the ID band to the imprint on the MAR, you would check the MAR sheet for
1. known allergies.
2. prn medications.
3. patient sex.
4. next dose time.

4. One of your patients requests a prn pain medication. When administering a prn pain medication it is important to check (Select all that apply)
1. side effects of previous doses.
2. date of the order.
3. number of doses given.
4. time last dose was given.

(656) 5. One of your patients needs a rectal suppository. You know to (Select all that apply)
1. warm the suppository before insertion.
2. chill the suppository before insertion if soft.
3. unwrap the suppository before insertion.
4. place the patient in prone position for insertion.

(658, 661) 6. One patient has been receiving an antibiotic for several days. You would evaluate its effectiveness by (Select all that apply)
1. checking the vital sign trends.
2. assessing the blood count for decrease in WBCs.
3. checking for decrease in signs and symptoms of the infection.
4. checking the culture and sensitivity report for the drug's ability to kill the organism.

(652) 7. One patient requires instillation of eye drops. Two safety factors you check when administering eye medications are
1. the medication does not blur the patient's vision or sting.
2. the drops fall directly on the eye and do not run out.
3. "ophthalmic" appears on the bottle and the medication is still in date.
4. the eye is not red and does not have a discharge.

8. An order that reads "1 tablet sub-ling prn chest pain" means
   1. administer one tablet orally.
   2. give one table sublingually each night.
   3. have patient place the tablet under the tongue when chest pain occurs.
   4. place one tablet on the tongue as needed for chest pain.

9. An order that is written, "Erythromycin 300 mg PO tid" means give erythromycin
   1. 300 mg orally three times a day.
   2. 300 mg orally twice a day.
   3. 300 mg at night for three days.
   4. 1 tablet orally three times a day.

10. An order that is written, "Mylanta 15 mL PO pc and nightly" means give Mylanta
    1. 1 ounce before meals and at bedtime.
    2. 15 mL before meals and at bedtime.
    3. 2 teaspoons by mouth after meals and at bedtime.
    4. 15 mL by mouth after meals and at bedtime.

CRITICAL THINKING ACTIVITIES

1. What would you do if you poured up a dose of cough medicine and your patient then tells you she does not need it anymore and refuses to take it?

2. What would you do if your patient tells you that the pill you have for him to take does not look familiar and he wants to know why he is supposed to take it?

3. What would you do if the pill the patient is taking falls from the cup onto his covers as he is trying to put it in his mouth?

MEETING CLINICAL OBJECTIVES

Directions: The following suggested activities will help you meet the stated clinical practice objectives for the chapter. Review your school's clinical objectives for the week and outline a plan of activities that will help you meet them. If you are unsure how to meet them, consult with your instructor at the beginning of the clinical day.

1. Practice giving oral and topical medications using the five rights.

2. Actively seek experience in applying eye medications, transdermal patches, and topical ointments. Tell other nurses on your unit that you would like this experience.

3. Actively seek opportunity to administer a vaginal and rectal suppository or medication.

4. With a staff nurse or your instructor supervising, check out a scheduled (controlled drug) medication.

Student Name _____

STEPS TOWARD BETTER COMMUNICATION

VOCABULARY BUILDING GLOSSARY

Term	Pronunciation	Definition
ambiguous	am BIG u ous	not clear, uncertain
deviation	DE vi A tion	a change, or doing something different than planned
potent	PO tent	powerful, strong

COMPLETION

Directions: Fill in the blanks with the correct terms from the Vocabulary Building Glossary above to complete the sentence.

This is a very _____ drug. The directions for using it are

_____, so we had better check with the doctor. I do not want to make

any _____ from his plans.

WORD ATTACK SKILLS

In English, there are many small words that have important functions in communication and meaning, but are not pronounced clearly or distinctly in conversation. They are often shortened and run together with other words. The non-native English speaker may not even hear the sound and may miss some important meaning. The native English speaker usually understands the meaning, but sometimes must ask for clarification.

Contractions of the negative and the verb "to be" are very common in informal speech and written communication. Common examples are:

I am = I'm, he is = he's, you are = you're, we are = we're

Common examples of negative contractions are:

cannot = can't, will not = won't, is not = isn't, did not = didn't

When native English speakers are not sure what they hear, they will say, "Did you say you can or cannot go?"

There are other contractions in sound that occur only with pronunciation and are not written. Because they are spoken so quickly and softly by the native speaker, the English learner often does not even hear them, but they are important to the meaning.

Following are some examples of short words and pronouns that are often reduced in sound, and the way they may sound in common speech:

and	I will have bread and butter. You are up bright and early!	I'll have bread 'n' butter. You're up bright 'n' early!
or	Are you coming or going? Do you want tea or coffee?	Are ya coming 'r' going? Do ya want tea 'r' coffee?
as	Your hands are as cold as ice!	They're 'z cold uz ice!

to	I need to go to the bathroom.	I need t'go t'the bathroom.
	Let's walk to the bed	Le's walk t'th'bed.
can	Can you stand up?	C'n ya stand up?
	I don't think I can do it.	I don't think I c'n do it.
will	You will feel better tomorrow.	You'll feel better t'morrow.
	This will help you sleep.	This'll help ya sleep.
do	How do you do?	How d'ya do?
	Do you want me to raise the rail?	D'ya want me t'raise the rail?
them	Where do you want them?	Where d'ya want 'em?
	I can't find them.	I can't find 'em.
a, an	Could you help me give him a bath?	Could ya help me give'm 'bath?
	It has only been an hour.	It's only been 'n hour.
have	You were supposed to have taken your medications an hour ago.	You're supposed to've taken y'r meds 'n hour ago.
	What have you done with my clothes?	What've ya done with m'clothes?

When you are speaking with an elderly person, one who has a hearing loss, or a non-native English speaker, you will need to speak carefully, slowly, and distinctly to make sure he or she understands you. If you are a non-native English speaker, you will also need to listen carefully to know what the person is saying. You may have to ask him or her to repeat or clarify by repeating what you think you understood. The person can correct you if you were wrong.

COMMUNICATION EXERCISES

1. Practice saying the sentences above with careful pronunciation and then with the contracted pronunciation. Can you hear and feel the difference?

2. Pick a spot where you can listen to people in conversation, like a seat in the cafeteria, near a telephone, or where friends are talking while waiting for class to begin. Listen carefully to what the native English speakers are saying, and see if you can tell what sounds are omitted or substituted. Can you understand what they are saying? Can you supply in your head the words that were reduced? Write five of the reduced words you heard here.

PRONUNCIATION OF DIFFICULT TERMS

Directions: Practice pronouncing the following words.

buccal	BUC cal (BUC cle)
cerumen	ce RU men
fornix, fornices	FOR nix, FOR ni CES (plural)

Review the chapter key points, answer the study questions, and complete the critical thinking activities at the end of the chapter in the textbook.

CHAPTER

35 Administering Intradermal, Subcutaneous, and Intramuscular Injections

Answer Key: Textbook page references are provided as a guide for answering selected questions. A complete answer key was provided for your instructor.

TERMINOLOGY

A. Matching

Directions: Match the terms in Column I with the definitions in Column II.

		Column I		Column II
(664)	1.	_____ ampule	a.	Small bottle
(667)	2.	_____ bevel	b.	Formation of fibrous tissue
(666)	3.	_____ bleb	c.	Scale of measurement
(668)	4.	_____ cannula	d.	Visible elevation of the epidermis
(672)	5.	_____ core	e.	Hollow shaft
(672)	6.	_____ diluent	f.	Red, elevated wheals
(665)	7.	_____ fibrosis	g.	Glass container of medication
(666)	8.	_____ gauge	h.	Opening or interior diameter
(684)	9.	_____ gluteal	i.	Solid material or particles
(667)	10.	_____ lumen	j.	Fluid to dissolve solute
(672)	11.	_____ solute	k.	Pertaining to the buttocks (muscle)
(689)	12.	_____ urticaria	l.	Sticky or gummy
(664)	13.	_____ vial	m.	Small circular piece at the center
(668)	14.	_____ viscous	n.	Slanted part of needle tip

B. Completion

Directions: Fill in the blank(s) with the correct word(s) to complete the sentence.

(676) 1. Skin testing for reaction to various substances is performed using a(n) _____ injection.

(689) 2. If a patient is allergic to the medication, an injection may cause _____.

(665) 3. Medications that are given by injection are termed _____ medications as they do not enter the gastrointestinal tract.

(689) 4. Medications such as hydroxyzine pamoate (Vistaril) should be given by the _____ method of injection because it is very irritating to subcutaneous tissue.

(666)   5.   Very small amounts of medication such as adrenalin (Epinephrine) are given with a(n) _____ syringe.

(666)   6.   Absorption time for the medication given by _____ injection is slower than that given intramuscularly.

(674)   7.   When mixing two medications together in the same syringe, you must first check drug _____.

(666)   8.   A(n) _____ injection is administered at a 90 degree angle.

SHORT ANSWER

Directions: Write a brief answer for each question.

(665)   1.   Parenteral routes are used for medication administration for the following three reasons.

     a. _____

     b. _____

     c. _____

(665)   2.   When administering a parenteral injection, the nurse must take the following precautions:

     a. _____

     b. _____

     c. _____

(666)   3.   The preferred sites for subcutaneous injections are:

     _____

     _____

(679)   4.   Heparin is given subcutaneously in the _____ sites.

(681)   5.   When giving insulin and heparin, do not _____ before injecting the medication.

(683)   6.   An intramuscular injection can be safely given in the following sites:

     a. _____

     b. _____

     c. _____

     d. _____

     e. _____

(665)   7.   When patients are receiving repeated injections, you should _____.

(688)   8.   To clear the needle of medication and to keep medication from flowing back up into the subcutaneous tissues, _____ technique is often used for intramuscular injections.

Student Name_____

(688)   9. When giving injections to children it is important to provide
_____ before, during, and after the injection.

(689) 10. Z-track method of injection is used for medications that are very
_____ to the tissue.

(689) 11. Symptoms of anaphylactic shock include:

_____

_____

(685) 12. When administering an intramuscular injection, it is essential to
_____ before injecting to avoid
_____.

(666) 13. When a 5/8" needle is used for a subcutaneous injection, the angle of injection should be
_____.

(666) 14. Up to _____ mL of solution can be injected for an intramuscular injection safely.

(668) 15. When withdrawing medication from an ampule, a(n) _____
needle should be used.

(667) 16. Tuberculin syringes are calibrated to measure _____ of
a mL for giving very small doses.

(674) 17. Typical diluents for mixing drugs are _____ and
_____.

(674-675) 18. Because injected medications are irretrievable, it is especially important to check for
_____ before giving the injection.

(666) 19. Regarding absorption, _____ solutions are absorbed
more rapidly than those in a(n) _____ suspension.

(669) 20. Safety syringes are used to prevent _____ and the possibility of _____ illness.

(687) 21. Factors to consider when giving an intramuscular injection to an elderly patient are:

_____

_____

CORRELATION

Directions: Indicate the type of injection in Column II that correlates with the item in Column I.
(666-668)

Column I

1. _____ 1 1/2" 20 ga. needle
2. _____ 1/4" 27 ga. needle
3. _____ TB syringe with 1/4" needle
4. _____ must form a bleb
5. _____ placed in tissue above the muscle layer
6. _____ may be placed in the gluteus medius
7. _____ 3 cc of medication
8. _____ 20 U of U 100 insulin
9. _____ 5,000 U of heparin sodium
10. _____ tuberculin test

Column II

a. Intradermal injection
b. Subcutaneous
c. Intramuscular injection

APPLICATION OF THE NURSING PROCESS

Directions: Write a brief answer for each of the following questions.

(674-676) 1. Besides carefully checking the medication with the order before administration, list three patient assessments that should be made.

a. _____

b. _____

c. _____

(676) 2. R.O. has vomited several times. The physician orders an antiemetic for him. What might be an appropriate nursing diagnosis for this patient related to this situation?

_____

(676) 3. Write an expected outcome for the chosen nursing diagnosis.

_____

4. Indicate three nursing interventions that could be implemented along with giving the antiemetic medication to ease R.O.'s nausea and prevent vomiting.

a. _____

b. _____

c. _____

5. Write an evaluation statement that would indicate the expected outcome is being attained.

_____

Student Name _____

NCLEX-PN® EXAM REVIEW

*Directions: Choose the **best** answer(s) for each of the following questions.*

(669) 1. If the order reads "75 mg meperidine, 25 mg Promethazine IM on call," which syringe and needle would be the best choice for the injection if the patient is a normal-sized adult? Each medication is supplied with 50 mg/mL.
1. 2 mL syringe with 23 gauge 1" needle
2. 3 mL syringe with 20 gauge 2" needle
3. 3 mL syringe with 22 gauge 1 1/2" needle
4. 3 mL syringe with 23 gauge 5/8" needle

(666) 2. Heparin sodium 5,000 SC is ordered for an average-sized adult. Using a 25 gauge, 5/8" needle this medication should be injected at a(n) _____ angle. (Fill in the blank)

(690) 3. The proper technique for administering a Z-track injection is to
1. insert the needle at a 45 degree slant.
2. use a 3" needle at a 45 degree slant.
3. insert the needle at a 90 degree angle and pull the tissue laterally before removing the needle.
4. pull the tissue at the site laterally, then insert the needle at a 90 degree angle.

(673) 4. When drawing up medication from a vial, you would
1. hold the vial at a 15 degree angle, stopper down.
2. hold the vial absolutely vertically.
3. Inject an equivalent amount of air into the vial for the medication to be withdrawn.
4. with the vial stopper up, inject at least 1 mL of air before withdrawing the medication.

(666) 5. A sign that an intradermal injection has been successfully given is when
1. a pale area 1/2" in diameter occurs at the site.
2. a small bleb is evident at the injection site.
3. a reddened wheal occurs at the injection site.
4. an area of erythema occurs within 4 hours at the site.

(668) 6. When drawing medication from a glass ampule, a filter needle should be used because
1. fragments of glass could be in the medication.
2. ampules often contain precipitate material.
3. the medication and the diluent may not be thoroughly mixed.
4. the filter thoroughly mixes the medication upon injection.

7. If a patient begins to show signs of anaphylactic shock after an injection is given, you would call for help and (Select all that apply)
1. administer a corticosteroid injection.
2. transfer the patient to the critical care unit.
3. maintain an open airway and respiration.
4. stay with the patient while seeking assistance.

(687) 8. When using the leg for an intramuscular injection, the area landmarks include
1. the head of the greater trochanter.
2. the posterior iliac spine.
3. a hand's breadth below the end of the greater trochanter.
4. a hand's breadth below the groin crease.

(666)   9. Different types of injection cause solutions to be absorbed at different rates. The advantage of a subcutaneous injection over an intramuscular injection is that the solution is absorbed more _____. (Fill in the blank)

(674)   10. Many things can happen when drugs are mixed in a syringe. Adverse consequences may be (Select all that apply)
1. a change in color.
2. formation of a precipitate.
3. rendering of one or both medications inactive.
4. formation of an abscess at the injection site.

CRITICAL THINKING ACTIVITIES

1. If you are asked to give an injection to a patient at a place distant from a sharps biohazard container, what would you do with the syringe and exposed needle?

2. If you have drawn up a pain medication for a patient and then before you administer it the patient decides he does not want it after all (he wants pills instead), what would you do?

3. When do you perform the three checks of medication for your injectable medications? Be specific.

4. Describe how to correctly draw up two insulins in a syringe.

MEETING CLINICAL OBJECTIVES

Directions: The following suggested activities will help you meet the stated clinical practice objectives for the chapter. Review your school's clinical objectives for the week and outline a plan of activities that will help you meet them. If you are unsure how to meet them, consult with your instructor at the beginning of the clinical day.

1. Practice giving the various types of injections using a mannequin or injection pad in the skill laboratory if possible. If a skill laboratory is not available, practice drawing up and giving injections using an orange or rubber ball at home.

2. Practice palpating bony landmarks and correctly finding injection sites for all types of injections on five different people of varying sizes and weights.

3. Seek injection experience in the clinical setting by telling the nurses on the unit at the beginning of the day that you want injection experience.

4. Ask to be assigned to the outpatient surgery or ER department to obtain injection practice.

5. Correctly reconstitute drugs, draw up medications, and give all types of injections in the clinical area.

6. Combine two types of insulin and correctly administer the injection.

7. Follow standard precautions at all times.

8. Properly document injections administered.

Student Name_____

STEPS TOWARD BETTER COMMUNICATION

VOCABULARY BUILDING GLOSSARY

Term	Pronunciation	Definition
A. Individual Terms		
aqueous	A que ous (À' kwee us)	watery; prepared with water
apprehensive	AP re HEN sive	concerned or worried about something that is going to happen
beveled	BEV eled	slanted
calibrated	CAL i bra ted	measured exactly
compatible	com PAT i ble	capable of working together
dexterity	dex TER i ty	skill with your hands
hasten	HAs ten (hÀ' sen)	to hurry, to make occur more quickly
induration	IN du RA tion	hardening; an abnormally hard spot
reconstituted	RE con sti TU ted	renewed; returned to its original state (by adding liquid)
scored	SCORed	marked with a line that allows accurate breaking apart
vial	VI al	a small bottle
B. Phrases		
sloughing off	SLOUGH ing (SLUFF ing) off	shedding, falling off
needle stick	NEED le stick	process of sticking with a needle as in giving an injection; needle going through the skin

COMPLETION

Directions: Fill in the blank(s) with the correct term(s) from the Vocabulary Building Glossary above to complete the sentence.

1. Most injectable medications are prepared as a(n) _____ solution.

2. Many antibiotics come as a powder and must be correctly _____.

3. Injection needles have a(n) _____ tip to make going through the skin smoother and less painful.

4. It requires a certain amount of _____ to smoothly give an injection.

5. When medications are mixed in a syringe, they must be _____.

6. Many injectable medications now come in a unit-dose _____.

7. The majority of patients are at least a little _____ when they are to receive an injection.

8. The nurse must be careful not to cause a _____ to him- or herself when giving an injection to a patient.

Directions: Now for fun, substitute words from the Vocabulary Building Glossary for the underlined words in the following sentences.

1. The snake had <u>shed</u> its skin and the small boy picked it up <u>skillfully</u> and put it in a <u>small bottle</u> to keep it.

2. The woman was <u>worried</u> about drinking the <u>watery</u> lemonade, which had been <u>made</u> from a powder.

3. The pitcher had been <u>marked</u> and <u>measured</u> exactly.

4. The parents <u>hurried</u> to take the child to the doctor when they felt the <u>hard lump</u> on his leg.

5. The <u>slanted edge</u> of the mirrors <u>looked good</u> with the modern furniture in the room.

WORD ATTACK SKILLS

The words *vital, viable,* and *vial* look like they all come from the same root word. In fact, vital and viable do come from the same Latin roots (vitalis—of life, vita—life, vivere—to live), while vial comes from the Latin- and Greek-rooted word *phial.* (The "ph" and "v" sounds are very similar.) No wonder English is so difficult!

PRONUNCIATION OF DIFFICULT TERMS

Directions: Practice pronouncing the following words.

anaphylactic	an a phy LAC tic
diluent	DIL u ent
ecchymosis	EC chy MO sis
erythema	ER y THE ma
Mantoux	MAN toux (man' too)
parenteral	pa REN ter al
subcutaneous	SUB cu TA ne ous
tuberculin	tu BER cu lin
urticaria	UR ti CA ri a
viscous	VIS cous

COMMUNICATION EXERCISE

Write a script requesting experience in injection practice either from a nurse in a clinical setting or in out-patient surgery as suggested in the Clinical Activities 3 and 4 above. Be sure to clarify when and where you should go for the practice and whether you need to bring anything with you. Practice the dialogue with another student, then actually make the request. Were you satisfied with what you said and how you were understood? What would you do differently next time?

Student Name_____

GRAMMAR POINTS

Time Clauses

Sometimes it is necessary to explain a relationship in time between two events:

I was walking up the stairs when I fell.

This sentence is made up of a main (or independent) clause (I was walking up the stairs) and a dependent clause (when I fell).

- Time clauses begin with a time word such as when/while, before, and after.
- Time clauses have a subject and a verb like an independent clause.
- A time clause must be attached to a main clause to complete its meaning.

Main clause (can be used alone)	Time clause (must be used with a main clause)
1. I was walking up the stairs	when I fell.
2. D.M. learned to give himself injections	while he was in the hospital.
3. M.L. was eating	when her sister arrived.
4. The patient felt better	after she received the injection.
5. She was having a lot of pain	before the nurse gave her the injection.

- The time clause can come before or after the main clause. The meaning is the same.
- When the time clause comes first, it is followed by a comma.
  Before she had lunch, she took her medication.

A. Use the five sentences above. Write the sentences putting the time clause first.

B. Write five sentences of your own using time clauses. Check with a native speaker to see if the sentences are correct.

CULTURAL POINTS

Asking Questions

Teachers and employers in the United States are usually very happy to have their students and employees ask questions; in fact, they encourage it because it shows an interest in the subject or the job and a desire to understand, learn, and to do things correctly. The only time a superior or colleague might object to questions is when you have not studied or read the material or instructions and are taking the easy way to get the information by asking someone to give it to you. If you do not understand something, it is very important that you ask and people will usually be happy to help explain. It often will save a company time and money to have the employee understand the correct way to do something. In the health care field, it can often save lives as well.

Asking questions and double or triple checking is especially important when administering medications. If you do not understand how to measure or administer a medication, be sure to ask. Your supervisors and co-workers, and especially the patients, will appreciate your care and concern.

Review the chapter key points, answer the study questions, and complete the critical thinking activities at the end of the chapter in the textbook.

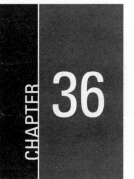

CHAPTER 36

Administering Intravenous Solutions and Medications

Answer Key: Textbook page references are provided as a guide for answering selected questions. A complete answer key was provided for your instructor.

TERMINOLOGY

A. Matching

Directions: Match the terms in Column I with the definitions in Column II.

	Column I		Column II
(718)	1. _____ antineoplastic	a.	Slow introduction of fluid into a vein
(718)	2. _____ autologous	b.	Tube-like chamber that will hold 100 mL of fluid
(704)	3. _____ bore		
(698)	4. _____ burette	c.	Puncture of a vein
(702)	5. _____ embolus (catheter)	d.	Introduction of blood components into the bloodstream
(694)	6. _____ infusion		
(701)	7. _____ lumens	e.	Channels within a tube
(698)	8. _____ transfusion	f.	Piece of catheter that has broken off and is obstructing blood flow
(705)	9. _____ venipuncture		
		g.	Internal diameter
		h.	Related to self (own)
		i.	Destroy or alter growth of malignant cells

B. Completion

Directions: Fill in the blank(s) with the correct term(s) from the terms list in the chapter in the textbook to complete the sentence.

(696) 1. The IV solution $D_5 1/2$ NS is _____ and will pull fluid into the vascular compartment.

(696) 2. The IV solution 0.45% saline is a(n) _____ solution and allows fluid to be drawn from the vascular space into the tissues.

(696) 3. Ringer's lactate IV solution is _____ and keeps fluids stable within the body.

(699) 4. When the IV will not continue to flow, chances are that the site has

_____ .

(698)   5.   _____ tubing is used to infuse viscous IV solutions and delivers 10 gtt/mL.

(698)   6.   When an IV must run very slowly, _____ tubing is used that delivers 60 drops per mL.

(701)   7.   In order for intravenous fluids to be infused, a(n) _____ must be in place.

SHORT ANSWER

Directions: Write a brief answer for each question.

(694)   1.   Four purposes for administering intravenous therapy are to:

   a.   _____

   b.   _____

   c.   _____

   d.   _____

(706)   2.   List the seven guidelines related to intravenous therapy in order of priority from the most important to the least important.

   a.   _____

   b.   _____

   c.   _____

   d.   _____

   e.   _____

   f.   _____

   g.   _____

(702-703)   3.   Four responsibilities of the nurse when caring for a patient undergoing IV therapy are:

   a.   _____

   b.   _____

   c.   _____

   d.   _____

(702)   4.   Signs of IV infiltration are:

   _____

(703)   5.   Describe corrective actions to be taken for each of the following complications of IV therapy.

   a.   infiltration _____

   _____

   b.   phlebitis _____

   _____

Student Name_____

    c.   speed shock_____

          _____

    d.   circulatory overload _____

          _____

    e.   air embolus_____

          _____

(723)   6. Signs and symptoms of a blood transfusion reaction are:

          _____

          _____

          _____

(723)   7. Describe actions to be taken if a transfusion reaction occurs.

          _____

          _____

(695)   8. The average adult needs _____ mL of fluids in a 24-hour period to replace fluids lost by elimination.

(720)   9. An intravenous solution of D_5W provides _____ calories.

(696)   10. When selecting an IV solution, it should be inverted 2–3 times and inspected for _____.

(698)   11. When setting the rate of flow for an IV infusion, the _____ must be checked for the tubing before calculating the flow rate.

(698)   12. The advantage of the IV piggyback system attached to the main IV infusion for medication administration is that _____.

(698)   13. The only intravenous fluid used in conjunction with blood administration is _____.

(698-699) 14. Intermittent intravenous devices are used for patients who:

    a.   _____

    b.   _____

(699)   15. When an intermittent intravenous device is in place it must be _____ regularly.

(699)   16. When infusing fluids by infusion pump, the pump should be checked for proper function at least every _____.

(700)   17. The three types of short-term intravenous cannulas inserted into a peripheral vein are:

    a.   _____

    b.   _____

    c.   _____

(701)   18. A central venous catheter is positioned in the _____ or the right _____.

(701) 19. A PICC catheter is used when the type of IV therapy requires a(n) _____.

(701) 20. When a PICC or MLC is in place in an extremity, you must not _____ on that arm.

(701) 21. A rule regarding subclavian central lines is that: _____

(701) 22. When an infusion port is in place, only _____ needles are used to infuse solutions.

(704) 23. IV fluids for adults are best administered at a rate of _____ mL/hour.

(705) 24. When the vein chosen for an IV site is not easily palpable, it may be necessary to: _____

(710) 25. When choosing an IV insertion site, the rule is to pick the most _____.

(714) 26. A medication that is **never** given as an IV bolus is _____.

(699) 27. To ensure you are meeting the JCAHO 2003 National Safety Goals regarding IV pump alarms, when your patient has an IV pump you should: _____

APPLICATION OF THE NURSING PROCESS

Directions: Write a brief answer for each question.

(702-703) 1. Four assessment responsibilities of the nurse when the patient is undergoing intravenous therapy are:

    a. _____
    b. _____
    c. _____
    d. _____

(703) 2. Two very important assessments to make before starting the infusion of an IV medication are:

    a. _____
    b. _____

(703) 3. One nursing diagnosis that is appropriate for every patient who is receiving an intravenous infusion is: _____

(704) 4. An expected outcome for the patient who is receiving intravenous fluids because of NPO status would be: _____

Student Name _____

(704) 5. Implementation of intravenous therapy requires calculation of IV flow rates. Calculate the correct flow rate for the following IV orders:

    a. 1000 mL D_5RL at 125 mL/hr. Drop factor: 15 gtt/mL
        Correct flow rate: _____

    b. 250 mL D_5W with 20 mEq potassium chloride over 3 hours. Drop factor: 60 gtt/mL
        Correct flow rate: _____

    c. 1000 mL NS q10h. Drop factor 15 gtt/mL
        Correct flow rate: _____

    d. 1000 cc $D_5$1/2 NS q8h. Drop factor 10 gtt/mL
        Correct flow rate: _____

    e. 500 cc D_5W at 80 cc/hr. Drop factor 10 gtt/mL
        Correct flow rate: _____

(710-711) 6. Managing IV therapy means keeping the IV solution running. When at the bedside, you would observe:

    a. _____

    b. _____

    c. _____

    d. _____

(723) 7. Evaluation data that would indicate that intravenous fluid infusion is hydrating the patient would be:

_____

(723) 8. When a blood product is given by intravenous infusion, evaluation criteria indicating success of the transfusion would be:

_____

NCLEX-PN® EXAM REVIEW

*Directions: Choose the **best** answer(s) for each of the following questions.*

(710) 1. Your patient is to receive intravenous therapy for at least a week. If all of the following sites are suitable, which is the preferred site in this situation?
    1. the antecubital space
    2. the plantar aspect of the lower arm
    3. the dorsum of the hand
    4. above the wrist and below the elbow

(711) 2. The order for the patient reads "D_5W 1000 cc to follow the container that is hanging presently." There are 50 mL left in the container hanging. You should
    1. hang the new container now before the old one runs dry.
    2. wait until another 25 mL have infused before hanging the new container.
    3. hang the new container when the remaining fluid has infused.
    4. hang the new container when there are 10 mL left in the container.

(704) 3. The next IV order for the patient reads "1000 cc D_5W with 20 mEq of KCl to run over 10 hours." The drop factor is 10 gtt/mL. The correct flow rate per minute is _____ gtt/min. (Fill in the blank)

(705) 4. The patient complains that the IV site is stinging. It is not reddened or warm to the touch. He has been up and about and the flow rate has increased from where it was set. You should first
   1. stop the infusion.
   2. take the vital signs.
   3. reset the drip rate.
   4. change the IV site.

(700) 5. The patient will need intravenous therapy for at least a week. You would change the IV cannula every
   1. 24 hours.
   2. 48–72 hours.
   3. 12 hours.
   4. 4 days.

(705) 6. While checking on the patient, you see that his IV is not running. To troubleshoot you might (Select all that apply)
   1. lower the container to see if there is a blood return.
   2. discontinue the infusion and restart at a new IV site.
   3. undo the dressing and rotate the needle or cannula.
   4. attempt to aspirate a clot from the IV cannula.

(714) 7. The patient's IV is changed to an intermittent intravenous access for antibiotic administration. You go to hang a piggyback and the first thing you do is
   1. attach the tubing to the PRN device.
   2. flush the cannula with normal saline.
   3. change the IV site to the other hand.
   4. set the flow rate for the piggyback infusion.

(714-715) 8. After the piggyback infusion is finished, you would first
   1. flush the cannula with normal saline.
   2. attach the next piggyback medication tubing.
   3. disconnect the piggyback tubing.
   4. cleanse the port on the PRN device with alcohol.

(704) 9. Your patient is receiving TPN through a central line. His TPN solution is behind schedule when you come on duty. You would
   1. increase the flow rate to "catch up."
   2. leave the flow rate alone.
   3. notify the physician that the solution is behind schedule.
   4. adjust the flow rate to that which is ordered.

(487) 10. During the first several days of TPN administration, it is especially important to check the patient's
   1. urine output.
   2. mental status.
   3. electrolyte status.
   4. blood glucose level.

Student Name_____

CRITICAL THINKING ACTIVITIES

1. Your elderly patient needs a peripheral IV started. Although his vein was difficult to stabilize, you attempted to insert the cannula. You were unsuccessful. What can you do to ensure the best chance of success with the next attempt?

2. Your patient's peripheral IV has stopped running. There is no redness, edema, or pain at the IV site. What steps would you take to assess and reestablish patency of the site?

3. You meet resistance when you try to flush your patient's PRN lock. What would you do?

MEETING CLINICAL OBJECTIVES

Directions: The following suggested activities will help you meet the stated clinical practice objectives for the chapter. Review your school's clinical objectives for the week and outline a plan of activities that will help you meet them. If you are unsure how to meet them, consult with your instructor at the beginning of the clinical day.

1. If a skill laboratory is available:
   a. practice changing IV fluid containers with a peer observing your technique. Practice until you are comfortable with the procedure.
   b. practice adding medications to an IV fluid container and calculating the flow rate. Have a peer observe the procedure.
   c. practice adjusting the flow rate with the roller clamp. Practice until you can smoothly and quickly adjust the rate.

2. For each assigned clinical patient who has an IV, calculate the flow rate from the order sheet.

3. Have a staff nurse or your instructor show you how to set up an IV infusion pump.

4. Go with a staff nurse whenever he or she goes to "troubleshoot" an infusion pump.

5. Seek opportunities to change IV solutions in the clinical setting by telling the nurses on the unit that you desire this experience and asking them to call you whenever a solution is to be changed while you are there. Remember to check the order yourself and to follow the five rights.

6. Observe other nurses starting IV lines in the clinical setting. Practice IV starts in the skill lab using an IV arm or seek this practice through the clinical facility education department.

7. Ask for experience in helping to monitor a patient receiving a blood product.

STEPS TOWARD BETTER COMMUNICATION

VOCABULARY BUILDING GLOSSARY

Term	Pronunciation	Definition
A. Individual Terms		
ascertain	as cer TAIN	make certain, find out for sure
chevron	CHEV ron	a wide "V" shape
discrepancy	dis CREP an cy	errors; things that do not match or fit
mimic	MIM ic	to look and act like

runaway	RUN a way	out of control, going too fast
taut	TAUT	tight, under tension
tonicity	to NI ci ty	state of tissue tone or tension; referring to body fluid pressure/ concentration

B. Phrases

criss cross	CRISS cross	make an "X" shape
piggyback	PIG gy BACK	something riding (or following) on another larger, more powerful object (or idea); example: a child riding on her father's shoulders
rule of thumb	RULE of THUMB	a general guideline that applies in most cases

COMPLETION

A. Directions: Fill in the blank(s) with the correct term(s) from the Vocabulary Building Glossary to complete the sentence.

1. Intravenous antibiotics are administered by _____, where a small bag of medication is added to the main IV line.

2. When the patient complains of soreness at an IV site, you must do your best to _____ what the problem is.

3. Proper documentation of each dose of medication administered prevents any _____ between what was given and the charges from the pharmacy.

4. A(n) _____ concerning an IV that has stopped running is that you never irrigate the cannula as this might force a clot into the bloodstream.

5. A(n) _____ IV fluid may cause fluid overload and is especially dangerous for an infant or an older adult.

B. Directions: Replace the underlined general vocabulary word with a word from the Vocabulary Building Glossary.

1. She followed the <u>guideline</u> in placing the <u>X's and V's</u> and <u>made sure</u> there were no <u>errors</u>.

2. The little boy <u>copied</u> his sister and carried his doll <u>on his</u> <u>shoulders</u>.

3. The nerves of the mother of the <u>out of control</u> juvenile were <u>under tension</u>.

PRONUNCIATION OF DIFFICULT TERMS

Directions: Practice pronouncing the following words.

antineoplastic	AN ti NE o PLAS tic
autologous	au TOL o gous
osmolality	os mo LAL i ty
subclavian	sub CLA vi an

Student Name _____

GRAMMAR POINTS

In order to clearly understand what patients and co-workers mean, learning the differences in past tenses is vitally important.

Past Time Clauses: Meaning and Order

Dependent time clauses using *when, while, before,* and *after* were discussed in Chapter 35. They describe the relationship in time between two events. The past time clause helps us understand which event happened first and which happened second.

Both Verbs in Simple Past

- If both verbs are in the simple past, the action in the when and after clause happened first. (It does not matter where the clause appears in the sentence.)

First Action	*Second Action*
When she received the IV,	her condition improved.
After her condition improved,	she went home.

First Action	*Second Action*
Her condition improved	**when she received the IV.**
She went home	**after her condition improved.**

- The action in a before clause happened second: (The order in the sentence does not matter.)

First Action	*Second Action*
He went home	**before his wound healed.**
His wound healed	**before he went home.**

Second Action	*First Action*
Before his wound healed,	he went home.

One Verb in Simple Past, One in Past Continuous/Progressive

- In *when* or *while* sentences, when one verb is in the simple past and one is in the past continuous (was ...-ing), **the action in the past continuous always starts first and lasts longer:**

First Action	*Second Action*
The fluid was infusing correctly	**when I left the room.**
While the fluid was infusing correctly,	**I left the room.**

First Action	*Second Action*
When I left the room,	the fluid was infusing correctly.

- Both *while* and *when* can introduce a past continuous time clause that means *during the time.*

First Action	*Second Action*
The nurse assessed the patient	**while she was taking vital signs.**

Both Verbs in Past Continuous

- When both verbs are in the past continuous, the activities are happening at the same time (simultaneously) in *while* or *when* sentences:

First Action	*Second Action*
The nurse was assessing the IV site	**while she was taking vital signs.**
While the solution was infusing,	the patient was sleeping comfortably.

Directions: Underline the action that was happening first.

1. The nurse observed the patient while checking the IV.

2. She checked the level of fluid remaining in the bag before disconnecting it.

3. The intravenous solution was leaking out of the bag when the patient pushed the call button.

4. Before making the subcutaneous pocket, the surgeon entered the subclavian vessel.

***Review the chapter key points, answer the study questions, and complete the
critical thinking activities at the end of the chapter in the textbook.***

CHAPTER 37

Care of the Surgical Patient

Answer Key: Textbook page references are provided as a guide for answering selected questions. A complete answer key was provided for your instructor.

TERMINOLOGY

A   Matching

Directions: Match the terms in Column I with the definitions in Column II.

Column I	Column II
(728) 1. _____ anesthesia	a. Voluntary
(729) 2. _____ autologous	b. To relieve pain or complication without curing
(726) 3. _____ elective	c. Care from decision to have surgery through the recovery period
(727) 4. _____ laser	d. Light amplification by the stimulated emission of radiation
(726) 5. _____ palliative	e. Loss of sensory perception
(727) 6. _____ perioperative care	f. Own; originating within an individual
(731) 7. _____ prosthesis	g. Artificial body part
(732) 8. _____ stasis	h. Stoppage of flow

B.   Completion

Directions: The following terms relate to complications of surgery. Briefly describe the complication.

(739)   1. Atelectasis _____

_____

(750)   2. Dehiscence _____

_____

(750)   3. Embolus _____

_____

(750)   4. Evisceration _____

_____

(751)   5. Hemorrhage _____

_____

(746)   6. Hypostatic pneumonia _____

_____

(750)   7. Aspiration pneumonia _____

_____

(746)   8. Thrombosis _____

_____

(750)   9. Thrombophlebitis _____

_____

C. Combining

Directions: Combine the correct suffix with the correct stem to complete each sentence correctly. Consult Table 37-1 and the appendix "Medical Terminology" at the back of the textbook or use your medical dictionary.

-ectomy   mammo-

-oma   orchio-

-ostomy   fibr-

-otomy   col-

-plasty   cholecyst-

-pexy   thorac-

1. A(n) _____ is the creation of an outlet from the colon.

2. A(n) _____ is the cutting into the chest cavity.

3. A(n) _____ is removal of the gallbladder.

4. A(n) _____ is the fixation of an undescended testicle into the scro-
    tum.

5. Removal of a(n) _____ is the removal of a fatty tumor.

6. A(n) _____ is often done after a mastectomy.

SHORT ANSWER

Directions: Write a brief answer for each question.

(726)   1. The three main reasons surgery is performed are to:

    a.   _____

    b.   _____

    c.   _____

Student Name _____

(728)   2.   The four types of anesthesia and an example of the type of procedure for which they may be used are:

      a. _____

      b. _____

      c. _____

      d. _____

(731)   3.   Six types of patients who would be considered at higher risk for surgery than others would be:

      a. _____

      b. _____

      c. _____

      d. _____

      e. _____

      f. _____

(730)   4.   How could you help to prepare the patient psychologically for surgery?

      _____

      _____

      _____

(727-728)   5.   Name two surgical innovations that have made surgery more precise and have reduced recovery time.

      a. _____

      _____

      b. _____

      _____

(729-730)   6.   Tasks you would complete during the immediate preoperative period to assess that the patient is ready for surgery are:

      _____

      _____

      _____

      _____

(731)   7.   L.M., a 76-year-old male, is scheduled for colon surgery in the morning. He tells you, "I hate the thought of being under anesthesia. I'm concerned that this cancer might be more serious than they think. I'm worried about my wife if I die. If I have to have a colostomy, how will I ever cope?" What would you choose as appropriate nursing diagnoses for L.M.?

      _____

      _____

      _____

(732)   8.   Write one expected outcome based on your nursing diagnoses for the planning phase of your care for L.M.

_____

_____

(732)   9.   Your preoperative nursing goals for the patient undergoing surgery would be:

a. _____

b. _____

c. _____

d. _____

(743)   10. Three tasks of the scrub nurse in the OR are:

a. _____

b. _____

c. _____

(743)   11. Three tasks of the circulating nurse in the OR are:

a. _____

b. _____

c. _____

(743)   12. The patient remains in the postanesthesia care unit (PACU) after surgery until:

_____

_____

TABLE ACTIVITY

Directions: For the following complications of surgery, fill in the one major sign or symptom of the complication.
(Table 37-4)

Complication	Sign or Symptom
Atelectasis	
Pneumonia (hypostatic or aspiration)	
Paralytic ileus	
Thrombophlebitis	
Urinary retention	
Urinary tract infection	
Wound infection	
Pulmonary embolus	
Hemorrhage and shock	
Wound dehiscence	
Fluid imbalance	

Student Name_____

SHORT ANSWER

Directions: Write a brief answer for each question.

(751)   1. Five points to cover for home care of the patient during discharge teaching include:

a. _____

b. _____

c. _____

d. _____

e. _____

(744)   2. It is essential to send home _____ for the patient being discharged to home care.

(745)   3. General goals for the postsurgery patient might be:

a. _____

b. _____

c. _____

d. _____

e. _____

APPLICATION OF THE NURSING PROCESS

Directions: Write a brief answer for each question.

Your assigned patient has just returned from the PACU after having a left thoracotomy. He has a chest tube to a disposable portable drainage unit with suction, a Foley catheter, an intravenous line, oxygen by cannula, a left lateral chest dressing, and is on pulse oximetry.

(744)   1. What specific assessments would you make as soon as you have received report and settled the patient in bed?

_____

_____

_____

_____

_____

_____

2. Your assessment reveals that the patient is in pain, has decreased breath sounds, cannot turn without assistance, and is very groggy from the anesthesia. Based on this information and the type of operation that was performed, what would be the nursing diagnoses for this patient?

_____

_____

3. Write an expected outcome for each nursing diagnosis:

_____

_____

_____

_____

4. What aspects of care for this patient would require some special planning, if any?

_____

_____

_____

_____

_____

5. What interventions would you mark on your work organization sheet for specific times during the shift?

_____

_____

6. List interventions to be included on the plan of care for the nursing diagnosis related to lung status.

_____

_____

_____

_____

_____

7. What evaluation data would you need to determine if the expected outcome for the nursing diagnosis related to lung status was being met?

_____

_____

8. Write three evaluation statements that would indicate that the expected outcome for the nursing diagnosis related to lung status was being met by these interventions.

a. _____

b. _____

c. _____

Student Name_____

NCLEX-PN® EXAM REVIEW

*Directions: Choose the **best** answer(s) for each of the following questions.*

(733)   1.   A female patient, age 56, is scheduled for major abdominal surgery. You are in charge of her care preoperatively. When teaching this patient to cough, you would advise her to (Select all that apply)
1.   sit with her back away from the mattress or chair.
2.   perform coughing every 15 minutes postoperatively.
3.   bend over to cough more effectively.
4.   take a deep breath before coughing.

(729)   2.   If a patient states that she is having second thoughts and is not sure she wants to have the surgery, you would
1.   assure her that everything will go well.
2.   ask her husband to speak to her to reassure her.
3.   tear up the surgical consent she signed.
4.   notify the surgeon right away of the situation.

(732)   3.   When teaching a patient to perform leg exercises, you would tell her that the purpose of the exercises is to
1.   ease the stiffness from being on the operating table.
2.   decrease pain from immobile extremities.
3.   increase venous return and decrease stasis.
4.   increase activity to help prevent atelectasis.

(736)   4.   When the transport person comes to take the patient to surgery, it is *most* important that you
1.   assist with the transfer of the patient to the stretcher.
2.   verify the patient's ID number with the chart and transport slip.
3.   tell the family how to get to the surgical waiting room.
4.   list the patient off the unit on the computer.

(743)   5.   In the operating room you observe the scrub nurse and the circulating nurse performing their functions. You note that a grounding pad is placed beneath the patient. The purpose of the pad is to
1.   allow electricity to penetrate the patient's body.
2.   provide safety by dissipating electricity from the cautery.
3.   illuminate the interior body cavity in which the surgeon is operating or inspecting.
4.   keep the surgical team from receiving electrical shocks.

(743-744)   6.   After the surgery, the patient is transferred to the PACU. Functions of the nurse in the PACU are to (Select all that apply)
1.   assist the patient to maintain a patent airway.
2.   keep the family posted on the patient's condition.
3.   maintain safety for the patient while unconscious.
4.   stimulate the patient to hasten return of consciousness.

(748) 7. The patient returns to your unit from the PACU. You prepare to give her immediate postoperative care. Once the patient has aroused completely from general anesthesia, most fluid is initially provided by the intravenous route. Ice chips only are given by mouth because
1. nausea persists for at least 24 hours.
2. a great deal of IV fluid is given in surgery.
3. GI motility is slowed by anesthesia.
4. hunger is not a problem in the first 48 hours.

(746) 8. It is very important to monitor the patient's urine output because
1. urinary tract infections are common at this stage.
2. decreased urine output may be a sign of shock.
3. a distended bladder is uncomfortable.
4. swelling may block the ureters or urethra.

(746) 9. You carefully monitor the patient for which of the following signs that might indicate internal hemorrhage and impending shock?
1. falling blood pressure, rapid pulse, and anxiety
2. copious, bloody drainage from the wound site
3. abdominal distention and lack of bowel sounds
4. increased amounts of blood-tinged urine

(746) 10. The patient is being monitored by pulse oximeter. Pulse oximetry readings will vary slightly depending on respiratory efforts. However, you know to report oximeter readings below _____
_____ immediately.
(Fill in the blank)

CRITICAL THINKING ACTIVITIES

1. Prioritize the following list of preoperative activities for the morning of surgery.
_____ Check the physician's orders.
_____ Check for a signed surgical consent form.
_____ Check that lab work is complete and on the chart.
_____ Have the patient empty the bladder.
_____ Check to see that preoperative medications ordered are available on the unit.
_____ Complete the preoperative checklist.
_____ Have the patient shower.
_____ Prepare the unit for the postoperative return of the patient.
_____ Give the preoperative medications.
_____ Document the patient's readiness for the OR.
_____ Transfer the patient to the OR.

2. What are the possible causes of a low urine output during the second postoperative day?

3. What actions would be necessary if your patient who had general anesthesia does not have any bowel sounds on the second postoperative day?

Student Name_____

MEETING CLINICAL OBJECTIVES

Directions: The following suggested activities will help you meet the stated clinical practice objectives for the chapter. Review your school's clinical objectives for the week and outline a plan of activities that will help you meet them. If you are unsure how to meet them, consult with your instructor at the beginning of the clinical day.

1. Ask to observe in the OR for a clinical day or two.

2. Prepare a patient for surgery and complete the preoperative checklist.

3. Ask to accompany an assigned patient to surgery and observe the operation.

4. Accompany a nurse who is receiving a patient back from surgery to observe the immediate postoperative assessment and care.

5. Perform a postoperative assessment and immediate postoperative care.

6. Assist a patient to perform postoperative turning, breathing, coughing, and leg exercises.

7. Begin discharge instruction for a surgical patient including wound care, diet, activity and rest, elimination, pain control, and medications.

STEPS TOWARD BETTER COMMUNICATION

VOCABULARY BUILDING GLOSSARY

Term	Pronunciation	Definition
A. Individual Terms		
allay	al LAY	to calm, reduce fears
elective	e LEC tive	voluntary
groggy	GROG gy	unsteady and with an unclear mind
grounded	GROUND ed	made an electrical connection with the earth to reduce chance of shock
hamper	HAM per	to make something hard to do
kink	kink	a sharp bend in a hose or pipe
predisposes	PRE dis PO ses	makes vulnerable, makes something more likely to happen
prior	PRI or	before
sharps	sharps	needles, scalpel blades, razors, or sharp instruments
vigilant	VIG i lant	watchful
B. Phrases		
significant other	sig NIF i cant OTH er	important loved one or spouse
up and about	up and about	able to be out of bed and walk around

COMPLETION

Directions: Circle the correct word in each sentence below.

1. The nurse's discussion with the patient <u>allayed/hampered</u> his fears about the surgery.

2. It is important to place the used <u>kinks/sharps</u> in the biohazard container.

3. When checking the patient an hour after surgery, he was <u>groggy/up and about</u>.

4. The electric cautery pad is placed beneath the patient during surgery so that the patient is <u>predisposes/grounded</u> properly.

5. Sedative medication is administered <u>elective/prior</u> to most surgical procedures.

PRONUNCIATION OF DIFFICULT TERMS

Directions: Practice pronouncing the following words.

atelectasis	a te LEC ta sis
antiembolic	an ti em BOL ic
dehiscence	de HIS cence
evisceration	e VIS er A tion
hemorrhage	HEM orrh age
paralytic ileus	par a LIT ic IL e us
perioperative	per i OP er a tive
prosthesis	pros THE sis
thrombophlebitis	throm bo phle BI tis

COMMUNICATION EXERCISES

1. Prepare an appropriate answer for L.M.'s concerns in the Short Answer #7 exercise above.

2. When you have prioritized the preoperative activities in Critical Thinking Activity #1, write what you will say to the patient as you prepare him for surgery.

3. Write what you will say to L.M. as you perform discharge teaching necessary for his postoperative home self-care.

Review the chapter key points, answer the study questions, and complete the critical thinking activities at the end of the chapter in the textbook.

CHAPTER

38 Providing Wound Care and Treating Pressure Ulcers

Answer Key: Textbook page references are provided as a guide for answering selected questions. A complete answer key was provided for your instructor.

TERMINOLOGY

A. Completion

Directions: Fill in the blank(s) with the correct term(s) from the terms list in the chapter in the textbook to complete the sentence.

(756) 1. One sign of inflammation around a wound is _____.

(761) 2. When eschar is present _____ of the wound is necessary.

(760) 3. The abdominal incision is swollen, painful, reddened, and warm, indicating the possible presence of a(n) _____.

(756) 4. Sometimes a(n) _____ forms after surgery, firmly connecting two surfaces of tissue.

(760) 5. The _____ from the wound was clear and nonodorous.

(760) 6. The patient unfortunately developed a(n) _____ between the rectum and vagina.

(759) 7. The presence of pus in a wound indicates a(n) _____.

(761) 8. Dark, tough tissue around or within a wound is called _____ and must be debrided.

(755) 9. If cellular blood supply is disrupted, _____ may occur.

(757) 10. When healing occurs by primary intention, the edges of the wound _____ reducing the chance of infection.

(756) 11. The process of _____ protects wounds against bacterial invasion.

(756) 12. Wounds around joints require maintaining joint mobility in order to prevent _____.

(759) 13. When blood collects beneath the skin, a(n) _____ forms.

(760) 14. _____ is an inflammation of the tissue surrounding the initial wound and is characterized by redness and induration.

(765)　15.　When there is a flat hemorrhagic spot in the skin, it is termed

_____.

(759)　16.　Drainage that is _____ is red.

(760)　17.　Drainage that contains both serum and blood is termed

_____.

(760)　18.　An abnormal passage between an internal organ and the outside of the body is a(n)

_____.

(759)　19.　Wound exudate composed of serum and pus is called

_____.

B.　Matching

Directions: Match the terms in Column I with the definitions in Column II.

	Column I		Column II
(759)	1. _____ adipose	a.	The skin
(764)	2. _____ binders	b.	Permanent, raised, enlarged scar
(755)	3. _____ fibrin	c.	Insoluble protein essential to clotting
(754)	4. _____ integument	d.	Monocyte that is phagocytic
(757)	5. _____ laceration	e.	Breakdown
(756)	6. _____ lysis	f.	Fatty
(756)	7. _____ macrophage	g.	Wide, elasticized, fabric bands used to decrease tension around a wound
(756)	8. _____ keloid	h.	Material used to sew a wound together
(761)	9. _____ suture	i.	A disruption in the skin or tissue

SHORT ANSWER

Directions: Write a brief answer for each question.

(756)　1.　The cardinal signs of the inflammatory process are:

a. _____

b. _____

c. _____

d. _____

e. _____

(755-757)　2.　Schematically or verbally describe in brief the process by which wounds heal.

_____

_____

_____

Student Name_____

(757, 759) 3. Give an example for each of the six factors that can affect wound healing.

    a. _____

    b. _____

    c. _____

    d. _____

    e. _____

    f. _____

(757, 759) 4. Wound healing is slower in the elderly because:

_____

_____

_____

(759) 5. If internal hemorrhage is extensive, hypovolemic shock may occur with the following signs and symptoms:

_____

_____

_____

(761) 6. The major purpose of a wound drain is to:

_____

(760) 7. Four signs and symptoms of a wound infection are:

    a. _____

    b. _____

    c. _____

    d. _____

(760) 8. If wound dehiscence and subsequent evisceration occurs, in order of priority for patient safety, you should:

_____

_____

_____

(778) 9. Local applications of heat are used to:

    a. _____

    b. _____

    c. _____

    d. _____

    e. _____

    f. _____

(778)   10.   Heat works to reduce pain by:

_____

(779)   11.   Cold reduces pain by:

_____

(779)   12.   Cold helps decrease swelling by:

_____

(779)   13.   Shivering may occur during a cold treatment as a result of the body:

_____

COMPLETION

Directions: Fill in the blank(s) with the correct word(s) from the chapter in the textbook to complete the sentence.

(755)   1.   _____ is a localized protective response brought on by injury or destruction of tissues.

(757)   2.   A wound with tissue loss heals by _____ intention.

(757)   3.   An abdominal wound left open and then later closed heals by _____ intention.

(756)   4.   If a(n) _____ forms, it will restrict joint movement.

(760)   5.   The microorganism most frequently present in wound infections is _____.

(760)   6.   The best way to prevent wound infection is to maintain _____ when performing _____ care.

(761)   7.   A yellow wound needs to be continually cleansed and should have a dressing that will _____ drainage and act to _____ the surface mechanically.

(761)   8.   A drainage device is emptied at the end of each shift and the drainage is measured and entered on the _____ record.

(762)   9.   The _____ side of a nonadherent dressing is applied to the wound.

(763)   10.   Superficial wounds heal faster when kept _____.

(763)   11.   _____ allow changing of the dressing without removing and reapplying tape.

(764)   12.   Tape on a dressing should be placed _____ to body action in the wound location.

Student Name _____

APPLICATION OF THE NURSING PROCESS

Directions: Write a brief answer for each question.

(765)   1.   How would you assess a surgical wound? What parameters would you include?

_____

_____

_____

(765)   2.   What methods would you use to assess a nonsurgical wound?

_____

_____

_____

(765)   3.   What other data would you need to determine whether the patient might have a wound infection?

_____

_____

_____

(766)   4.   Your patient was involved in a bicycle accident. She has a 1 1/2" x 1" area of missing subcutaneous tissue on her left thigh. The area is reddened around it and the wound is weeping serosanguineous fluid with cream-colored exudate. Her temperature is 101.4° F and her WBCs are 11,220μ. What would you list as the appropriate nursing diagnosis? What are the defining characteristics for this diagnosis?

_____

_____

_____

5.   Write an expected outcome for the above nursing diagnosis.

_____

6.   What interventions would you list on your nursing care plan for this nursing diagnosis?

_____

_____

_____

_____

_____

7.   What evaluation data would you need to determine if the expected outcome is being met?

_____

_____

_____

NCLEX-PN® EXAM REVIEW

*Directions: Choose the **best** answer(s) for each of the following questions.*

(276) 1. A patient was transferred to your hospital after a fall in the LTC facility. He has fractured his hip. You want to do everything possible to prevent pressure ulcer formation while he is recuperating from his hip repair. A factor that would increase this patient's risk of pressure ulcer formation is
   1. generalized edema.
   2. high fever.
   3. electrolyte imbalance.
   4. dry skin.

(763) 2. The patient has an area over the sacrum that is reddened and the color does not subside when he is repositioned. It is prudent to
   1. cleanse the area with hydrogen peroxide and dress with a non-adherent dressing.
   2. massage the area with lotion several times a day.
   3. place a hydrocolloid dressing over the reddened area.
   4. protect the reddened area with a thin dressing such as Opsite or Tegaderm.

(763) 3. He is incontinent the first day after his surgery. This is a risk factor for the development of skin breakdown and infection because of the added moisture and because
   1. greater pressure is exerted by a wet bed.
   2. shearing is more likely from wet sheets.
   3. the patient has to be repositioned for the bed to be changed.
   4. the moisture creates an environment suitable for the growth of microorganisms in a wound.

4. The patient entered the hospital with a reddened area containing an open, abraded area over the left hip. He states that it is painful. This is a _____ pressure ulcer.
   1. Stage I
   2. Stage II
   3. Stage III
   4. Stage IV

(757, 759) 5. Many factors aid healing. You assist the patient to specifically improve his healing ability by encouraging (Select all that apply)
   1. exercise and deep-breathing to increase oxygen.
   2. proper nutrition with adequate protein and vitamin C.
   3. increasing fluid intake to at least 2000 mL per day.
   4. resting as much as possible and keeping the incisional area still.

(768-770) 6. There are many points to keep in mind for a sterile dressing change. When changing the sterile dressing over the incision for the patient it is important to remember to (Select all that apply)
   1. place a discard bag close to the wound.
   2. refrain from talking while the wound is uncovered.
   3. change gloves after removing the old dressing.
   4. open supplies as you need them during the procedure.

(768-770) 7. When working with his closed wound drainage system, if it becomes 2/3 full, you should
   1. recompress the device and let it fill some more.
   2. wait until it is full to empty it.
   3. replace the entire device with another one.
   4. empty it and recompress the device.

Student Name _____

(779) 8. When providing hot and cold treatments for patients, several principles apply. A systemic effect of cold therapy is
   1. alteration of the pulse rate.
   2. shunting of blood from the periphery to the central organs.
   3. speeding up metabolic processes such as digestion and tissue building.
   4. numbing of the area of application.

(778) 9. Moist heat has the physiological effect of
   1. constricting the blood vessels.
   2. drawing fluid to the site of application.
   3. numbing the area treated.
   4. dilating the blood vessels.

(779) 10. When teaching the patient how to apply a cold pack, you would say which of the following?
   1. "Wrap the pack in thick cloth before applying it to the skin.
   2. "Use the ice pack continuously for the first 24 hours."
   3. "Leave the pack in place for 15 minutes out of each hour for the first 24 hours."
   4. "Only use the ice pack for 10 minutes four times a day."

(779) 11. When applying an ice pack, it is necessary to
   1. use a light cover on the pack.
   2. use small ice cubes.
   3. fill the pack and refreeze it.
   4. cover the pack with plastic wrap.

(779) 12. Safety factors involved in using an Aquathermia pad unit for a patient include (Select all that apply)
   1. securing the pad to the patient.
   2. using a thermometer to check the temperature of the pad.
   3. inspecting the plug and cord for cracks or fraying.
   4. instructing the patient not to sleep on the pad.

(779) 13. When giving a hot soak treatment, it is *most* important to
   1. soak only the affected area.
   2. test the temperature of the solution.
   3. position the patient comfortably.
   4. use only sterile equipment and solution.

(755-756) 14. A 28-year-old male is a patient at your clinic. He states that had a minor accident with his motorcycle 5 days ago. He sustained several scrapes and wounds. The wound on his calf has a pinkish-red center area that looks bumpy. This indicates that the wound is
   1. becoming infected.
   2. beginning to heal.
   3. needs to be debrided.
   4. is purulent.

(760) 15. When changing the dressing on the patient's right arm, you see that the dressing has a moist yellow-red stain on it. You would chart this as _____ drainage. (Fill in the blank)

CRITICAL THINKING ACTIVITIES

1. P.S. has an open wound on her right heel. It is 3 x 5 cm and has a blackened area in the center. It is reddened around the perimeter. How would you stage this pressure ulcer? How would you treat it?

2. List the equipment and supplies you would need to change a sterile dressing over a 4" abdominal incision that contains a Penrose wound drain.

3. B.W. has developed a cellulitis in the arm where he had an IV line. He is placed on antibiotics and told to use heat on it at home. How would you instruct B.W. to safely give his own heat treatments at home?

MEETING CLINICAL OBJECTIVES

Directions: The following suggested activities will help you meet the stated clinical practice objectives for the chapter. Review your school's clinical objectives for the week and outline a plan of activities that will help you meet them. If you are unsure how to meet them, consult with your instructor at the beginning of the clinical day.

1. Ask nurses on the units to which you are assigned to allow you to accompany them to see various types of wounds and observe dressing techniques.

2. Study the AHCPR Guideline booklet *Pressure Ulcers in Adults: Prediction and Prevention* to become more familiar with pressure ulcers and their care.

3. Practice sterile dressing changes in the skill lab or at home until you are comfortable and confident of your sterile technique.

4. Perform a wound irrigation.

5. Ask to be assigned to patients who have pressure ulcers for experience in providing care for these wounds.

6. Remove sutures or staples from a wound and apply Steri-Strips.

7. Give a heat treatment and a cold treatment to a patient and teach the patient how to do these treatments at home.

8. Question other nurses about ways to decrease the trauma of dressing changes on the skin of the elderly patient.

9. Seek assignment to patients who need sterile dressing changes.

STEPS TOWARD BETTER COMMUNICATION

VOCABULARY BUILDING GLOSSARY

Term	Pronunciation	Definition
A. Individual Terms		
adhere	ad HERE	to hold, stick to something
binder	BIND er	a wide band, usually cloth, to hold something to-gether
cardinal	CARD i nal	the most important, primary
cessation	ces SA tion	a stopping
frayed	FRAY ed	worn with loose threads at the edge
friable	FRI a ble	easily crumbled, broken
gauze	gauze	lightweight fabric with a loose, open mesh weave
hydrate	hy DRATE	keep moist or wet
immunocompromised	im mu no COM pro mised	poor immune response because of illness, drugs, poor physical condition
nonadherent	non ad HER ent	will not stick to another surface
nosocomial	no so CO mi al	originating in a hospital
numbing	NUM bing	lacking in feeling

Student Name _____

obese	o BESE	excessively overweight
occlusive	oc CLU sive	obstructing
radiant	RA di ant	diverging from a center
regeneration	re gen e RA tion	the natural renewal, regrowth
sloughing	SLOUGH (sluf) ing	the shedding or dropping off of dead tissue

B. Phrases

frost bite (frost nip)	FROST bite	a condition in which body tissue is exposed to low temperatures and begins to freeze
shearing forces	SHEAR ing forces	two surfaces sliding across each other in opposite directions

COMPLETION

Directions: Fill in the blank(s) with the correct term(s) from the Vocabulary Building Glossary to complete the sentence.

1. Often, IV fluids are essential to _____ the patient.

2. The nurse must check for a(n) _____ cord before plugging in a piece of electrical equipment.

3. The elderly often have very _____ skin.

4. Right lower quadrant pain is a(n) _____ sign of appendicitis.

5. An open wound often requires a(n) _____ type of dressing.

6. A lift sheet is used to turn a patient to prevent the consequences of _____ that occur if the patient is pulled across the sheets rather than lifted.

7. An abdominal _____ keeps a patient who has had major abdominal surgery more comfortable when out of bed.

8. It is a major nursing responsibility to prevent _____ infection in hospitalized patients.

9. A safety device when placed too tightly around a limb may result in _____ of the distal part of the extremity.

10. Safety devices that are placed improperly may cause a(n) _____ of blood flow in the body part.

VOCABULARY EXERCISE

Directions: Which of the words in the Vocabulary Building Glossary have you seen or heard used in another way in everyday speech? Give some examples; i.e., cardinal = a red bird: There were three cardinals at my bird feeder this morning.

_____

_____

_____

PRONUNCIATION OF DIFFICULT TERMS

Directions: Practice pronouncing the following words.

cellulitis	CELL u li tis
dehiscence	de HIS cence
ecchymosis	ec chy MO sis
erythema	er y THE ma
eschar	ES char(kar)
evisceration	E vis cer A tion
hypoallergenic	hy po al ler GEN ic
hypovolemic	hy po vo LE mic
purulent	PU ru lent
phagocytosis	pha go cy TO sis
sanguineous	san GUIN e ous
serosanguineous	ser o san GUIN e ous

The word débridement is given the French pronunciation "da BREED maw"

COMMUNICATION EXERCISES

1. Using the following as an example, explain to a patient or peer how to care for an abdominal wound at home.

   "When at home, Ms. T., I want you to change the dressing every day. Wash your hands well before touching the dressing or the wound. You can use a pair of these clean disposable gloves each time you do the dressing change. I usually prepare the tape strips before I start. This tape can be torn easily. I just stick it on the side of the table or the counter where I can reach it. I do that before I put on the gloves. You may want to shower before you change the dressing. Just tape a piece of plastic over the dressing. Try not to let the shower water run directly over that area. This way if the dressing gets a bit wet, you will be changing it anyway. With the gloves on, remove the old dressing and put it into a sealable plastic bag for disposal. Inspect the wound for redness, tenderness around it, increased drainage, or separation of the edges. If these occur, report them to the doctor. Clean around the wound with gauze squares moistened with saline. Clean from the center of the wound outward. That way you don't bring bacteria into the wound area. You can prepare those ahead of time as I just did also. Pat the area dry and attach a new dressing just like the old one."

2. Write out how you would explain to a mother how to care for her child's wound at home. Have a peer or your instructor critique your instructions.

Review the chapter key points, answer the study questions, and complete the critical thinking activities at the end of the chapter in the textbook.

CHAPTER 39 Promoting Musculoskeletal Function

Answer Key: Textbook page references are provided as a guide for answering selected questions. A complete answer key was provided for your instructor.

TERMINOLOGY

A.   Matching

Directions: Match the terms in Column I with the definitions in Column II.

		Column I		Column II
(793)	1.	_____ blanch	a.	Exertion of a pulling force
(788)	2.	_____ cast	b.	Bandage for supporting a body part
(784)	3.	_____ debilitating	c.	A stiff dressing used to immobilize a body part
(793)	4.	_____ dorsum	d.	Moving
(802)	5.	_____ hydrotherapy	e.	Artificial substitute for a body part
(784)	6.	_____ immobilization	f.	To become pale
(791)	7.	_____ kinetic	g.	Weakening
(793)	8.	_____ paresthesia	h.	Back
(808)	9.	_____ prosthesis	i.	Use of water to treat injury
(788)	10.	_____ sling	j.	To prevent movement
(784)	11.	_____ traction	k.	Tingling or burning sensation

B.   Completion

Directions: Fill in the blank(s) with the correct term(s) from the terms list in the chapter in the textbook to complete the sentence.

(789)   1.   When a cast becomes too tight due to swelling of an extremity, the physician will _____ it to relieve the pressure.

(808)   2.   The young man had been in a diving accident and was _____, having no use of his arms or legs.

(786)   3.   Often, while a patient is in leg traction, the doctor will order _____ exercises to strengthen muscles and prevent atrophy.

(807)   4.   The patient had paralysis of the legs after the accident and was _____.

(787)   5. A traction bed often requires a(n) _____ from which to hang the traction apparatus.

(789)   6. A(n) _____ cast may be needed to immobilize a part of the trunk and one or both legs.

(793)   7. After the stroke, G.R. had right-sided _____ and could not walk unassisted.

(793)   8. The accident left I.B. with _____ and he had no use of his left arm or leg.

(789)   9. For skin traction, sometimes adhesive _____ is used to attach the traction to the skin.

(787) 10. A(n) _____ hung over the bed is used so the patient in traction can reposition him- or herself.

(787) 11. A splint is used to _____ a body part.

SHORT ANSWER

Directions: Write a brief answer for each question.

(785)   1. In what ways does inactivity affect respiratory exchange and airway clearance?

_____

_____

_____

(793)   2. To perform a neurovascular assessment on an immobilized extremity, you would

_____

_____

_____

(789)   3. H.D. has just had a long leg cast applied. Describe the care of this cast during the drying period.

_____

_____

_____

(790-791) 4. Describe the special features of each of the following specialty beds and the advantages of each.

  a. Air-fluidized bed

  _____

  _____

  b. Low air-loss bed

  _____

  _____

Student Name_____

    c.   Continuous lateral-rotation bed

       _____

       _____

    d.   CircOlectric bed

       _____

       _____

(791)   5. Five pressure relief devices used to help prevent skin injury for immobilized patients are:

    a. _____

    b. _____

    c. _____

    d. _____

    e. _____

(798-799) 6. Four principles or guidelines for applying an elastic or roller bandage are:

    a. _____

    b. _____

    c. _____

    d. _____

   7. List one nursing action to prevent each of the following potential complications of immobility:

    a.   Thrombus formation:_____

       _____

    b.   Atelectasis: _____

       _____

    c.   Constipation: _____

       _____

    d.   Joint contracture: _____

       _____

    e.   Renal stones:_____

       _____

    f.   Skin breakdown:_____

       _____

    g.   Boredom: _____

       _____

(786) 8. How can you promote adequate nutrition for the immobilized elderly patient who is anorexic?

_____

_____

_____

(787) 9. Traction is used to maintain parts of the body in _____.

(788) 10. When moving a patient in the bed, you must be careful to avoid a(n) _____ injury to the skin.

(787) 11. Two main aspects of nursing care for the patient in traction are to keep the weights _____ and to keep the patient in _____.

(787) 12. It is very important that the weight of traction be _____ when the patient is moved in the bed.

(787) 13. For traction to be maximally effective, the ropes must _____.

(788) 14. When traction is being used, it is important to maintain a balance between traction pull and _____.

(788) 15. Countertraction force is provided by the _____ of the patient and the _____ of the bed.

(788) 16. Dents in a cast can lead to _____ and consequent _____.

(788) 17. When a cast is to be applied, the patient is told to expect a feeling of _____, especially with a plaster of paris cast.

(788) 18. It is critical that the cast be protected from _____ pressure while drying.

(788) 19. When handling the cast while it is drying, use the _____ rather than the fingertips.

(789) 20. When the patient has a spica cast, never use the _____ to help turn the patient.

(802) 21. When transferring a patient with a mechanical lift, never leave the person _____.

(805) 22. Walkers are helpful to patients who are _____ or tend to lose _____.

(805) 23. The height of the walker is correct if the person grasping the hand grips is standing upright with the elbow bent _____ degrees.

(805) 24. A very important point in teaching a patient to use crutches is to teach NOT to:

_____

(805) 25. Crutches need to be adjusted to the individual patient both in _____ and from the _____ to the _____.

Student Name _____

789)   26. The advantage of an external fixator over traction is that the patient has more

_____ .

787)   27. When applying a first aid splint to an extremity, a very important principle is to handle the injured part gently and not to _____ of the extremity in any way.

APPLICATION OF THE NURSING PROCESS

Directions: Write a brief answer for each question.

793)   1. M.B. has been immobilized with a Thomas splint with Pearson attachment on her left leg after she fractured it in an automobile accident. Your beginning-of-shift assessment of M.B. would include:

_____

_____

_____

_____

793)   2. Your nursing diagnosis related to M.B.'s main problem would be:

_____

793-794) 3. Another nursing diagnosis for every patient who is immobilized by traction is:

_____

4. One expected outcome for the nursing diagnosis in #2 would be:

_____

786)   5. Three nursing interventions to prevent boredom for M.B. while she is immobilized are:

a. _____

b. _____

c. _____

808)   6. How would you evaluate the effectiveness of the traction and immobilization treatment for M.B.?

_____

_____

808)   7. Write two evaluation statements that would assist in evaluating whether M.B. was meeting the expected outcome in #4.

a. _____

b. _____

NCLEX-PN® EXAM REVIEW

*Directions: Choose the **best** answer(s) for the following questions.*

(785) 1. A 46-year-old male was injured in an industrial accident and has suffered a fractured left leg and left wrist. His wrist is treated with a cast and the leg is placed in skeletal traction. Because of immobilization of his leg, the patient is at risk for (Select all that apply)
1. pressure ulcer.
2. venous thrombosis.
3. generalized edema.
4. foot drop.

(785) 2. You encourage the patient recovering from a fractured leg to deep-breathe, cough, and use his incentive spirometer to prevent
1. pulmonary embolus.
2. bronchoconstriction.
3. hypostatic pneumonia.
4. delayed healing.

(788) 3. Another aspect of caring for a patient while he is in skeletal traction is to
1. use aseptic technique for pin care.
2. exercise the leg in traction passively.
3. remove the traction while showering him.
4. lift the weights to remove pressure while moving him.

4. To make the patient's bed while he is in skeletal traction you would (Select all that apply)
1. roll him from one side to the other.
2. make the bed from top to bottom.
3. only change the top sheet.
4. obtain a helper to assist with the linen change.

(789) 5. The patient with a fractured left wrist, although right handed, will have self-care deficits while he is recovering. He will especially need assistance with (Select all that apply)
1. toileting.
2. eating.
3. combing his hair.
4. bathing.

(789) 6. Your patient, an 8-year-old male, has fractured his leg. The leg is placed in a cast. When instructing his mother about repositioning the new cast, you tell her to
1. lift the leg with a sling to move it.
2. have the boy move the cast.
3. use the flat palm of the hand to lift the cast.
4. wait until the cast is completely dry.

(792-793) 7. While assessing the patient with a leg cast, an indication that swelling is occurring and the cast is becoming too tight would be
1. the cast is hot to the touch.
2. the area distal is a dusky color and cold.
3. capillary refill distally is 10–15 seconds.
4. the patient complains of discomfort.

Student Name _____

(798-799) 8. It is discovered that the patient sprained his wrist when he broke his leg. An elastic bandage wrap is ordered. You would be sure to (Select all that apply)
1. pull the bandage tightly around the extremity.
2. elevate the extremity before beginning to wrap it.
3. slightly overlap each turn of the bandage.
4. use a circular technique from the wrist up the arm.

(808) 9. The patient is given some exercises to do while his leg fracture is healing. The purpose of the exercises is to
1. help the bone heal.
2. prevent boredom.
3. increase circulation.
4. prevent loss of muscle tone.

(807) 10. The cast is dry and he is started on crutch walking. You explain that when going up stairs he is to
1. first move the crutches up onto the stair.
2. move the good leg up onto the stair and then the crutches and the bad leg.
3. move the bad leg and one crutch onto the stair and then move the other leg and crutch.
4. move the good leg and opposite crutch up onto the stair and then move the bad leg and other crutch up.

(787) 11. There are many points to be followed when applying a first aid splint to an extremity. One is to

_____

_____ to prevent pressure wounds. (Fill in the blank)

CRITICAL THINKING ACTIVITIES

1. L.K., age 46, is going to be immobilized for several weeks while his injuries heal. Design an activity program to help prevent boredom and depression.

2. How would you handle the situation if your new amputee states that she has no interest in learning to wrap her stump properly?

3. How would you explain to an elderly patient who has had a stroke and has hemiparesis how using a walker can both protect her safety and provide more independence for her?

MEETING CLINICAL OBJECTIVES

Directions: The following suggested activities will help you meet the stated clinical practice objectives for the chapter. Review your school's clinical objectives for the week and outline a plan of activities that will help you meet them. If you are unsure how to meet them, consult with your instructor at the beginning of the clinical day.

1. Actively seek assignment to patients with problems of immobility so that experience is gained in caring for patients with casts, traction, prostheses, paralysis, and so forth.

2. Whenever there is a special bed in use on the unit, ask the staff nurse to explain its use and any special nursing care or problems associated with the bed's use.

3. Observe a physical therapist adjusting crutches for a patient and when teaching crutch walking.

4. Practice transferring a person with hemiparesis into and out of a wheelchair safely and smoothly. Have a peer role play the patient.

5. Ask a staff nurse to teach you to use a mechanical lift if one is available on your unit.

6. Any time someone asks for help in transferring a patient to or from a stretcher, if possible, go and assist so that you learn all the tricks of performing this procedure efficiently and safely. Observe exactly where a slide or roller board is placed or how a lift sheet is utilized.

7. Apply an elastic bandage to a patient's extremity.

STEPS TOWARD BETTER COMMUNICATION

VOCABULARY BUILDING GLOSSARY

Term	Pronunciation	Definition
A. Individual Terms		
buoyancy	BUOY an cy	ability to float
debilitating	de BIL i TA ting	making weak
diminished	de MIN ished	made less, decreased
diversionary	di VER sion ar y	distracting, to put attention in another place
disintegrate	dis IN te grate	to fall apart; break into small pieces
gait	GAIT	the way a person walks
groundless	GROUND less	without basis in fact; with no reason
kinetic	ki NET ic	moving
longitudinally	lon gi TUD in al ly	along the length of something
regress	re GRESS	to go back; return to an earlier state
trapeze	tra PEZE	a horizontal bar hung by ropes (often used as a swing for acrobats)
B. Phrases		
oscillating saw	OS cil la ting saw	an electrical saw that goes back and forth, not around
pen pal	PEN pal	a person you know only through letters; someone you write to regularly
work things through	work things through	to think and talk about a problem or feelings, and come to a resolution

COMPLETION

Directions: Fill in the blank(s) with the correct term(s) from the Vocabulary Building Glossary to complete the sentence.

1. The nurse tried to plan some _____ activities for the boy in traction who stated he was very bored and was really hurting.

2. The leg was swelling and the cast was becoming tight, so the cast was bivalved _____ down the leg.

3. The 6-year-old with the fractured leg in skeletal traction began to _____ and started wetting the bed.

Student Name _____

4. After several weeks, the area around the toes of the walking cast began to
   _____ and it had to be replaced.

5. The nurse used a diagram to help teach the patient the proper _____
   to use when crutch walking.

6. The motor vehicle accident and resulting fractures and injuries ended up being very
   _____ for the patient.

VOCABULARY EXERCISES

These words may be used as a verb or a noun.

	Verb	*Noun*
Hamper	to make difficult	a basket or container for food or clothing
Dictate	to tell someone what to do, say, or write	a rule or regulation
Stress	to emphasize, or consider important	anxiety; mental or physical strain caused by pressure

Directions: Use each word above in a sentence first as a noun and then as a verb.

1. a. (Noun) _____
   b. (Verb) _____
2. a. (Noun) _____
   b. (Verb) _____
3. a. (Noun) _____
   b. (Verb) _____

PRONUNCIATION OF DIFFICULT TERMS

Directions: Practice pronouncing the following words.

atelectasis	a te lec ta sis
hemiplegia	hem i PLE gi a
hemiparesis	HEM i par E sis
paraplegic	par a PLE gic
prosthesis	pros THE sis
quadriplegic	QUAD ri PLE gic

COMMUNICATION EXERCISE

Directions: Practice these questions for neurovascular assessment with a peer.

Do you feel any tingling or numbness?

Where does it hurt? Describe the pain—is it sharp, or dull, constant, or intermittent? When does it hurt? How much does it hurt?

CULTURAL POINTS

In the United States today, a great deal of emphasis is placed on rehabilitation. Amputees are fitted with prostheses with the goal of enabling them to return to as normal a life a possible. People who use wheelchairs may participate in sports such as basketball, and the Americans with Disabilities Act (ADA) makes more buildings, job sites, and outdoor areas accessible to them. Amputees have run across the country and climbed mountains. These are exceptional people, but they show that they can succeed in spite of the physical difficulties they have. Their success may have more to do with their own attitudes and how people treat them than their actual physical status. This is something to remember as you deal with patients.

How are people with physical limitations treated in your native country? Are they encouraged to return to normal life and given training and assistance? Many countries may not have the finances to remove all physical barriers, but are there social and emotional barriers still in place?

Have you known a person with such a disability? Have you ever talked with him or her about it? What are the problems the person faces? What is his or her philosophy in dealing with the problem?

To raise your own awareness of the difficulties a person with physical limitations might face, even temporarily while in a cast or wheelchair, pay attention for one day or even a morning. Notice what might be difficult for you if you were on crutches, in a wheelchair, had only use of one hand, or were unable to see clearly. Could you navigate stairs, step off the curb, reach your car, push the elevator button, use the soft-drink machine, open the door, cross the street, leave your house? How would it affect what you could and could not do? How would it change your life?

Review the chapter key points, answer the study questions, and complete the critical thinking activities at the end of the chapter in the textbook.

CHAPTER 40

Common Physical Care Problems of the Elderly

Answer Key: Textbook page references are provided as a guide for answering selected questions. A complete answer key was provided for your instructor.

TERMINOLOGY

A. Matching

Directions: Match the terms in Column I with the definitions in Column II.

<table>
<tr><th colspan="3">Column I</th><th>Column II</th></tr>
<tr><td>(817)</td><td>1. _____</td><td>beta-carotene</td><td>a. Unusually low blood pressure when standing</td></tr>
<tr><td>(816)</td><td>2. _____</td><td>cataracts</td><td>b. Difficulty swallowing</td></tr>
<tr><td>(815)</td><td>3. _____</td><td>dysphagia</td><td>c. Ability to focus on far and near objects</td></tr>
<tr><td>(816)</td><td>4. _____</td><td>glaucoma</td><td>d. Age-related decreased ability to focus on near objects</td></tr>
<tr><td>(817)</td><td>5. _____</td><td>presbycusis</td><td>e. Excess fluid in eye that exerts pressure on the optic nerve</td></tr>
<tr><td>(816)</td><td>6. _____</td><td>presbyopia</td><td></td></tr>
<tr><td>(818)</td><td>7. _____</td><td>polypharmacy</td><td>f. Clouding of the lens of the eye</td></tr>
<tr><td>(813)</td><td>8. _____</td><td>postural hypotension</td><td>g. Substance found in orange vegetables and fruits and dark green, leafy vegetables</td></tr>
<tr><td>(816)</td><td>9. _____</td><td>visual accommodation</td><td>h. Inability to hear high-pitched sounds and spoken words</td></tr>
<tr><td>(818)</td><td>10. _____</td><td>over-the-counter</td><td>i. Use of multiple medications</td></tr>
<tr><td></td><td></td><td></td><td>j. Drugs that can be purchased at the pharmacy without a prescription</td></tr>
</table>

B. Completion

Directions: Fill in the blank(s) with the correct term(s) from the terms list in the chapter in the textbook to complete the sentence.

(812)   1. At the onset of menopause, some women take _____ to decrease the unpleasant symptoms.

(814)   2. Often, urinary incontinence can be corrected by _____ and without surgery.

(816)   3. A disease that often robs the elderly of their vision is _____.

(814)   4. One technique used in bladder retraining is _____,
where the patient is assisted to void just before times when incontinence has been known to
occur.

(815)   5. When an elderly, inactive person experiences a change in bowel pattern that includes passage
of small amounts of liquid stool, _____ should be sus-
pected.

SHORT ANSWER

Directions: Write a brief answer for each question.

(811)   1. Five age-related common physical care problems to be considered when assessing an elderly
patient are:

a. _____

b. _____

c. _____

d. _____

e. _____

(814)   2. Describe how chronic urinary incontinence might affect a person both physically and psychologically.

_____

_____

_____

(811)   3. Three ways to promote mobility in the elderly are:

a. _____

b. _____

c. _____

(814)   4. Four ways to prevent falls in the home are:

a. _____

b. _____

c. _____

d. _____

(812)   5. Identify four factors affecting the elderly that may lead to an alteration in nutrition.

a. _____

b. _____

c. _____

d. _____

Student Name_____

(817)   6. List four techniques that will facilitate communication and safety for the patient with a sensory deficit.

        a. _____

        b. _____

        c. _____

        d. _____

(818)   7. Identify five reasons the older adult is prone to the problem of polypharmacy.

        a. _____

        b. _____

        c. _____

        d. _____

        e. _____

(813)   8. Describe how a chronic respiratory disease can affect an elderly person's mobility.

        _____

        _____

(813)   9. Describe the ways in which decreased activity on the part of an elderly person may affect his or her mobility.

        _____

        _____

        _____

(814) 10. List the five factors you consider the most important for safety in the home for an elderly person.

        a. _____

        b. _____

        c. _____

        d. _____

        e. _____

(811) 11. Diseases that interfere with _____ or _____ contribute to activity intolerance and immobility.

(812) 12. Four accessible activities that can promote mobility in the elderly are:

        a. _____

        b. _____

        c. _____

        d. _____

(812)   13.   To protect against osteoporosis, all adults should engage in
_____ exercise and take in sufficient
_____ .

(813)   14.   One factor to consider in promoting mobility among the elderly is that most
would rather risk _____ than be placed in a
_____ .

(813)   15.   Approximately one _____ of people over 65 years old and _____
of those over 80 fall each year.

(813)   16.   With each additional _____ taken, the risk of falls is
increased.

(813)   17.   Elderly patients need to be moved slowly out of bed to prevent possible
_____ .

(814)   18.   When an elderly person who lives alone is discharged home, it is wise to make a referral for a
home health team member to assess the home for _____ .

(814)   19.   If an elderly person has some difficulty with balance, the person should be told not to reach
for objects _____ level.

(814)   20.   When incontinence occurs, the _____ should be sought.

(815)   21.   For the person who does experience urinary incontinence, odor can be reduced by encouraging the person to _____ to dilute the urine.

(815)   22.   The ill older adult who is on bed rest, receiving pain medication, and not eating a normal
diet is at high risk for _____ .

(815)   23.   The primary dietary guidelines for the elderly are to reduce the
_____ and _____
intake and to increase _____ in the diet.

(816)   24.   Three visual changes that occur with aging because of decreased blood supply to the retina are:

     a.   _____

     b.   _____

     c.   _____

(817)   25.   When a patient has considerable visual deficit, it is important to identify yourself when
_____ or _____
the room.

(817)   26.   For the person with a visual deficit, it is also important to refrain from
_____ personal belongings without permission or ex-
planation.

(817)   27.   Hearing deficits are usually intensified by the presence of
_____ .

(818)   28.   The problem of polypharmacy often occurs because the older adult with multiple health
problems sees multiple _____ .

(814)   29.   The goal of prompted voiding is to _____
_____ .

(816)   30.   The percentage of the daily calories that should be protein in the diet of the person over age
51 is _____ .

Student Name_____

TABLE ACTIVITY

Directions: Use a separate sheet of paper to list three contributing factors for each physical care problem of the elderly.

(Table 40-1)

Physical Care Problem	Contributing Factors
Impaired mobility	
Alteration in elimination	
Alteration in nutrition	
Sensory deficit—vision	
Sensory deficit—hearing	
Polypharmacy	

NCLEX-PN® EXAM REVIEW

*Directions: Choose the **best** answer(s) for the following questions.*

(815) 1. A 78-year-old female has a stasis ulcer on her right leg. As her home health nurse you visit to change her dressing. During the visit you perform other assessments. Since the patient is mostly immobile because she needs to keep the right leg elevated and because she is taking pain medication, it is especially important to assess her
   1. mental status.
   2. urinary status.
   3. bowel status.
   4. heart status.

(821) 2. When you asked the patient with the stasis ulcer if she is taking her antibiotics for the infection in her leg, the patient replies, "Yes, but I have so many pills, I'm not sure I'm taking them at the right times." What would be a good method to assist her to take her pills correctly?
   1. Have a neighbor come in and give her the pills at different times during the day.
   2. Set up a seven-day medicine planner for her that you can refill during your nursing visits.
   3. Have her daughter call and remind her when to take her pills.
   4. Write out a list of the medications and the times that each is to be taken.

(818, 821) 3. When listing the patient's medications, you find that she has two very similar blood pressure medications prescribed by different doctors. To remedy the problem of polypharmacy you would recommend that she
   1. give each doctor she sees a list of her medications.
   2. make certain that she knows exactly what each prescription is supposed to treat.
   3. obtain all her prescription medications from one pharmacy.
   4. ask her daughter to monitor her prescriptions for her.

(815) 4. A patient indicates she is not eating much as it is difficult to cook. Nursing interventions that might be appropriate in this case are (Select all that apply)
   1. ask her best friend to prepare meals for her.
   2. ask her daughter to bring her several microwave meals.
   3. suggest using supplements such as Ensure to maintain her nutrition.
   4. ask the social worker to set up Meals on Wheels service for her.

(813) 5. Your patient has hypertension, asthma, hypothyroidism, and osteoarthritis which are chronic conditions. Her _____ _____ may become worse due to her decreased mobility. (Fill in the blank)

(814) 6. An alert, well-groomed, 82-year-old resident of the long-term care facility has been experiencing bladder incontinence since she had pneumonia. She seems quite depressed and you suspect that this development has seriously affected her
   1. self-esteem.
   2. attitude toward others.
   3. personality.
   4. mental acuity.

7. The first thing that should be done when beginning a bladder retraining program for a patient is
   1. planning scheduled toileting times.
   2. decreasing her fluid intake.
   3. tracking when incontinence occurs.
   4. placing her in adult diapers.

8. When considering a teaching session for a patient about the bladder retraining program, you would plan to (Select all that apply)
   1. eliminate outside noise and distractions.
   2. use printed materials along with explaining the process.
   3. quickly present the material so as not to cause fatigue.
   4. speak distinctly in a very loud voice.

(815) 9. A patient has been having some difficulty with constipation from decreased appetite and antibiotic therapy. To assist her with this problem, you would encourage her to (Select all that apply)
   1. increase roughage with fresh fruits and vegetables.
   2. take a laxative each night at bedtime.
   3. attempt to evacuate the bowels at the same time each day.
   4. choose more breads and pastas at meals.

Student Name_____

10. A patient has moderate macular degeneration. To decrease the possibility of falls at night, you would
   1. keep a very bright light burning in her room.
   2. ask her to call for assistance to the bathroom.
   3. keep her cane within reach of the bed.
   4. have an attendant stay with her at night.

(812) 11. There are various drugs used to treat osteoporosis. Besides Fosamax and Actonel, another drug that may be used to arrest osteoporosis in the elderly is _____ _____. (Fill in the blank)

(813) 12. A leading cause of hospitalization and placement in long-term care is
   1. cardiac disease.
   2. diabetes.
   3. hip fracture.
   4. pneumonia.

(813) 13. A medicine that may contribute to falls in the elderly is
   1. Thorazine.
   2. Miacalcin.
   3. Flonase.
   4. ampicillin.

(814) 14. Many common physical problems affect the elderly. A common physical care problem in the elderly that has been reported to cost billions of dollars for nursing home care is

   _____. (Fill in the blank)

(814) 15. An herbal approach to reduce prostate swelling is
   1. saw palmetto.
   2. St. John's wort.
   3. evening primrose.
   4. ginkgo biloba.

(815-816) 16. Patients with dysphagia can choke easily. After eating, patients with dysphagia should be placed in

   _____ position for 45–60 minutes following eating. (Fill in the blank)

(816) 17. Glaucoma is a common eye disorder that is characterized by
   1. a clouding of the lens.
   2. inability to focus on near objects.
   3. an accumulation of excess fluid inside the eye.
   4. a yellowing of the sclera.

(817) 18. Antioxidants that may help protect against macular degeneration include
   1. calcium and vitamin C.
   2. calcium and vitamin D.
   3. vitamin C and vitamin B.
   4. vitamin C and vitamin E.

(817) 19. Presbycusis is characterized by the inability to hear
   1. low-frequency sounds.
   2. high-frequency sounds.
   3. mid-frequency sounds.
   4. vowel sounds.

(821) 20. Strategies to increase compliance in self-medication administration include which of the following (Select all that apply)
   1. the use of color-coded medication bottles.
   2. periodically counting the remaining pills.
   3. an alarm clock.
   4. cueing with daily events.

CRITICAL THINKING ACTIVITIES

1. Your home care patient is having a difficult time obtaining adequate nutrition. She has family 2 hours away, but lives alone. She has limited mobility, but can walk short distances. How would you go about assisting her to obtain better nutrition?

2. Perform a safety assessment of an elder relative or friend's home. What hazards did you find?

3. Describe ways you might assist an elderly adult who has a visual deficit stay independent.

MEETING CLINICAL OBJECTIVES

Directions: The following suggested activities will help you meet the stated clinical practice objectives for the chapter. Review your school's clinical objectives for the week and outline a plan of activities that will help you meet them. If you are unsure how to meet them, consult with your instructor at the beginning of the clinical day.

1. Work with an elderly patient on a bladder retraining program.

2. Develop a teaching plan to assist the elderly patient who has a small appetite increase his or her nutritional intake with appropriate foods.

3. Assess each elderly patient assigned for signs of polypharmacy.

STEPS TOWARD BETTER COMMUNICATION

VOCABULARY BUILDING GLOSSARY

Term	Pronunciation	Definition
A. Individual Terms		
address (verb)	ad DRESS	to deal with; to treat a problem
chore	CHORE	work, a routine job to be done that is not fun
clutter	CLUT ter	objects scattered around, not neat
cueing	CUE ing	giving a reminder
engaged	en GAGEd	turned on, put into active use
enhance	en HANCE	to improve, to add to in order to make better
imperative	im PER a tive	necessary; urgent
inclement	in CLEM ent	refers to bad or severe conditions, especially weather
odoriferous	o dor IF er ous	smelly; having a strong odor
prudently	PRU dent ly	carefully; with good judgment
B. Phrase		
coupled with	COUP led with	together with; joined with

COMPLETION

A. Directions: Fill in the blank(s) with the correct term(s) from the Vocabulary Building Glossary to complete the sentence.

1. It was difficult for D.R. to _____ the problem of the high cost of the new prescription since she is on a fixed income.

Student Name _____

2. It is _____ to stop S.P. from driving, as he has suffered a stroke and becomes confused easily.

3. Signs were posted at the entrance to the dining room of the assisted living facility for _____ the residents as to the day, date, and season.

4. Having lots of _____ such as old boxes and magazines stacked all over tends to lead to accidents in the home of the older adult.

5. Having someone with whom to eat meals can greatly _____ both the appetite and quality of living of the older adult.

6. The older adult who remains _____ in the community by doing volunteer work tends to be healthier.

B. Directions: Substitute words from the Vocabulary Building Glossary above for the underlined words in the paragraph below.

Together with the mud from the bad weather we were having, cleaning up the mess was quite a job. With good judgment, I took care of the problem by using help to clean up the smelly mess. The situation was improved by reminding my helper that it was necessary to finish early.

PRONUNCIATION OF DIFFICULT TERMS

Directions: Practice pronouncing the following words.

dysphagia	dys PHA gi a
orthostatic hypotension	OR tho STAT ic HY po TEN sion
presbycusis	pres by CU sis
presbyopia	pres by O pi a
rehabilitative	RE ha BIL i ta tive

COMMUNICATION EXERCISES

1. Write out the questions you would ask a patient to get information about current prescriptions, over-the-counter drugs, and any vitamins and herbal preparations being taken (See textbook Chapter 40). Practice asking the questions with a partner.

2. Write an explanation you would give a patient about how to use a medication reminder system you have developed. Practice it with a partner who will play the role of the patient and ask questions for clarification.

3. With a partner, write a short dialogue in which you assess an elderly patient's activity, nutrition, medications, and elimination habits during a home visit with the patient. Write your questions and the patient's possible responses.

Review the chapter key points, answer the study questions, and complete the critical thinking activities at the end of the chapter in the textbook.

CHAPTER 41

Common Psychosocial Care Problems of the Elderly

Answer Key: Textbook page references are provided as a guide for answering selected questions. A complete answer key was provided for your instructor.

TERMINOLOGY

A. Matching

Directions: Match the terms in Column I with the definitions in Column II.

Column I	Column II
(828) 1. _____ behavior modification	a. A morbid sadness, dejection, or melancholy
(824) 2. _____ delirium	b. Increase in symptoms of confusion or agitation as sunlight fades
(824) 3. _____ dementia	c. Permanent impairment of memory, intellectual functioning, and ability to problem-solve
(829) 4. _____ depression	d. Intervention used to change agitated behavior by giving positive feedback for desired behaviors and negative feedback for undesired behaviors
(829) 5. _____ electroconvulsive therapy (ECT)	e. Electric shock to the brain in an effort to change symptoms of severe depression
(824) 6. _____ nocturnal delirium	f. Re-examine the past to promote socialization and mental stimulation
(826) 7. _____ reminiscence	g. Encourage active socialization patterns with a group
(826) 8. _____ resocialization	h. Acute confusional state that can occur as a result of an underlying biologic or psychologic cause

B. Completion

Directions: Fill in the blank(s) with the correct term(s) from the terms list in the chapter in the textbook to complete the sentence.

(823)   1.   The lapses in memory that occur as people get older are termed
_____.

(823)   2.   Making lists of things is one way to cope with _____.

    375

(826)   3. Stimulating the senses while introducing factual information is used during
_____ therapy.

(829)   4. The _____ are one class of an-
tidepressants that have proven helpful in treating depression in the elderly.

(826)   5. Sharing family photos is a technique used for _____
therapy.

IDENTIFICATION

Directions: Identify the condition for which each of the following symptoms/signs occurs. Use "delirium," "dementia," or "depression." Symptoms/signs may occur with more than one condition.

(Table 41-2)

1. Resolves with treatment _____

2. Impaired memory for recent events _____

3. Sparse, repetitive speech _____

4. Sudden onset _____

5. Despair, worry _____

6. Coherent speech _____

7. Poor prognosis _____

8. Inability to perform activities of daily living (ADLs) _____

9. Changes in sleep-wake cycle _____

10. Self-neglect _____

11. Intact remote memory _____

12. Decreased ability to concentrate_____

SHORT ANSWER

Directions: Write a brief answer for each question.

(825)   1. Identify four principles of nursing care for the patient with cognitive impairment.

      a. _____

      b. _____

      c. _____

      d. _____

(829)   2. Explain the interrelationship of alcohol abuse, suicide, and depression in the elderly patient.

_____

_____

_____

_____

Student Name _____

(830-832) 3. List five crimes commonly occurring to the elderly along with one intervention that could possibly prevent the crime.

    a. _____

    _____

    b. _____

    _____

    c. _____

    _____

    d. _____

    _____

    e. _____

    _____

(830) 4. Identify the four main categories of elder abuse with an example for each one.

    a. _____

    b. _____

    c. _____

    d. _____

(832) 5. Identify two future psychosocial issues for the elderly population.

    a. _____

    b. _____

(824) 6. When assessing significant changes in mental functioning in an elderly person, you should:

    _____

    _____

    _____

(824) 7. When assessing an elderly person, you should exercise _____ and allow enough time for the person to _____.

(824) 8. Five factors that can contribute to an altered mental state in the elderly are:

    a. _____

    b. _____

    c. _____

    d. _____

    e. _____

(824) 9. Signs of confusion include:

    _____

    _____

(824) 10. Dementia is characterized by a slow, insidious onset that affects:

_____

_____

(825) 11. When a plan of care with therapy to decrease confusion and disorientation is implemented, it is very important that _____.

(825) 12. The desired effects of drugs when used for patients with dementia are to:

_____

_____

(826) 13. Family support is essential when one member is suffering from dementia because the family members are subject to:

_____

_____

_____

(826) 14. Families who are caring for a member with dementia should be encouraged to take advantage of _____ opportunities in their community.

(827) 15. Three characteristics for each stage of Alzheimer's disease are:

a. Early stage: _____

_____

b. Middle stage: _____

_____

c. Late stage: _____

_____

(827) 16. Aggressive behavior may also occur as a self-protective response to

_____.

(828) 17. When agitation and hostility become a problem, physical restraints are only used

_____.

(828) 18. For the patient with paranoia, developing _____ is the most important goal to accomplish.

(828) 19. Identify three interventions to decrease wandering.

a. _____

b. _____

c. _____

(828) 20. The underlying principle for developing interventions for the patient experiencing "sundown syndrome" is to _____.

(829) 21. Three strategies to improve nutritional status of the patient with dementia are:

a. _____

b. _____

c. _____

Student Name_____

(829)   22.   Signs of depression in the elderly may be slightly different and could include:

_____

_____

(829)   23.   Alcoholism should be considered if the elderly person has some of the following signs and symptoms:

_____

_____

_____

(829)   24.   It is especially important to protect the depressed patient from self-injury after _____ has been initiated.

(830)   25.   Signs of potential suicide are:

_____

_____

TABLE ACTIVITY

Directions: Fill in the following table with the cause, signs and symptoms, methods of diagnosis, and treatment for Alzheimer's disease.

(Table 41-5)

Alzheimer's Disease
Cause
Signs and Symptoms
Diagnosis
Treatment

NCLEX-PN® EXAM REVIEW

*Directions: Choose the **best** answer(s) to the following questions.*

(830) 1. A 79-year-old female lives with her son. She has come into the clinic for the second time with bruises and abrasions she claims came from a fall. She seems unkempt and says she has difficulty grooming and dressing because of the severe arthritis in her hands. She is very thin. You know that in order to assess her for elder abuse it is necessary to first
   1. confront her with the facts.
   2. establish a confidential, trusting relationship.
   3. remove her from her current living situation.
   4. say you do not believe the injuries are from a fall.

(830) 2. If there seems to be a likelihood of elder abuse involved in a patient's injuries, you know
   1. definite proof is necessary before calling the authorities.
   2. it must be corroborated by a third person.
   3. legally, it must be reported to the authorities.
   4. nothing can be done if she denies abuse occurred.

(826) 3. Sometimes elder abuse can be avoided by
   1. admonishing the elder to "do as she is told."
   2. making weekly visits to the home.
   3. obtaining help for the caregiver with daily care.
   4. medicating the elder to improve behavior.

(831) 4. Your neighbor shares with you that two of his elderly friends have been victims of telemarketing crime lately. He asks for advice on how to avoid this. You tell him
   1. refrain from answering the phone in the evening.
   2. not to put his telephone number on forms requesting it.
   3. give only a false credit card number to a phone solicitor.
   4. not to order anything over the telephone; ask for written information.

(824) 5. Your female patient, age 82, is displaying signs of confusion. There are many causes of confusion in the elderly, many of which are physiological rather than a problem with the brain. Before assuming that her confusion is related to mental causes, you should check

   _____

   _____ status. (Fill in the blank)

(826) 6. A patient's confusion is worsening. Reality orientation is part of her therapy. Which one of the following would be part of reality orientation?
   1. displaying memory aids such as a clock and calendar
   2. singing favorite songs with a group
   3. relating a favorite past experience to the group
   4. helping serve refreshments after an activity

Student Name _____

(828) 7. A patient's confusion becomes worse at about 5:00 P.M. One intervention that may help decrease her confusion is to
1. institute creative therapy activities in the late afternoon.
2. reduce stimulation in the environment.
3. reward positive behaviors.
4. use a security vest to keep her in the chair.

(829) 8. Your male patient, age 80, drinks a lot of alcohol. He is on several medications for his heart disease and hypertension. One danger of alcoholism—in addition to interaction with medication—is
1. loss of income.
2. increased anxiety.
3. loss of insurance.
4. inadequate nutrition.

(829) 9. When assessing him, in addition to determining his alcohol pattern, you should look for signs of underlying _____ _____. (Fill in the blank)

(829) 10. If the patient shows signs of both alcohol abuse and depression, it is *most* important to assess for
1. social isolation.
2. suicidal intent.
3. accident potential.
4. gastrointestinal bleeding.

(825) 11. Delirium in the elderly is often characterized by a(n)
1. gradual onset.
2. rapid onset.
3. poor prognosis.
4. intact remote memory.

(826) 12. A psychosocial approach for confusion/disorientation that reexamines the past to promote socialization and mental stimulation is
1. validation therapy.
2. remotivation therapy.
3. reminiscence.
4. resocialization.

(827) 13. Early-stage Alzheimer's disease is characterized by which of the following? (Select all that apply)
1. mild short-term memory loss
2. suspicion
3. difficulty learning new things
4. mild depression

(825) 14. Complaints of vague aches and pains, fatigue, and "just not feeling good" may be indicative of what condition in the elderly?
1. delirium
2. confusion
3. depression
4. dementia

(830) 15. The elderly may experience many types of abuse and neglect. Intentionally withholding medication from an elder would be considered _____ _____. (Fill in the blank)

(829) 16. Clues to alcoholism may include which of the following? (Select all that apply)
1. mental alertness.
2. insomnia.
3. gastritis.
4. anemia.

(829) 17. Three conditions that are interrelated and have similar risk factors associated with loss are
1. alcohol abuse, suicide, and dementia.
2. drug abuse, suicide, and delirium.
3. alcohol abuse, suicide, and depression.
4. alcohol abuse, depression, and elder abuse.

(829) 18. A primary nursing intervention for a depressed patient *after* he or she has initiated antidepressive therapy is
   1. protection for other people.
   2. avoidance of contact with other depressed patients.
   3. protection from self-injury.
   4. avoidance of overly concerned family members.

(830) 19. Elder abuse is often related to
   1. caregiver stress and unresolved family conflicts.
   2. caregiver stress and economic problems.
   3. belligerent behaviors of the older person.
   4. uneducated caregivers.

(831-832) 20. Many organizations promote education and provide assistance for the elderly. An organization that is instrumental in helping elders achieve the goal of increasing healthy life after age 65 is the

_____.

(Fill in the blank)

CRITICAL THINKING ACTIVITIES

1. It has been 2 years since V.E.'s husband died. She has not been able to shake her depression and has become more withdrawn in the past month. She comes to the clinic for monitoring of her diabetes. What plan could you devise to assist B.E. to deal with her depression?

2. You suspect that J.P. is being abused by the grandson with whom he lives. Identify signs that might contribute to your suspicion. How would you approach J.P. about this issue?

3. What three things do you feel should be done to address the challenges that will face the elderly in another 10 years?

MEETING CLINICAL OBJECTIVES

Directions: The following suggested activities will help you meet the stated clinical practice objectives for the chapter. Review your school's clinical objectives for the week and outline a plan of activities that will help you meet them. If you are unsure how to meet them, consult with your instructor at the beginning of the clinical day.

1. Assess each elderly patient assigned for signs of depression.

2. Formulate a teaching plan for the elderly members of a church group regarding ways to avoid crimes against them. Include specific measures.

3. Your patient is in the middle stage of Alzheimer's disease. Write a care plan to deal with her cognitive impairment and need for assistance with ADLs.

Student Name_____

STEPS TOWARD BETTER COMMUNICATION

VOCABULARY BUILDING GLOSSARY

Term	Pronunciation	Definition
A. Individual Terms		
adaptation	a dap TA tion	change to function in a new way; adjustment
advocacy	AD vo ca cy	supporting or working for a person or an issue
condescending	CON de SCEND ing	having a self-important or superior attitude
distraction	di STRAC tion	turning the attention to something else
implications	im pli CA tions	suggestions
inflicted	in FLIC ted	forced upon someone
insidious	in SID i ous	something bad or harmful that is not easily seen
manifestation	man i FES TA tion	an example; a sign
pose	POSE	to present or put forward
retaliation	re TAL i A tion	doing something bad to someone because of what they did; striking back
scams	SCAMS	schemes or plans to make money by deceiving people
symptomatic	symp to MA tic	based on symptoms
undetected	un de TEC ted	not seen or discovered
unkempt	un KEMPT	messy; deficient in order and neatness
B. Phrases		
go to sleep for the last time	go to SLEEP for the LAST time	to die in one's sleep
one-stop-shopping	one-stop-shop ping	everything needed is available at one place
out to get them	out to GET them	threatening them; intending harm or danger
solely attributable to	SOLE ly at TRIB u ta ble to	caused only by one thing
the graying of America	the GRAY ing of a MER i ca	the increasing number of older people in United States (because of better health care)
white collar crime	WHITE COL lar crime	criminal acts through a business or office involving paper or money schemes; not physical crime like taking a purse, or breaking into a house

COMPLETION

Directions: Underline the words from the Vocabulary Building Glossary in the following sentences, and fill in the blanks correctly with one of the words below.

advocacy   condescending   implication   unkempt   pose

1. The scams inflicted on the _____ woman were undetected.

2. _____ for respite care is very welcome for caregivers.

3. Retaliation may be symptomatic when a caregiver is angry and can _____ an insidious danger to a patient.

4. A(n) _____ attitude is sometimes a manifestation of low self-esteem.

5. The use of distraction and adaptation is a(n) _____ that the nurse understand how to deal with the patient's outburst.

WORD ATTACK SKILLS

Directions: Look at these words composed of a stem and suffix.

adaptation   manifestation
distraction   retaliation
implication

-ation—is a suffix added to a verb to create a noun. The meaning of the noun is an action or process connected with the verb.

Verb	Meaning	Noun	Meaning
adapt	to change to fit the situation	adaptation	a change to suit the situation
distract	to put attention on something else	distraction	an action that puts the attention on something else
imply	to suggest indirectly	implication	an indirect suggestion
manifest	to exhibit, to show	manifestation	a sign showing or displaying something
retaliate	to respond to an action with another similar action	retaliation	a direct response to an action with a similar action

PRONUNCIATION OF DIFFICULT TERMS

Directions: Practice pronouncing the following words and phrases with a peer.

benign senescent forgetfulness	be NIGN se NES cent for GET ful ness
electroconvulsive therapy	e LEC tro con VUL sive ther a py
remotivation therapy	re mo ti VA tion THER a py
resocialization therapy	re SO cial i ZA tion THER a py
reminiscence	rem i NIS cense
selective serotonin reuptake inhibitors	se LEC tive ser o TON in re UP take in HIB i tors

Student Name_____

COMMUNICATION EXERCISE

Dealing with the possibility of elder abuse is a sensitive issue. The following is an example of how this issue might be approached with the patient mentioned in Critical Thinking Exercise #2 above.

Nurse: "How do you like living with your grandson, J.P.?"

J.P.:   "I guess it's OK."

Nurse: "Young people don't always understand what it is like to be older. Sometimes they become impatient with older people."

J.P.:   "You can say that again."

Nurse: "Has that happened to you?"

J.P.:   "He is always wanting me to hurry, and he asks another question before I can get out an answer to his first one. I move rather slowly, and that irritates him too."

Nurse: "I noticed these marks on your upper arm, J.P. Do you know how those happened?"

J.P.:   "I'm not sure. Sometimes he will grab my arm and pull me along when he is a hurry to get to the car."

Nurse: "Are there other ways in which he becomes impatient with you?"

J.P.:   "I stumbled and fell one day when he kind of had a hold of me and was dragging me into the house. I don't think he meant to hurt me."

Nurse: "I'll talk to him about giving you time to do things, J.P. I don't want you to get really hurt."

Directions: Write a dialogue explaining to a family the effects of alcohol on medications and the chronic health conditions (hypertension and gastritis) of their father. Be ready to answer their questions, objections, and denials. Compare your dialogue with your partner's, combine the two dialogues into one, and practice the dialogue together.

CULTURAL POINTS

Does your native country or cultural community have any of the problems of the elderly that are described in this chapter? If not, why do you think it is different? If you do, how are they handled? Have you seen any of these problems in your own family? What about your grandparents? If they had any of these problems, how were they cared for and what were the family and society attitudes about the problems? Would things be different today? Talk about these questions in a group, preferably with people from different cultures. Compare your attitudes. What similarities and differences do you find? Notes for discussion:

Review the chapter key points, answer the study questions, and complete the critical thinking activities at the end of the chapter in the textbook.

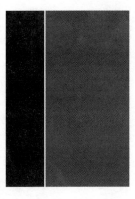

Skills Performance Checklists

These checklists were developed to assist in evaluating the competence of students in performing the nursing interventions presented in the text *Fundamental Concepts and Skills for Nursing*. The checklists are perforated for easy removal and reference. Students can be evaluated with an "S" for satisfactory or a "U" for unsatisfactory performance rating by putting a check in the appropriate column for each step. Specific instruction or feedback can be provided in the "Comments" box.

Skill 15-1   Postmortem Care

Student:_____

Date: _____

	S	U
1. Carries out Standard Steps A, B, C, D, and E as need indicates.	❑	❑
2. Prepares equipment and provides privacy.	❑	❑
3. Washes hands and dons gloves.	❑	❑
4. Positions body supine, in proper alignment, with head slightly elevated.	❑	❑
5. Replaces dentures as appropriate, closes mouth and secures it; closes eyes.	❑	❑
6. Removes jewelry and clothing and prepares items to be returned to family.	❑	❑
7. Cleans body appropriately and combs hair.	❑	❑
8. Removes or secures all tubes and lines, and changes dressings.	❑	❑
9. Dresses body in clean gown and straightens room. Drapes body with sheet.	❑	❑
10. Allows viewing time for family; remains in room to offer emotional support.	❑	❑
11. Follows agency procedure for tagging body and preparing it in a shroud.	❑	❑
12. Removes gloves and washes hands.	❑	❑
13. Transports the body to the morgue.	❑	❑
14. Documents the procedure.	❑	❑

Successfully completed   ❑

Needs practice and retesting ❑

Comments:

Instructor: _____

Skill 16-1 Handwashing

Student:_____

Date: _____

	S	U
1. Stands away from sink to prevent contaminating uniform.	❑	❑
2. Uses constantly running water.	❑	❑
3. Wets hands.	❑	❑
4. Soaps hands sufficiently to provide lather.	❑	❑
5. Washes entire surfaces of hands and wrists vigorously using friction.	❑	❑
6. Interlaces fingers to wash spaces between them; rubs back and forth.	❑	❑
7. Washes for at least 15 seconds.	❑	❑
8. Rinses hands well with fingers pointing down.	❑	❑
9. Dries hands thoroughly.	❑	❑
10. Turns off water without contaminating hands.	❑	❑

For Alcohol Hand Rub

	S	U
11. Dispenses sufficient hand rub agent to thoroughly cover hands.	❑	❑
12. Rubs cleansing agent over all aspects of hands and fingers.	❑	❑
13. Continues to rub until all signs of the agent are gone and hands are dry.	❑	❑

Successfully completed ❑

Needs practice and retesting ❑

Comments:

Instructor: _____

Skill 16-2 Using Personal Protective Equipment: Gown and Mask

Student:_____

Date: _____

	S	U
1. Correctly puts on gown.	❏	❏
2. Places mask to cover nose and mouth and secures it correctly.	❏	❏
3. Dons protective eyewear.	❏	❏
4. Dons shoe covering and head cover if indicated.	❏	❏
5. Dons nonsterile gloves and pulls gloves over gown cuffs.	❏	❏
6. Removes PPEs in correct order.	❏	❏
7. Correctly disposes of PPEs without contaminating self.	❏	❏
8. Washes hands.	❏	❏

Successfully completed ❏

Needs practice and retesting ❏

Comments:

Instructor: _____

Skill 17-1   Performing a Surgical Hand Scrub

Student: _____

Date: _____

	S	U
1. Removes jewelry.	❏	❏
2. Adjusts water to correct temperature and force.	❏	❏
3. Wets hands and arms from above elbows to fingertips, keeping hands higher than elbows.	❏	❏
4. Applies soaping agent or uses soap-impregnated brush or sponge pad. Works up a lather.	❏	❏
5. Cleans nails on each hand while holding the scrub brush/pad in other hand.	❏	❏
6. Starts scrubbing at fingertips with a circular motion scrubs each finger, between fingers, palm and back of hand using light to moderate friction; scrubs wrist and up the arm to 2" above the elbow.	❏	❏
7. Scrubs each arm for approximately 2–2 1/2 minutes. Times the scrub by the clock.	❏	❏
8. Rinses each hand and arm thoroughly, keeping the hands pointed up and allowing water to run from the fingertips down off of the elbow area.	❏	❏
9. Turns off water using foot or knee control.	❏	❏
10. Dries hands with a sterile towel without contaminating sterile field or scrubbed hands.	❏	❏
11. Drops used towel into proper receptacle.	❏	❏

OR

	S	U
12. Dispenses waterless hand cleanser into palm of one hand.	❏	❏
13. Rubs cleanser into skin covering all areas of opposite hand and arm to 2" above the elbow.	❏	❏
14. Keeps rubbing until hands and arms are dry.	❏	❏
15. Dispenses waterless hand cleanser into palm of other hand.	❏	❏
16. Rubs cleanser into skin covering all areas of second hand and arm to 2" above the elbow.	❏	❏
17. Continues to rub until hand and arm are dry.	❏	❏

Successfully completed ❏

Needs practice and retesting ❏

Comments:

Instructor: _____

Skill 17-2   Opening Sterile Packs and Preparing a Sterile Field

Student:_____

Date: _____

	S	U
1. Carries out Standard Steps A, B, C, D, and E as indicated for the procedure.	❑	❑
2. Clears a working surface.	❑	❑
3. Removes outer wrap.	❑	❑
4. Opens pack with proper aseptic technique.	❑	❑
5. Arranges items on the sterile field.	❑	❑
6. Adds supplies or equipment to the field correctly.	❑	❑
7. Performs procedure.	❑	❑
8. Carries out Standard Steps X, Y, and Z.	❑	❑

Successfully completed   ❑

Needs practice and retesting ❑

Comments:

Instructor: _____

Skill 17-3   Sterile Gloving and Ungloving

Student:_____

Date: _____

	S	U
1. Obtains pair of sterile gloves of correct size; washes hands.	❑	❑
2. Peels open outer wrapper and positions inner glove package on flat surface.	❑	❑
3. Opens the inner glove package exposing the gloves without contaminating them.	❑	❑
4. Picks up the first glove by the folded-over cuff.	❑	❑
5. Inserts hand into glove without touching the outside of the glove to any part of the skin or other unsterile object; keeps hands above waist level.	❑	❑
6. Picks up the second glove by placing gloved fingers under the cuff; slips hand into the glove being careful not to allow bare skin to touch the other gloved hand.	❑	❑
7. Slides cuffs over the wrists; adjusts the fingers inside the gloves.	❑	❑

Ungloving

8. Grasps the outside surface of one glove at the top of the palm and pulls glove off while rolling it inside out.	❑	❑
9. Holds removed glove in palm of other hand; slips bare fingers under the cuff of the remaining glove and slides the glove down over the hand, rolling it inside-out as it is removed. Does not contaminate hands.	❑	❑
10. Disposes of the contaminated gloves.	❑	❑
11. Washes the hands.	❑	❑

Successfully completed   ❏

Needs practice and retesting ❏

Comments:

Instructor: _____

Skill 18-1   Positioning the Patient

Student:_____

Date: _____

	S	U
1. Carries out Standard Steps A, B, C, D, and E as need indicates.	❑	❑
2. Prepares the patient for the position change.	❑	❑
3. Prepares bed: proper working height, bed flat, near side rail down, wheels locked.	❑	❑

Supine Position

	S	U
4. Places patient supine in center of bed in good alignment.	❑	❑
5. Positions pillow under head and shoulders.	❑	❑
6. Uses pillows, trochanter rolls, and footboard as needed to maintain correct body alignment and prevent pressure on heels.	❑	❑
7. Supports arms and hands with pillows as needed; positions hands in proper alignment using splints as needed.	❑	❑

Fowler's and Semi-Fowler's Position

	S	U
8. Elevates head of bed to correct angle.	❑	❑
9. Uses pillows, towel rolls, and supports as needed to maintain alignment and prevent pressure necrosis.	❑	❑

Side-Lying Position

	S	U
10. With patient flat in bed, moves patient toward the far side of the bed.	❑	❑
11. Rolls patient into a semi-side–lying position so that weight is not on trochanter.	❑	❑
12. Adjusts patient's alignment.	❑	❑
13. Places pillow under head and neck with ear flat.	❑	❑
14. Tucks rolled pillow at back to support in position.	❑	❑
15. Positions arm next to mattress.	❑	❑
16. Supports upper arm with pillow.	❑	❑
17. Flexes upper knee and supports leg with pillow(s).	❑	❑

Sims' Position

18. While in side-lying position, moves patient further to far side of bed and rolls partially onto abdomen. ❏ ❏
19. Positions arms correctly and supports as needed. ❏ ❏
20. Readjusts pillows to provide support for leg. ❏ ❏

Prone Position

21. With bed flat and patient on back, moves to far side of the bed. ❏ ❏
22. Correctly places pillow on the abdomen, and positions arms close to body with hands tucked under hips. ❏ ❏
23. Rolls patient towards self onto the abdomen; readjusts alignment and centers in the bed. ❏ ❏
24. Turns head to side and places pillow. ❏ ❏
25. Supports flexed arms at the shoulders. ❏ ❏
26. Supports lower legs. ❏ ❏
27. Lowers the bed and restores the unit. ❏ ❏
28. Carries out Standard Steps X, Y, and Z. ❏ ❏
29. Documents positioning. ❏ ❏

Successfully completed ❏

Needs practice and retesting ❏

Comments:

Instructor: _____

Skill 18-2   Moving the Patient Up in Bed

Student:_____

Date: _____

	S	U
1. Carries out Standard Steps A, B, C, D, and E as indicated.	❑	❑
2. Positions bed: locks wheels, raises bed to correct working height in flat position, lowers near side rail, places pillow upright against headboard.	❑	❑
3. Instructs patient if patient can assist.	❑	❑
4. Positions patient on back with knees flexed and arms across chest if patient is unable to help.	❑	❑
5. Shifts patient up in bed using proper body mechanics.	❑	❑

For Lift (Draw) Sheet:

	S	U
6. Obtains assistant to help.	❑	❑
7. Places lift (draw) sheet under patient, fan-folded close to patient.	❑	❑
8. Places pillow upright at head of bed to protect head.	❑	❑
9. On count of three both nurses slide lift sheet and patient toward head of bed using correct body mechanics.	❑	❑
10. Carries out Standard Steps X, Y, and Z.	❑	❑

Successfully completed ❑

Needs practice and retesting ❑

Comments:

Instructor: _____

Skill 18-3   Passive Range-of-Motion Exercises

Student:_____

Date: _____

	S	U
1. Carries out Standard Steps A, B, C, D, and E as indicated.	❑	❑
2. Prepares the bed: wheels locked, bed at proper working height.	❑	❑
3. Positions patient in supine position and drapes.	❑	❑
4. Performs passive range-of-motion (ROM) exercises for the head and neck.	❑	❑
5. Performs passive ROM on the near upper extremity, using correct movements and appropriate number of repetitions:		
a. Arm flexion, extension.	❑	❑
b. Shoulder abduction, adduction, internal rotation, external rotation.	❑	❑
c. Elevation and depression of shoulders.	❑	❑
d. Wrist.	❑	❑
e. Fingers.	❑	❑
6. Performs passive range of motion on the near lower extremity, using correct movements and appropriate number of repetitions:		
a. Leg flexion and extension.	❑	❑
b. Hip abduction and adduction.	❑	❑
c. Hip internal rotation and external rotation.	❑	❑
d. Ankle.	❑	❑
e. Foot dorsiflexion and plantarflexion.	❑	❑
f. Toes.	❑	❑
7. Raises side rail; moves to opposite side of bed.	❑	❑
8. Lowers side rail and performs passive ROM on upper extremity, using correct movements and appropriate number of repetitions.	❑	❑
9. Performs passive ROM on lower extremity, using correct movements and appropriate number of repetitions.	❑	❑
10. Places patient in position of comfort.	❑	❑
11. Carries out Standard Steps X, Y, and Z.	❑	❑

Successfully completed   ❑

Needs practice and retesting ❑

Comments:

Instructor: _____

Skill 18-4 Transferring the Patient to a Wheelchair

Student:_____

Date: _____

	S	U
1. Carries out Standard Steps A, B, C, D, and E as need indicates.	❑	❑
2. Positions the wheelchair appropriately, locks wheels, and raises foot rests.	❑	❑
3. Assists patient to sit at side of bed using correct body mechanics.	❑	❑
4. Assists patient with robe and slippers.	❑	❑
5. Assists patient to stand, pivot, and sit, using correct body mechanics, including a helper if needed.	❑	❑
6. Places feet on foot rests.	❑	❑
7. Provides for patient safety while sitting up.	❑	❑
8. Returns patient to bed after appropriate interval to prevent overtiring.	❑	❑
9. Carries out Standard Steps X, Y, and Z.	❑	❑

Successfully completed   ❑

Needs practice and retesting ❑

Comments:

Instructor: _____

Skill 18-5   Transferring the Patient to a Stretcher

Student:_____

Date: _____

	S	U
1. Carries out Standard Steps A, B, C, D, and E as need indicates.	❑	❑
2. Has enough staff present for safe transfer.	❑	❑
3. Prepares patient and bed for the transfer procedure, including elevating bed, lowering side rail, locking wheels, covering patient, and removing any obstructions.	❑	❑
4. Positions any tubes so they will not be pulled or dislodged during transfer.	❑	❑
5. Performs the transfer with the assistance of other staff:		
a. Uses pull sheet.	❑	❑
b. Places stretcher firmly against open side of bed and locks wheels.	❑	❑
c. Utilizes correct body mechanics.	❑	❑
6. Fastens safety belt securely over patient and elevates stretcher side rails.	❑	❑
7. Provides for patient comfort.	❑	❑
8. Remakes or straightens bed before patient's return.	❑	❑
9. Carries out Standard Steps X, Y, and Z.	❑	❑

Successfully completed   ❑

Needs practice and retesting ❑

Comments:

Instructor: _____

Skill 18-6   Ambulating the Patient and Breaking a Fall

Student:_____

Date: _____

	S	U
1. Carries out Standard Steps A, B, C, D, and E as need indicates.	❑	❑
2. Sits the patient on the side of the bed.	❑	❑
3. Places patient's feet firmly on the floor.	❑	❑
4. Places gait belt around patient's waist if one is available.	❑	❑
5. Safely assists patient to a standing position using proper body mechanics.	❑	❑
6. Allows patient to stabilize and gain balance.	❑	❑
7. Checks and corrects patient's posture; provides support with near hand holding gait belt.	❑	❑
8. Walks at patient's side, matching gait, while safely stabilizing patient.	❑	❑

Should Patient Begin to Fall

	S	U
9. When patient begins to fall, assumes broad stance, and grasps patient's body at waist or under the axilla. Grasp gait belt if one is on patient.	❑	❑
10. Extends near leg against the patient, bracing patient's body and slides patient down the leg to the floor while bending own knees.	❑	❑
11. Examines patient for any sign of injury sustained in the fall.	❑	❑
12. Calls for additional help to assist the patient back to bed.	❑	❑

To Return to Bed While Ambulating

	S	U
13. After ambulating, walks patient to the side of the bed, positions patient with legs at edge of mattress and while facing patient, assists patient to safely sit on side of bed.	❑	❑
14. Carries out Standard Steps X, Y, and Z.	❑	❑

Successfully completed   ❏

Needs practice and retesting ❏

Comments:

Instructor: _____

Skill 19-1   Administering a Bed Bath and Perineal Care

Student:_____

Date: _____

		S	U
1.	Carries out Standard Steps A, B, C, D, and E as need indicates.	❑	❑
2.	Prepares the environment for the bath.	❑	❑
3.	Offers bedpan or urinal.	❑	❑
4.	Raises bed to comfortable working height. Lowers rail and positions patient close to side of bed.	❑	❑
5.	Drapes patient with bath blanket or top sheet.	❑	❑
6.	Removes bed linen and disposes of soiled linen not to be reused.	❑	❑
7.	Raises rail while preparing the bath water; checks temperature of water.	❑	❑
8.	Removes gown without exposing patient.	❑	❑
9.	Washes and dries the face using separate corner of mitt for each eye.	❑	❑
10.	Washes and dries the arms and axillae, protecting the bedding.	❑	❑
11.	Washes and dries the chest using circular motions.	❑	❑
12.	Washes and dries the abdomen. Keeps patient draped.	❑	❑
13.	Washes and dries the legs with long firm strokes; places towel lengthwise under the leg.	❑	❑
14.	Soaks feet in basin; washes and dries the feet.	❑	❑
15.	Changes water when it becomes cool or soapy.	❑	❑
16.	Washes and dries the back, buttocks and anal area; changes water.	❑	❑
17.	Washes or permits patient to wash the perineal area; uses gloves.	❑	❑
18.	Assists patient into clean gown or pajamas.	❑	❑
19.	Completes personal care.	❑	❑
20.	Lowers bed, raises rail, and restores unit.	❑	❑
21.	Cleans and stores equipment.	❑	❑
22.	Documents the procedure.	❑	❑

Successfully completed   ❏

Needs practice and retesting ❏

Comments:

Instructor: _____

Skill 19-2   Administering Oral Care to the Unconscious Patient

Student:_____

Date: _____

	S	U
1. Carries out Standard Steps A, B, C, D, and E as need indicates.	❑	❑
2. Turns patient onto the side.	❑	❑
3. Attaches oral suction device to tubing and turns on suction.	❑	❑
4. Dons gloves.	❑	❑
5. Cleanses mouth and teeth thoroughly.	❑	❑
6. Flosses teeth.	❑	❑
7. Rinses mouth as needed.	❑	❑
8. Lubricates lips.	❑	❑
9. Removes gloves.	❑	❑
10. Cleans and stores equipment.	❑	❑
11. Repositions patient, lowers bed, and restores unit.	❑	❑
12. Documents procedure.	❑	❑

Successfully completed   ❑

Needs practice and retesting ❑

Comments:

Instructor: _____

Skill 19-3   Denture Care

Student:_____

Date: _____

	S	U
1. Washes hands and dons clean gloves.	❑	❑
2. Removes dentures and places in emesis basin.	❑	❑
3. Places washcloth or towels in bottom of sink.	❑	❑
4. Cleans dentures thoroughly.	❑	❑
5. Rinses dentures.	❑	❑
6. Replaces dentures in mouth or stores in denture cup with fresh water.	❑	❑
7. Removes gloves and washes hands.	❑	❑
8. Documents procedure.	❑	❑

Successfully completed   ❑

Needs practice and retesting ❑

Comments:

Instructor: _____

Skill 19-4 Shampooing Hair

Student:_____

Date: _____

	S	U
1. Carries out Standard Steps A, B, C, D, and E as need indicates.	❏	❏
2. Raises the bed, lowers the near side rail, and moves patient to near side of bed.	❏	❏
3. Drapes the patient.	❏	❏
4. Brushes or combs tangles from hair.	❏	❏
5. Positions shampoo tray and places drainage receptacle beneath spout of tray.	❏	❏
6. Obtains warm water in pitcher maintaining patient safety.	❏	❏
7. Moistens hair and applies shampoo.	❏	❏
8. Works shampoo into hair massaging scalp thoroughly.	❏	❏
9. Rinses hair.	❏	❏
10. Repeats shampoo process if needed.	❏	❏
11. Applies conditioner if needed; rinses thoroughly.	❏	❏
12. Wraps head in towel, dries face and shoulders.	❏	❏
13. Removes shampoo tray and drainage receptacle.	❏	❏
14. Towel-dries hair or uses hair dryer.	❏	❏
15. Repositions patient for comfort.	❏	❏
16. Finishes arranging hair.	❏	❏
17. Lowers bed, raises rail, and restores unit.	❏	❏
18. Cleans and stores equipment.	❏	❏
19. Documents the procedure.	❏	❏

Successfully completed ❏

Needs practice and retesting ❏

Comments:

Instructor: _____

Skill 20-1   Making an Unoccupied Bed

Student:_____

Date: _____

	S	U
1. Carries out Standard Steps A, B, C, D, and E as need indicates.	❏	❏
2. Raises bed and lowers side rail.	❏	❏
3. Loosens linens, removes spread and/or blanket, and folds them for reuse.	❏	❏
4. Removes the sheets and pillowcases and places them in laundry hamper or bag.	❏	❏
5. Moves mattress to the head of the bed.	❏	❏
6. Makes bed on one side, mitering corners of sheet and bed covers.	❏	❏
7. Positions drawsheet correctly if used.	❏	❏
8. Makes other side of the bed, mitering the corners.	❏	❏
9. Bed is tight and smooth with a cuff at the top of the covers.	❏	❏
10. Provides a toe pleat if needed.	❏	❏
11. Changes pillowcases without contaminating them and replaces pillows.	❏	❏
12. Lowers the bed to lowest position, raises side rails as need indicates, attaches the call light, and places personal items within reach.	❏	❏
13. Removes the soiled linens without contaminating uniform.	❏	❏
14. Completes bed-making within allotted time.	❏	❏
15. Carries out Standard Steps X, Y, and Z.	❏	❏

Successfully completed   ❏

Needs practice and retesting ❏

Comments:

Instructor: _____

Skill 20-2   Making an Occupied Bed

Student:_____

Date: _____

	S	U
1. Carries out Standard Steps A, B, C, D, and E as need indicates.	❑	❑
2. Raises the bed to working height and raises far side rail before turning the patient.	❑	❑
3. Loosens top covers and removes spread and/or blanket, folds and places them over a chair for reuse if unsoiled.	❑	❑
4. Places bath blanket over the patient and removes the top sheet.	❑	❑
5. Assists patient to a side-lying position on the far side of the bed.	❑	❑
6. Loosens bottom linens and rolls each piece of linen close to the patient.	❑	❑
7. Positions clean bottom sheet, fan folded beneath edge of rolled dirty linen.	❑	❑
8. Makes near side of the bed with the bottom linens, mitering the corner at the top and bottom of the mattress.	❑	❑
9. Positions drawsheet correctly if used.	❑	❑
10. Raises the side rail before going to the other side of the bed.	❑	❑
11. Assists patient to move to the other side of the bed.	❑	❑
12. Lowers side rail and loosens bottom linens and removes them; places soiled linens in hamper or bag.	❑	❑
13. Tightens, smoothes, and tucks bottom linens in on near side of the bed, mitering the top corner.	❑	❑
14. Positions patient in center of bed in supine position, places top sheet, removes bath blanket, and places spread.	❑	❑
15. Smoothes top linens, tucks in and miters the bottom corners, and forms top cuff.	❑	❑
16. Makes room for toes.	❑	❑

17. Changes pillowcases without contaminating them and replaces pillows. ❑ ❑

18. Lowers the bed to lowest position, raises side rails as need indicates, attaches the call light, and places personal items within reach. ❑ ❑

19. Removes the soiled linens without contaminating uniform. ❑ ❑

20. Completes bed-making within allotted time. ❑ ❑

21. Carries out Standard Steps X, Y, and Z. ❑ ❑

Successfully completed ❑

Needs practice and retesting ❑

Comments:

Instructor: _____

Skill 20-3   Applying a Protective Device

Student:_____

Date: _____

	S	U
1. Carries out Standard Steps A, B, C, D, and E as need indicates.	❑	❑
2. Explains the purpose and need for the device to the patient and family.	❑	❑
3. Applies the security device correctly.	❑	❑
4. Checks for correct application.	❑	❑
5. Secures device correctly with a half-bow knot.	❑	❑
6. Verbalizes need to check on patient at specific intervals.	❑	❑
7. Verbalizes need to remove device and exercise joints and muscles every 2 hours.	❑	❑
8. Documents reason for use of restraint, other measures attempted, and correct application of device.	❑	❑
9. Carries out Standard Steps X, Y, and Z.	❑	❑

Successfully completed   ❑

Needs practice and retesting ❑

Comments:

Instructor: _____

Skill 21-1 Measuring the Temperature with an Electronic Thermometer

Student:_____

Date: _____

	S	U
1. Carries out Standard Steps A, B, C, D, and E as need indicates.	❑	❑
2. Places probe cover over probe.	❑	❑
3. Places thermometer probe in patient's mouth with thermometer turned on.	❑	❑
4. Waits until machine indicates temperature reading is complete.	❑	❑
5. Disposes of probe cover.	❑	❑
6. Turns off unit by returning probe to base.	❑	❑
7. Records temperature.	❑	❑
8. Carries out Standard Steps X, Y, and Z.	❑	❑

Successfully completed ❑

Needs practice and retesting ❑

Comments:

Instructor: _____

Skill 21-2 Measuring the Temperature with a Tympanic Thermometer

Student:_____

Date: _____

	S	U
1. Carries out Standard Steps A, B, C, D, and E as need indicates.	❑	❑
2. Readies tympanic thermometer unit and places probe cover over the probe.	❑	❑
3. Inspects ear canal and places probe in auditory canal.	❑	❑
4. Steadies tympanic thermometer unit.	❑	❑
5. Reads tympanic temperature accurately and removes probe from ear.	❑	❑
6. Discards probe cover.	❑	❑
7. Returns probe to base of tympanic thermometer unit.	❑	❑
8. Records tympanic temperature accurately.	❑	❑
9. Carries out Standard Steps X, Y, and Z.	❑	❑

Successfully completed ❑

Needs practice and retesting ❑

Comments:

Instructor: _____

Skill 21-3   Measuring the Radial Pulse

Student:_____

Date: _____

	S	U
1. Carries out Standard Steps A, B, C, D, and E as need indicates.	❑	❑
2. Locates radial pulse using pads of fingers.	❑	❑
3. Counts radial pulse accurately for 30 seconds.	❑	❑
4. Records radial pulse rate accurately.	❑	❑
5. Reports any abnormalities.	❑	❑
6. Carries out Standard Steps X, Y, and Z.	❑	❑

Successfully completed   ❑

Needs practice and retesting   ❑

Comments:

Instructor: _____

Skill 21-4   Measuring an Apical Pulse

Student:_____

Date: _____

	S	U
1. Carries out Standard Steps A, B, C, D, and E as need indicates.	❑	❑
2. Exposes chest and correctly locates apex of heart area.	❑	❑
3. Listens and counts apical pulse rate accurately for 60 seconds.	❑	❑
4. Records the apical pulse rate accurately.	❑	❑
5. Carries out Standard Steps X, Y, and Z.	❑	❑

Successfully completed   ❑

Needs practice and retesting ❑

Comments:

Instructor: _____

Skill 21-5   Measuring Respirations

Student:_____

Date: _____

	S	U
1. Carries out Standard Steps A, B, C, D, and E as need indicates.	❑	❑
2. Counts the respirations accurately noting rate, depth, and character.	❑	❑
3. Records the respiratory rate accurately.	❑	❑
4. Carries out Standard Steps X, Y, and Z.	❑	❑

Successfully completed   ❑

Needs practice and retesting ❑

Comments:

Instructor: _____

Skill 21-6   Measuring the Blood Pressure

Student:_____

Date: _____

	S	U
1. Carries out Standard Steps A, B, C, D, and E as need indicates.	❑	❑
2. Positions patient and allows to rest for 5 minutes before taking BP.	❑	❑
3. Applies appropriate size cuff to arm correctly.	❑	❑
4. Palpates brachial pulse; inflates cuff until brachial pulse disappears; deflates cuff.	❑	❑
5. Places stethoscope diaphragm over brachial pulse and inflates cuff to a point 30 mm Hg above point where pulse disappeared.	❑	❑
6. Slowly deflates cuff while listening for Korotkoff's sounds.	❑	❑
7. Identifies accurate systolic and diastolic blood pressure measurement.	❑	❑
8. Records systolic and diastolic blood pressure.	❑	❑
9. Repeats procedure if uncertain readings are accurate.	❑	❑
10. Carries out Standard Steps X, Y, and Z.	❑	❑

Successfully completed   ❑

Needs practice and retesting ❑

Comments:

Instructor: _____

Skill 22-1 Performing a Physical Examination

Student:_____

Date: _____

	S	U
1. Carries out Standard Steps A, B, C, D, and E as need indicates.	❑	❑
2. Obtains a through history.	❑	❑
3. Prepares the patient for the physical examination.	❑	❑
4. Weighs and measures the patient.	❑	❑
5. Takes the vital signs.	❑	❑
6. Examines each body system: head and neck, skin and extremities, chest, heart and lungs, abdomen.	❑	❑
7. Obtains needed specimens.	❑	❑
8. Performs visual acuity and hearing test if required.	❑	❑
9. Documents findings.	❑	❑
10. Carries out Standard Steps X, Y, and Z.	❑	❑

Successfully completed ❑

Needs practice and retesting ❑

Comments:

Instructor: _____

Skill 22-2   Performing a Neurologic Check

Student:_____

Date: _____

	S	U
1. Carries out Standard Steps A, B, C, D, and E as need indicates.	❑	❑
2. Asks appropriate questions to determine mental orientation and cognition.	❑	❑
3. Examines pupils for size; tests pupil constriction in each eye separately.	❑	❑
4. Tests patient's ability to follow a finger to the cardinal points.	❑	❑
5. Tests motor reflexes and ability to follow commands by asking patient to perform certain maneuvers with the extremities.	❑	❑
6. Tests extremity muscle strength by having patient push against hands with the feet and by grasping fingers in each hand.	❑	❑
7. For comatose patient: checks response to a stimulus appropriately.	❑	❑
8. Calculates Glasgow Coma Scale score.	❑	❑
9. Carries out Standard Steps X, Y, and Z.	❑	❑

Successfully completed   ❑

Needs practice and retesting ❑

Comments:

Instructor: _____

Skill 24-1 Phlebotomy and Obtaining Blood Samples with a Vacutainer System

Student:_____

Date: _____

	S	U
1. Carries out Standard Steps A, B, C, D, and E as need indicates.	❏	❏
2. Washes hands and dons latex gloves.	❏	❏
3. Selects an appropriate venipuncture site and positions the tourniquet; has patient form a fist with the hand.	❏	❏
4. Cleanses the area thoroughly.	❏	❏
5. Punctures the site and gathers needed blood samples.	❏	❏
6. Releases the tourniquet.	❏	❏
7. Withdraws the needle and applies a dry gauze pad and pressure to the site.	❏	❏
8. When bleeding has stopped, applies an adhesive bandage.	❏	❏
9. Disposes of used equipment properly; removes gloves and washes hands.	❏	❏
10. Places labels on tubes and prepares them for transport to the laboratory with the requisition slips.	❏	❏
11. Documents the procedure.	❏	❏

Successfully completed ❏

Needs practice and retesting ❏

Comments:

Instructor: _____

Skill 24-2   Performing Capillary Blood Tests: Blood Glucose or Hemoglobin

Student:_____

Date: _____

	S	U
1. Carries out Standard Steps A, B, C, D, and E as need indicates.	❑	❑
2. Prepares the hand and finger for the test.	❑	❑
3. Washes hands and puts on gloves.	❑	❑
4. Prepares the fingerstick site.	❑	❑
5. Turns on the machine and prepares the lancet.	❑	❑
6. Checks that the machine is set properly.	❑	❑

For Glucometer (Follows Directions for Type of Machine)

	S	U
7. Inserts a test strip into the machine.	❑	❑
8. Performs the fingerstick.	❑	❑
9. Correctly obtains drop of blood.	❑	❑
10. Places drop of blood on test strip.	❑	❑
11. Applies cotton ball or gauze to finger to stop bleeding.	❑	❑
12. Notes the reading on the screen and documents it.	❑	❑

For Hemoglobin Test

	S	U
13. After step 6, performs the fingerstick, wipes away the first drop of blood with gauze pad; gathers second drop in capillary collection device.	❑	❑
14. Gently wipes the flat back side of the test stick on the clean gauze pad.	❑	❑
15. Places cotton ball or gauze firmly against puncture site to stop bleeding.	❑	❑
16. Places capillary collection device in the machine.	❑	❑
17. Reads and documents the result.	❑	❑

For Both Tests

	S	U
18. Turns off the machine and properly disposes of used equipment.	❑	❑
19. Applies bandage to puncture site as needed.	❑	❑
20. Removes gloves and washes hands.	❑	❑

Successfully completed ❏

Needs practice and retesting ❏

Comments:

Instructor: _____

Skill 24-3   Performing a Urine Dipstick Test

Student:_____

Date: _____

	S	U
1. Carries out Standard Steps A, B, C, D, and E as need indicates.	❑	❑
2. Fills out report slip with patient information.	❑	❑
3. Obtains a urine specimen.	❑	❑
4. Washes hands and dons gloves.	❑	❑
5. Wets a dipstick correctly.	❑	❑
6. Times and reads the series of tests accurately.	❑	❑
7. Notes the test results on the report slip.	❑	❑
8. Disposes of urine and used equipment appropriately.	❑	❑
9. Removes gloves and washes hands.	❑	❑
10. Delivers the report slip to the person who ordered the test.	❑	❑

Successfully completed   ❑

Needs practice and retesting   ❑

Comments:

Instructor: _____

Skill 24-4 Obtaining Culture Specimens: Throat and Wound

Student:_____

Date: _____

	S	U
1. Carries out Standard Steps A, B, C, D, and E as need indicates.	❑	❑
2. Labels culture tube with patient's name and date.	❑	❑
3. Fills out requisition slip.	❑	❑

Throat

	S	U
4. Readies light to visualize throat.	❑	❑
5. Washes hands and dons gloves.	❑	❑
6. Withdraws sterile swab from culture tube.	❑	❑
7. Asks patient to tip head back and open the mouth; instructs to sing a low note "ah."	❑	❑
8. Depresses tongue with tongue blade and without contaminating the swab, inserts it and rotates it around the tonsil area and the back wall, touching areas of exudate of inflammation.	❑	❑
9. Withdraws swab without contaminating the specimen.	❑	❑
10. Places swab into culture tube without contaminating it.	❑	❑

Wound Culture

	S	U
11. With clean hands, dons gloves.	❑	❑
12. Removes wound dressing and disposes of it properly.	❑	❑
13. Cleanses area around wound.	❑	❑
14. Removes gloves, washes hands, and prepares dressing supplies.	❑	❑
15. Dons gloves and removes swab from culture tube.	❑	❑
16. Obtains specimen(s) from wound correctly from base of active drainage area.	❑	❑
17. Places swab into culture tube without contaminating it.	❑	❑
18. Crushes transport medium vial area and pushes swab into contact with the medium.	❑	❑
19. Closes container and places it in a sealed plastic bag if required.	❑	❑
20. Removes gloves, washes hands, and continues with application of sterile dressing.	❑	❑

21. Removes gloves and washes hands.	❏	❏
22. Transports or sends specimen to lab within 30 minutes. (Refrigerates if transport is delayed.)	❏	❏
23. Documents procedure.	❏	❏
24. Carries out Standard Steps X, Y, and Z.	❏	❏
25. If anerobic culture is needed, obtains specimen from deep within the wound where oxygen is not present and prevents oxygen from affecting specimen.	❏	❏

Successfully completed ❏

Needs practice and retesting ❏

Comments:

Instructor: _____

Skill 24-5 Obtaining a Stool Specimen for Occult Blood Testing, and Ova and Parasites

Student:_____

Date: _____

	S	U
1. Carries out Standard Steps A, B, C, D, and E as need indicates.	❑	❑
2. Labels specimen container with patient's name and date.	❑	❑
3. Fills out requisition slip.	❑	❑
4. Washes hands and dons gloves.	❑	❑
5. Takes stool specimen to bathroom or dirty utility room.	❑	❑
Specimen for Stool Culture		
6. Opens jar containing culture medium, keeping lid interior sterile.	❑	❑
7. With sterile swab, obtain stool the size of a bean and place it into the culture medium; replace lid on container.	❑	❑
Specimen for Ova and Parasites		
8. With tongue blades, transfers a portion from middle of stool to the specimen container.	❑	❑
9. Readies specimen for the lab and sends it immediately.	❑	❑
Test for Occult Blood		
10. Opens front window(s) of specimen card.	❑	❑
11. Transfers small amount of stool with wooden stick to area within window. Obtains stool from middle, interior portion of specimen.	❑	❑
12. Opens occult blood specimen card back window.	❑	❑
13. Places two drops of reagent on the stool smear and one drop on the control area for each window.	❑	❑
14. Waits 30 seconds and reads results.	❑	❑
15. Disposes of test card in biohazard container.	❑	❑
16. Removes gloves and washes hands.	❑	❑
17. Documents procedure and disposition of specimen.	❑	❑
18. Carries out Standard Steps X, Y, and Z.	❑	❑

Successfully completed   ❏

Needs practice and retesting ❏

Comments:

Instructor: _____

Skill 24-6 Assisting with a Pelvic Examination and Pap Test (Smear)

Student:_____

Date: _____

	S	U
1. Carries out Standard Steps A, B, C, D, and E as need indicates.	❑	❑
2. Labels slide or thin prep container with patient's name and date.	❑	❑
3. Fills out requisition slip.	❑	❑
4. Sets up the table and equipment.	❑	❑
5. Readies patient and positions on table with appropriate draping.	❑	❑
6. Passes equipment to examiner.	❑	❑
7. Dons gloves and applies fixative to the slide or places lid on thin prep container.	❑	❑
8. Removes gloves and washes hands.	❑	❑
9. Assists patient after examination to arise from the table.	❑	❑
10. Prepares specimen for laboratory and sends to lab.	❑	❑
11. Restores the examination room and disposes of used equipment and supplies properly.	❑	❑
12. Documents procedure as necessary.	❑	❑

Successfully completed ❑

Needs practice and retesting ❑

Comments:

Instructor: _____

Skill 25-1   Measuring Intake and Output

Student:_____

Date: _____

	S	U
1. Explains procedure and gives instructions to patient about recording I & O.	❑	❑
2. Provides container for collecting urine and places measuring container in bathroom.	❑	❑
3. Records fluid intake throughout the shift.	❑	❑
4. Measures and records output throughout the shift.	❑	❑
5. At end of shift, empties collection containers, measures output and records it.	❑	❑
6. Cleans or replaces collection containers.	❑	❑
7. Calculates IV intake and records it.	❑	❑
8. Calculates total intake and total output for shift.	❑	❑
9. Enters amounts in correct columns on 24-hour I & O record.	❑	❑
10. Determines if I & O are within normal limits.	❑	❑
11. Compares amounts from previous 2 or 3 days to determine if a fluid imbalance is developing.	❑	❑
12. Places new I & O shift recording sheet in room.	❑	❑

Successfully completed   ❑

Needs practice and retesting ❑

Comments:

Instructor: _____

Skill 27-1   Assisting a Patient with Feeding

Student:_____

Date: _____

	S	U
. Carries out Standard Steps A, B, C, D, and E as need indicates.	❏	❏
. Checks diet tray for correct diet.	❏	❏
. Positions the patient and the tray correctly.	❏	❏
. Protects the patient's clothing and the bedding.	❏	❏
. Opens the containers and prepares the food for eating.	❏	❏
. Asks patient about preferences for order of eating foods.	❏	❏
. Feeds slowly and without impatience.	❏	❏
. Offers fluids as patient desires.	❏	❏
. Wipes mouth at intervals.	❏	❏
0. Encourages patient to self-feed a few bites, if able.	❏	❏
1. Removes tray when meal is finished.	❏	❏
2. Offers mouth care and handwashing if needed.	❏	❏
3. Explains how to feed a patient who is blind or how to set up the tray and plate and to instruct the patient who is self-feeding.	❏	❏
4. Documents amount and types of food eaten.	❏	❏
5. Carries out Standard Steps X, Y, and Z.	❏	❏

Successfully completed   ❏

Needs practice and retesting ❏

Comments:

Instructor: _____

Skill 27-2   Inserting a Nasogastric Tube

Student:_____

Date: _____

	S	U
1. Carries out Standard Steps A, B, C, D, and E as indicated.	❑	❑
2. Checks airflow through each nostril.	❑	❑
3. Positions patient with HOB at 30–90 degrees.	❑	❑
4. Provides basin, tissues, and water with straw for patient as appropriate.	❑	❑
5. Puts on gloves.	❑	❑
6. Measures distance to insert tube correctly.	❑	❑
7. Prepares tube for insertion.	❑	❑
8. Inserts tube correctly.	❑	❑
9. Verifies correct placement of tube.	❑	❑
10. Secures tube to patient.	❑	❑
11. Attaches tube to suction at proper setting.	❑	❑
12. Positions tube in most functional position.	❑	❑
13. Removes gloves and washes hands.	❑	❑
14. Makes patient comfortable and restores unit.	❑	❑
15. Assesses tube function.	❑	❑
16. Documents procedure.	❑	❑

Successfully completed   ❑

Needs practice and retesting ❑

Comments:

Instructor: _____

Skill 27-3   Using a Feeding Pump

Student:_____

Date: _____

	S	U
1. Checks the order for type and amount of feeding.	❑	❑
2. Carries out the Standard Steps.	❑	❑
3. Washes hands and puts on gloves.	❑	❑
4. Elevates head of bed to at least 30 degrees. Keeps bed elevated.	❑	❑
5. Sets up feeding pump and tubing.	❑	❑
6. Verifies tube's placement location.	❑	❑
7. Primes tubing and attaches it to NG or PEG tube.	❑	❑
8. Sets flow rate and turns on pump.	❑	❑
9. Observes infusion for several minutes.	❑	❑
10. Removes gloves and washes hands.	❑	❑
11. Assesses patient for signs of complications periodically.	❑	❑
12. Checks stomach residual every 4 hours.	❑	❑
13. Documents tube status, stomach residual, and feeding.	❑	❑

Successfully completed   ❑

Needs practice and retesting ❑

Comments:

Instructor: _____

Skill 27-4   Administering a Nasogastric/ Duodenal Tube Feeding or Feeding Via a PEG Tube

Student:_____

Date: _____

	S	U
1. Carries out the Standard Steps A, B, C, D, and E as indicated.	❑	❑
2. Elevates HOB to 30–90 degrees.	❑	❑
3. Puts on gloves.	❑	❑
4. Prepares feeding.	❑	❑
5. Attaches syringe and verifies tube placement.	❑	❑
6. Checks for residual feeding for gastrostomy tube.	❑	❑
7. Pinches off tube and pours formula into syringe or hooks up gavage bag; regulates flow correctly.	❑	❑
8. Prevents air from entering the tube.	❑	❑
9. For continuous feeding: sets up feeding pump and sets rate correctly.	❑	❑
10. Follows formula with 1–2 ounces water to clear the tube.	❑	❑
11. Removes syringe or connecting tubing and clamps the tube for intermittent feeding.	❑	❑
12. Washes equipment appropriately.	❑	❑
13. Removes gloves and washes hands.	❑	❑
14. Monitors lab values and weight daily.	❑	❑
15. Documents the procedure.	❑	❑
16. Carries out Standard Steps X, Y, and Z.	❑	❑

Successfully completed ❑

Needs practice and retesting ❑

Comments:

Instructor: _____

Skill 28-1   Using a Pulse Oximeter

Student:_____

Date: _____

	S	U
1. Carries out Standard Steps A, B, C, D, and E as indicated.	❑	❑
2. Turns on oximeter and checks calibration.	❑	❑
3. Chooses appropriate site for sensor, cleans site, and applies sensor and secures it.	❑	❑
4. Checks machine function and sets alarms.	❑	❑
5. Read beginning saturation level and record it.	❑	❑
6. Note and record saturation level every hour or according to agency protocol.	❑	❑
7. Immediately report saturation level below 90%.	❑	❑
8. Rotate site of probe per protocol.	❑	❑
9. When discontinuing measurements, take final reading and record it.	❑	❑
10. Remove sensor, and prepare machine for next use.	❑	❑
11. Document discontinuation of pulse oximetry.	❑	❑

Successfully completed   ❑

Needs practice and retesting ❑

Comments:

Instructor: _____

Skill 28-2   Administering the Heimlich Maneuver

Student:_____

Date: _____

	S	U
1. Verifies that person is choking.	❑	❑
2. Positions self to deliver appropriate thrusts.	❑	❑
3. Places hands in correct position.	❑	❑
4. Repeats thrust sequence until foreign body is expelled or person becomes unconscious.	❑	❑

For Unconscious Person

	S	U
5. Calls for help.	❑	❑
6. Positions person on ground.	❑	❑
7. Opens airway, checks for breathing, looks for debris in mouth and uses finger sweep if debris is present.	❑	❑
8. Attempts to ventilate.	❑	❑
9. If ventilation unsuccessful, repositions head and attempts to ventilate again.	❑	❑
10. Positions hands correctly for thrusts.	❑	❑
11. Delivers thrusts.	❑	❑
12. Checks mouth for debris and uses finger sweep if debris is visualized.	❑	❑
13. Opens airway and attempts to ventilate.	❑	❑
14. Repeats sequence as needed.	❑	❑

For Conscious Infant

	S	U
15. Positions infant with head lower than trunk straddling arm; supports chest and jaw.	❑	❑
16. Delivers five back blows correctly.	❑	❑
17. Turns infant and delivers chest thrusts.	❑	❑
18. Repeats sequence until object is dislodged.	❑	❑

For Unconscious Infant

	S	U
19. Places infant on hard surface and attempts to visualize object; removes with finger sweep if debris or object is present.	❑	❑
20. Opens airway and attempts to ventilate.	❑	❑

21. If unable to ventilate, repositions head and attempts to ventilate again. ❑ ❑
22. If unable to ventilate, repositions infant for back blow and chest thrust sequence. ❑ ❑
23. Performs tongue-jaw lift after each sequence to attempt visualization of object in mouth; removes object or debris, if present, with finger sweep. ❑ ❑
24. Activates EMS if obstruction not relieved within 1 minute. ❑ ❑

Successfully completed ❑

Needs practice and retesting ❑

Comments:

Instructor: _____

Skill 28-3   Cardiopulmonary Resuscitation

Student:_____

Date: _____

	S	U
1. Shakes victim and shouts; activate EMS if unresponsive.	❑	❑
2. Positions victim supine and opens airway.	❑	❑
3. Looks, listens, and feels for air movement.	❑	❑
4. Forms seal and delivers two slow breaths, allowing for adequate exhalation between breaths.	❑	❑
5. Repositions head and attempts ventilation again if first breath is unsuccessful.	❑	❑
6. Performs Heimlich maneuver if needed.	❑	❑
7. Checks carotid pulse.	❑	❑
8. Positions hands on sternum correctly.	❑	❑
9. Performs chest compressions correctly.	❑	❑
10. Opens airway and delivers two slow breaths at appropriate intervals.	❑	❑
11. Checks carotid pulse after first minute and then every 5 minutes.	❑	❑
12. Continues rescue breathing or CPR sequence as needed until relieved or unable to continue.	❑	❑

Successfully completed   ❑

Needs practice and retesting ❑

Comments:

Instructor: _____

Skill 28-4   Administering Oxygen

Student:_____

Date: _____

	S	U
1. Carries out Standard Steps A, B, C, D, and E as indicated.	❑	❑
2. Connects flowmeter and attaches humidifier and tubing.	❑	❑
3. Positions ordered oxygen therapy device properly on patient.	❑	❑
4. Adjusts oxygen flow to rate ordered.	❑	❑
5. Instructs patient and visitors regarding safety precautions.	❑	❑
6. Documents use of oxygen.	❑	❑

Successfully completed   ❑

Needs practice and retesting ❑

Comments:

Instructor: _____

Skill 28-5   Nasopharyngeal Suctioning

Student:_____

Date: _____

	S	U
1. Carries out Standard Steps A, B, C, D, and E as indicated.	❑	❑
2. Connects tubing to suction source; sets suction pressure correctly.	❑	❑
3. Opens and prepares equipment and supplies.	❑	❑
4. Dons sterile gloves.	❑	❑
5. Attaches catheter to connecting tubing maintaining sterile technique.	❑	❑
6. Moistens catheter and introduces via the nares.	❑	❑
7. Suctions patient for no more than 10 seconds using aseptic technique.	❑	❑
8. Rinses suction catheter.	❑	❑
9. Suctions other naris.	❑	❑
10. Rinses catheter.	❑	❑
11. Asks patient to cough.	❑	❑
12. Suctions oropharynx and mouth.	❑	❑
13. Rinses catheter and suction tubing.	❑	❑
14. Disposes of catheter or cleanses and stores catheter aseptically.	❑	❑
15. Auscultates lungs.	❑	❑
16. Documents procedure.	❑	❑

Successfully completed   ❑

Needs practice and retesting ❑

Comments:

Instructor: _____

Skill 28-6   Endotracheal and Tracheostomy Suctioning

Student:_____

Date: _____

	S	U
1. Carries out Standard Steps A, B, C, D, and E as indicated.	❑	❑
2. Attaches connecting tubing, turns on suction, and checks pressure.	❑	❑
3. Opens supplies and dons sterile gloves.	❑	❑
4. Pours solution.	❑	❑
5. Connects catheter to tubing with sterile technique.	❑	❑
6. Preoxygenates patient.	❑	❑
7. Moistens catheter.	❑	❑
8. Suctions patient via endotracheal or tracheostomy tube using sterile technique.	❑	❑
9. Suctions for no more than 10 seconds.	❑	❑
10. Reattaches patient to oxygen source.	❑	❑
11. Allows rest period between suctioning.	❑	❑
12. Rinses catheter and tubing.	❑	❑
13. Disposes of catheter and gloves properly.	❑	❑
14. Auscultates lungs to verify success of suctioning.	❑	❑

For Sleeved Catheter

	S	U
15. Adapts procedure for suctioning with sleeved catheter, omitting moistening the catheter.	❑	❑
16. Properly rinses catheter after suctioning.	❑	❑
17. Documents procedure.	❑	❑
18. Carries out Standard Steps X, Y, and Z.	❑	❑

Successfully completed   ❑

Needs practice and retesting   ❑

Comments:

Instructor: _____

Skill 28-7 Providing Tracheostomy Care

Student:_____

Date: _____

	S	U
1. Carries out Standard Steps A, B, C, D, and E as indicated.	❑	❑
2. Opens supplies and pours solutions.	❑	❑
3. Using gloves, unlocks the inner cannula and removes it; places it in cleansing solution.	❑	❑
4. Cleans the inner cannula maintaining aseptic technique.	❑	❑
5. Dries the cannula, reinserts it, and locks it in place.	❑	❑
6. Removes old dressing and cleans tracheostomy.	❑	❑
7. Replaces tube ties or holder, if soiled, following safety precautions.	❑	❑
8. Applies new precut or folded dressing.	❑	❑
9. Carries out Standard Steps X, Y, and Z.	❑	❑

Successfully completed ❑

Needs practice and retesting ❑

Comments:

Instructor: _____

Skill 29-1   Placing and Removing a Bedpan

Student:_____

Date: _____

	S	U
1. Carries out Standard Steps A, B, C, D, and E as need indicates.	❑	❑
2. Correctly places bedpan under the patient and positions patient.	❑	❑
3. Provides tissue and call light.	❑	❑
4. Removes the bedpan without spilling the contents.	❑	❑
5. Assists the patient to cleanse the perineal area if needed.	❑	❑
6. Measures and records the urine output.	❑	❑
7. Cleans the equipment.	❑	❑
8. Allows patient to wash the hands.	❑	❑
9. Removes gloves and washes own hands.	❑	❑
10. Carries out Standard Steps X, Y, and Z.	❑	❑

Successfully completed   ❑

Needs practice and retesting ❑

Comments:

Instructor: _____

Skill 29-2 Applying a Condom Catheter

Student:_____

Date: _____

	S	U
1. Carries out Standard Steps A, B, C, D, and E as need indicates.	❑	❑
2. Washes and dries genital area; trims pubic hair as necessary.	❑	❑
3. Applies condom catheter and smoothes out adhesive surface for good adherence.	❑	❑
4. Leaves a 1 1/2 in. space at tip of penis.	❑	❑
5. Connects the condom catheter to a drainage tube.	❑	❑
6. Attaches drainage bag.	❑	❑
7. Checks to see that catheter has not become twisted, preventing urine flow.	❑	❑
8. Carries out Standard Steps X, Y, and Z.	❑	❑

Successfully completed ❑

Needs practice and retesting ❑

Comments:

Instructor: _____

Skill 29-3   Catheterizing the Female Patient

Student:_____

Date: _____

	S	U
1. Carries out Standard Steps A, B, C, D, and E as need indicates.	❑	❑
2. Positions and drapes patient.	❑	❑
3. Opens catheter tray and positions it appropriately while maintaining sterile technique.	❑	❑
4. Dons sterile gloves correctly.	❑	❑
5. Prepares tray for use maintaining sterility.	❑	❑
6. Tests balloon and deflates it.	❑	❑
7. Holds labia open throughout cleaning and catheterization.	❑	❑
8. Lubricates and inserts catheter correctly, maintaining sterility.	❑	❑
9. Inflates balloon.	❑	❑
10. Cleanses perineum and removes equipment.	❑	❑
11. Secures the catheter to thigh.	❑	❑
12. Positions drainage bag and tubing correctly.	❑	❑
13. Carries out Standard Steps X, Y, and Z.	❑	❑

Successfully completed   ❑

Needs practice and retesting ❑

Comments:

Instructor: _____

Skill 29-4 Catheterizing the Male Patient

Student:_____

Date: _____

	S	U
1. Carries out Standard Steps A, B, C, D, and E as need indicates.	❑	❑
2. Positions and drapes patient.	❑	❑
3. Opens catheter tray and positions it appropriately maintaining sterile technique.	❑	❑
4. Dons sterile gloves correctly.	❑	❑
5. Prepares tray for use maintaining sterility.	❑	❑
6. Tests balloon on catheter and deflates it.	❑	❑
7. Cleanses penis correctly using forceps.	❑	❑
8. Lubricates and inserts catheter maintaining sterility.	❑	❑
9. Inflates balloon, positions catheter correctly.	❑	❑
10. Cleans up used supplies and cleans and dries perineal area of patient.	❑	❑
11. Secures catheter to abdomen or thigh.	❑	❑
12. Hangs drainage bag correctly and positions tubing to promote best drainage.	❑	❑
13. Carries out Standard Steps X, Y, and Z.	❑	❑

Successfully completed ❑

Needs practice and retesting ❑

Comments:

Instructor: _____

Skill 29-5   Performing Intermittent Bladder Irrigation and Instillation

Student:_____

Date: _____

	S	U
1. Carries out Standard Steps A, B, C, D, and E as need indicates.	❑	❑
2. Positions and drapes patient.	❑	❑
3. Opens irrigation tray and positions it appropriately while maintaining sterile technique.	❑	❑
4. Pours irrigation solution or prepares solution for instillation.	❑	❑
5. Determines amount of urine in drainage bag.	❑	❑
6. Dons sterile gloves correctly.	❑	❑
7. Clamps connecting tubing or disconnects tubing from catheter maintaining aseptic technique.	❑	❑
8. Draws up solution and instills it into the catheter port.	❑	❑
9. Uses 30–50 cc of solution for each irrigation; instills total amount of fluid ordered.	❑	❑
10. Allows fluid to flow back after appropriate period of time.	❑	❑
11. For irrigation, continues to irrigate 3–4 times.	❑	❑
12. Withdraws syringe and cleanses the port with a fresh antiseptic swab.	❑	❑
13. Cleans up used supplies.	❑	❑
14. Carries out Standard Steps X, Y, and Z.	❑	❑

Successfully completed   ❑

Needs practice and retesting ❑

Comments:

Instructor: _____

Skill 30-1 Administering an Enema

tudent:_____

ate: _____

	S	U
Carries out Standard Steps A, B, C, D, and E as need indicates.	❑	❑
Positions the patient appropriately.	❑	❑
Prepares the enema, clears air from tubing, and lubricates tip.	❑	❑
Positions bedpan or bedside commode; places underpad beneath patient.	❑	❑
Dons gloves and gently inserts the rectal tip correct distance.	❑	❑
Positions fluid no higher than 18" or squeezes plastic bottle to instill the solution.	❑	❑
Regulates flow according to patient's amount of discomfort.	❑	❑
Clamps tubing before withdrawing the tip.	❑	❑
Assists patient onto bedpan, bedside commode, or to toilet.	❑	❑
0. Instills correct amount of solution for total enema.	❑	❑
1. Assists patient to clean anal area if needed.	❑	❑
2. Carries out Standard Steps X, Y, and Z.	❑	❑

Successfully completed ❑

Needs practice and retesting ❑

Comments:

Instructor: _____

Skill 30-2   Changing an Ostomy Appliance

Student: _____

Date: _____

	S	**U**
1. Carries out Standard Steps A, B, C, D, and E as need indicates.	❑	❑
2. Measures stoma and prepares appliance.	❑	❑
3. Dons gloves and empties old pouch.	❑	❑
4. Removes old appliance.	❑	❑
5. Cleanses skin and stoma.	❑	❑
6. Changes gloves and prepares skin for new appliance.	❑	❑
7. Applies pouch smoothly.	❑	❑
8. Firmly attaches appliance and closes pouch; attaches belt and tape if needed.	❑	❑
9. Removes gloves and washes hands.	❑	❑
10. Assists patient to replace gown or clothing.	❑	❑
11. Carries out Standard Steps X, Y, and Z.	❑	❑

Successfully completed ❑

Needs practice and retesting ❑

Comments:

Instructor: _____

Skill 31-1 Operating a Transcutaneous Electrical Nerve Stimulator (TENS) Unit

Student:_____

Date: _____

	S	U
1. Carries out Standard Steps A, B, C, D, and E as need indicates.	❑	❑
2. Correctly applies the electrodes to the skin.	❑	❑
3. Attaches the electrodes to the stimulator unit.	❑	❑
4. Turns on TENS unit.	❑	❑
5. Explains sensations that should be felt.	❑	❑
6. Explains how to increase and decrease the amplitude of the TENS unit.	❑	❑
7. Turns off unit and removes electrodes when treatment has ended.	❑	❑
8. Assists in cleaning the skin and rearranging clothing.	❑	❑
9. Assesses how patient tolerated the procedure.	❑	❑
10. Document the treatment and results.	❑	❑

Successfully completed   ❑

Needs practice and retesting ❑

Comments:

Instructor: _____

Skill 31-2 Setting Up (or Monitoring) a Patient-Controlled Analgesia (PCA) Pump*

Student:_____

Date: _____

	S	U
1. Carries out Standard Steps A, B, C, D, and E as need indicates.	❏	❏
2. Assembles the equipment.	❏	❏
3. Starts an IV if one does not exist.	❏	❏
4. Assembles the PCA ordered medication vial and tubing.	❏	❏
5. Flushes air from system.	❏	❏
6. Connects the primed IV set and PCA tubing.	❏	❏
7. Inserts vial into PCA pump correctly.	❏	❏
8. Plugs the PCA pump into a power source.	❏	❏
9. Sets the PCA pump according to ordered parameters.	❏	❏
10. Opens all slide clamps.	❏	❏
11. Reviews for patient how to use the pump.	❏	❏
12. Assesses the patient frequently for ability to use the pump and for effectiveness and side effects of the medication.	❏	❏
13. Documents use of pump, effectiveness, and any side effects.	❏	❏

*LPNs/LVNs are not licensed to set up PCA pumps in some states.

Successfully completed   ❏

Needs practice and retesting ❏

Comments:

Instructor: _____

Skill 34-1   Administering Oral Medications

Student:_____

Date: _____

	S	U
1. Carries out Standard Steps A, B, C, D, and E as need indicates.	❑	❑
2. Verifies that MAR orders have been compared with physician's orders.	❑	❑
3. Takes medication cart to patient's room.	❑	❑
4. Verifies patient is ready to receive medications.	❑	❑
5. Performs first check of medications to be given, cross-checking the drug name, dosage, route ordered, date and time to be given, and expiration date of the drug.	❑	❑
6. Performs a second check of each medication.	❑	❑
7. Verbalizes signs and symptoms of adverse effects and any special precautions for each medication to be given.	❑	❑
8. Pours liquid medications correctly.	❑	❑
9. Identifies the patient using two identifiers, by checking the ID band, comparing name and hospital number to information imprinted on MAR or card.	❑	❑
10. Checks each medication a third time and tells the patient what the medication is for.	❑	❑
11. Pours water for use of patient in taking the medications.	❑	❑
12. Positions patient properly and assesses vital signs as indicated.	❑	❑
13. Administers medications, observing patient taking them.	❑	❑
14. Documents medication doses taken.	❑	❑
15. Repeats the process for the next patient.	❑	❑
16. Returns the unit-dose cart and supplies to the central area.	❑	❑

Successfully completed   ❑

Needs practice and retesting ❑

Comments:

Instructor: _____

Skill 34-2   Instilling Eye Medications

Student:_____

Date: _____

	S	U
1. Carries out Standard Steps A, B, C, D and E as need indicates. (Checks medication; washes hands thoroughly.)	❑	❑
2. Positions patient properly for procedure.	❑	❑
3. Exposes the conjunctival sac and instills correct number of drops of medication, or amount of ointment, into the sac.	❑	❑
4. Occludes lacrimal duct for 1–2 minutes.	❑	❑
5. Cautions patient not to clamp eye tightly shut.	❑	❑
6. For ointment, has patient roll eye around.	❑	❑
7. Cleanses excess medication off of eyelid.	❑	❑
8. Carries out Standard Steps X, Y, and Z.	❑	❑

Successfully completed   ❑

Needs practice and retesting ❑

Comments:

Instructor: _____

Skill 34-3   Administering Topical Skin Medications

Student:_____

Date: _____

	S	U
1. Carries out Standard Steps A, B, C, D, and E as need indicates. (Checks medications three times.)	❑	❑
To Apply Lotion		
2. Prepares work surface and shakes lotion.	❑	❑
3. Moistens gauze or cotton balls using aseptic technique.	❑	❑
4. Applies the liquid to the affected area by patting.	❑	❑
5. Discards gauze or cotton balls correctly, recaps medicine.	❑	❑
For Application of Cream or Ointment		
6. Applies the medication with a gloved finger or a tongue blade correctly.	❑	❑
7. Applies dressing if ordered.	❑	❑
For Antianginal Ointment		
8. Measures correct amount of ointment using paper measuring guide.	❑	❑
9. Applies paper to the patient's skin distributing the ointment beneath the paper gently.	❑	❑
10. Removes all old ointment from previous site.	❑	❑
11. Washes hands after removing gloves.	❑	❑
12. Carries out Standard Steps X, Y, and Z.	❑	❑

Successfully completed ❑

Needs practice and retesting ❑

Comments:

Instructor: _____

Skill 34-4   Administering Medication Through a Feeding Tube

Student:_____

Date: _____

	S	U
1. Carries out Standard Steps A, B, C, D, and E as need indicates.	❑	❑
2. Checks each medication three times and assesses all necessary parameters.	❑	❑
3. Crushes medications that can be safely crushed and administered; mixes each medication with 5–15 mL of warm water.	❑	❑
4. Correctly identifies the patient.	❑	❑
5. Correctly positions the patient.	❑	❑
6. Dons gloves and prepares tube for medication administration.	❑	❑
7. Administers each medication with at least 10 mL of water between them.	❑	❑
8. Irrigates with 15–30 mL of water after last medication.	❑	❑
9. Clamps or plugs tube for 30 minutes before reattaching to suction or restarts feeding at appropriate time.	❑	❑
10. Leaves HOB up for 30–60 minutes.	❑	❑
11. Cleans up equipment, removes gloves, and washes hands.	❑	❑
12. Restores the unit.	❑	❑
13. Documents procedure.	❑	❑

Successfully completed   ❑

Needs practice and retesting   ❑

Comments:

Instructor: _____

Skill 35-1 Administering an Intradermal Injection

Student:_____

Date: _____

	S	U
1. Carries out Standard Steps A, B, C, D, and E as need indicates.	❑	❑
2. Checks the medication twice with the MAR.	❑	❑
3. Draws up the medication correctly.	❑	❑
4. Properly identifies the patient.	❑	❑
5. Rechecks the medication using the five rights.	❑	❑
6. Dons gloves and cleanses the injection area.	❑	❑
7. Gives injection that forms bleb.	❑	❑
8. Carries out Standard Steps X, Y, and Z.	❑	❑

Successfully completed ❑

Needs practice and retesting ❑

Comments:

Instructor: _____

Skill 35-2 Administering a Subcutaneous Injection

Student:_____

Date: _____

	S	U
1. Carries out Standard Steps A, B, C, D, and E as need indicates.	❑	❑
2. Prepares the medication checking it with the MAR twice.	❑	❑
3. Properly identifies the patient using two identifiers.	❑	❑
4. Checks the medication with the MAR adhering to the five rights.	❑	❑
5. Dons gloves and selects appropriate site.	❑	❑
6. Cleanses site and administers injection correctly.	❑	❑
7. Removes needle quickly and massages site if appropriate.	❑	❑
8. Carries out Standard Steps X, Y, and Z.	❑	❑

Successfully completed ❑

Needs practice and retesting ❑

Comments:

Instructor: _____

Skill 35-3   Administering an Intramuscular Injection

Student:_____

Date: _____

	S	U
1. Carries out Standard Steps A, B, C, D, and E as need indicates.	❑	❑
2. Verifies the medication with the MAR twice (right drug, dose, route, time).	❑	❑
3. Draws up the medication correctly.	❑	❑
4. Properly identifies the patient using two identifiers.	❑	❑
5. Rechecks the medication using the five rights.	❑	❑
6. Chooses appropriate location and utilizes correct landmarks for site.	❑	❑
7. Dons gloves, cleanses area, and gives injection correctly.	❑	❑
8. Removes needle quickly and massages area.	❑	❑
9. Carries out Standard Steps X, Y, and Z.	❑	❑

Successfully completed   ❑

Needs practice and retesting ❑

Comments:

Instructor: _____

Skill 36-1 Starting the Primary Intravenous Solution

Student:_____

Date: _____

	S	U
1. Carries out Standard Steps A, B, C, D, and E as need indicates.	❑	❑
2. Checks the IV solution with the order.	❑	❑
3. Checks solution for sterility and expiration date.	❑	❑
4. Attaches correct IV administration set efficiently without contaminating it.	❑	❑
5. Clears tubing of air without wasting solution.	❑	❑
6. Places time tape label on container and marks it correctly.	❑	❑
7. Reverifies IV solution and additives, if any, with MAR.	❑	❑
8. Verifies patient identity correctly using two identifiers.	❑	❑
9. Chooses appropriate IV site for infusion.	❑	❑
10. Prepares the IV site properly.	❑	❑
11. Dons gloves and inserts IV cannula or needle.	❑	❑
12. Removes tourniquet and attaches IV tubing; begins infusion.	❑	❑
13. Observes for any problems with infusion.	❑	❑
14. Applies a sterile dressing to IV site; secures tubing to the patient.	❑	❑
15. Regulates IV flow as ordered.	❑	❑
16. Carries out Standard Steps X, Y, and Z.	❑	❑

Successfully completed   ❑

Needs practice and retesting ❑

Comments:

Instructor: _____

Skill 36-2   Adding a New Solution to the Intravenous Infusion

Student:_____

Date: _____

	S	U
1. Carries out Standard Steps A, B, C, D, and E as need indicates.	❑	❑
2. Checks the solution for sterility and expiration date.	❑	❑
3. Compares label with order.	❑	❑
4. Places a time tape on the solution.	❑	❑
5. Properly identifies patient before adding solution using two identifiers.	❑	❑
6. Checks solution and additives with order for third time.	❑	❑
7. Removes IV tubing from completed bag and spikes new bag of IV solution.	❑	❑
8. Removes air bubbles that occurred in tubing.	❑	❑
9. Readjusts flow rate to prescribed rate.	❑	❑
10. Disposes of empty container.	❑	❑
11. Adds infused solution amount on intake and output record.	❑	❑
12. Records the added fluid on the parenteral infusion record.	❑	❑
13. Carries out Standard Steps X, Y, and Z.	❑	❑

Successfully completed ❑

Needs practice and retesting ❑

Comments:

Instructor: _____

Skill 36-3　Administering Intravenous Piggyback Medication

Student:_____

Date: _____

	S	U
1. Carries out Standard Steps A, B, C, D, and E as need indicates.	❑	❑
2. Checks medication with MAR and assesses for allergies.	❑	❑
3. Calculates flow rate if not indicated on label.	❑	❑
4. Hooks up the IVPB administration set to the small bag or bottle.	❑	❑
5. Clears the tubing of air.	❑	❑
6. Reverifies the drug and dosage with MAR; follows five rights.	❑	❑
7. Properly identifies patient using two identifiers and reverifies allergies.	❑	❑
8. Connects IVPB properly using aseptic technique.	❑	❑
9. Adjust the flow rate to correct flow.	❑	❑
10. Monitors the patient for adverse reaction.	❑	❑
11. Documents the IVPB on the MAR.	❑	❑
12. Disposes of equipment when IVPB infusion is complete.	❑	❑
13. Notes amount infused on I & O record.	❑	
14. Carries out Standard Steps X, Y, and Z.	❑	❑

Successfully completed　　❑

Needs practice and retesting　❑

Comments:

Instructor: _____

Skill 36-4 Administering Medication Via a PRN Lock

Student:_____

Date: _____

	S	U
1. Carries out Standard Steps A, B, C, D, and E as need indicates.	❑	❑
2. Prepares the IV medication correctly, checking the medication with the order; checks medication with MAR twice (drug, dose, time, route).	❑	❑
3. Properly identifies patient using two identifiers and reverifies allergies.	❑	❑
4. Selects an appropriate site for insertion.	❑	❑
5. Dons gloves and inserts IV cannula with cap or PRN lock.	❑	❑
6. Flushes with 2 mL of normal saline.	❑	❑
7. Secures the lock with a transparent dressing or other sterile dressing.	❑	❑
8. Verifies drug with MAR again adhering to five rights.	❑	❑
9. Cleanses the injection cap of the lock before inserting a needle.	❑	❑
10. Properly injects the medication into the PRN lock.	❑	❑
11. Flushes the lock with 2 mL of normal saline.	❑	❑
12. Documents medication administration and insertion of PRN lock.	❑	❑
13. Carries out Standard Steps X, Y, and Z.	❑	❑

Successfully completed ❑

Needs practice and retesting ❑

Comments:

Instructor: _____

Skill 36-5   Administration of Medication with a Volume-Controlled Set

Student:_____

Date: _____

	S	U
1. Carries out Standard Steps A, B, C, D, and E as need indicates.	❑	❑
2. Checks the medication with the MAR order twice (drug, dose, route, time).	❑	❑
3. Prepares the medication and draws it up in a syringe.	❑	❑
4. Properly identifies the patient using two identifiers; reverifies the medication with the MAR using the five rights.	❑	❑
5. Checks patient allergies.	❑	❑
6. Cleanses the injection cap on the burette and adds the medication to the correct amount of IV solution.	❑	❑
7. Labels the burette and mixes the medication and solution.	❑	❑
8. Opens lower clamp and adjusts the rate of flow.	❑	❑
9. As soon as burette empties, reopens top clamp to continue the IV infusion.	❑	❑
10. Documents medication administration.	❑	❑
11. Carries out Standard Steps X, Y, and Z.	❑	❑

Successfully completed   ❑

Needs practice and retesting ❑

Comments:

Instructor: _____

Skill 36-6   Administration of Blood Products

Student:_____

Date: _____

	S	U
Carries out Standard Steps A, B, C, D, and E as need indicates.	❑	❑
Verifies size of IV catheter in place.	❑	❑
Obtains blood using proper procedure.	❑	❑
Double-checks the blood with another nurse.	❑	❑
Attaches the "Y" administration set and sets up normal saline solution.	❑	❑
Spikes the blood component bag correctly.	❑	❑
Properly identifies the patient and checks the blood identification bracelet with the transfusion record numbers. Uses two identifiers.	❑	❑
Dons gloves and connects the blood component to the administration set.	❑	❑
Obtains baseline vital signs.	❑	❑
0. Primes administration set with normal saline.	❑	❑
1. Begins the blood administration, remains with patient for first 5 minutes, and checks the patient every 15 minutes for first half hour.	❑	❑
2. Monitors vital signs every 30 minutes.	❑	❑
3. Flushes line with normal saline at end of infusion.	❑	❑
4. Carries out Standard Steps X, Y, and Z.	❑	❑

Successfully completed   ❑

Needs practice and retesting ❑

Comments:

Instructor: _____

Skill 37-1   Performing a Surgical Prep

Student:_____

Date: _____

	S	U
1. Carries out Standard Steps A, B, C, D, and E as indicated.	❑	❑
2. Trims hair close to the skin before clipping or using depilatory or antibacterial soap.	❑	❑
3. Clips hair close to skin.	❑	❑

OR

	S	U
4. Dons gloves.	❑	❑
5. Works up a soapy lather.	❑	❑
6. Holds skin taut while shaving.	❑	❑
7. Washes off all loose hair.	❑	❑
8. Strokes with razor in same direction as hair growth.	❑	❑
9. Scrubs from center outward.	❑	❑
10. Rinses and dries area.	❑	❑
11. Removes and discards gloves.	❑	❑
12. Carries out Standard Steps X, Y, and Z.	❑	❑

Successfully completed   ❑

Needs practice and retesting ❑

Comments:

Instructor: _____

Skill 37-2 Applying Antiembolism Stockings

Student:_____

Date: _____

	S	U
1. Carries out Standard Steps A, B, C, D, and E as indicated.	❏	❏
2. Measures leg correctly for type of stocking ordered.	❏	❏
3. Prepares legs for application of stockings.	❏	❏
4. Applies each stocking correctly.	❏	❏
5. Smoothes out any wrinkles.	❏	❏
6. Carries out Standard Steps X, Y, and Z.	❏	❏

Successfully completed ❏

Needs practice and retesting ❏

Comments:

Instructor: _____

Skill 38-1   Sterile Dressing Change

Student:_____

Date: _____

	S	U
. Carries out Standard Steps A, B, C, D, and E as indicated.	❑	❑
. Loosens tape or binder, puts on gloves, and removes old dressing.	❑	❑
. Inspects dressing and places it in discard bag.	❑	❑
. Removes and discards gloves; washes hands.	❑	❑
. Prepares dressing supplies, maintaining asepsis.	❑	❑
. Dons sterile gloves.	❑	❑
. Cleans around the wound with sterile technique.	❑	❑
. Applies medication if ordered.	❑	❑
. Applies sterile dressing with sterile technique.	❑	❑
0. Removes gloves and secures dressing; washes hands.	❑	❑
1. Carries out Standard Steps X, Y, and Z.	❑	❑

Successfully completed   ❑

Needs practice and retesting ❑

Comments:

Instructor: _____

Skill 38-2   Wound Irrigation

Student:_____

Date: _____

	S	U
1. Carries out Standard Steps A, B, C, D, and E as indicated.	❑	❑
2. Exposes wound using aseptic technique.	❑	❑
3. Prepares irrigation set and places underpad appropriately; places basin to catch irrigation fluid.	❑	❑
4. Dons sterile gloves.	❑	❑
5. Irrigates wound with sterile technique.	❑	❑
6. Dries skin around wound before applying dressing.	❑	❑
7. Applies sterile dressing.	❑	❑
8. Removes and discards gloves; washes hands.	❑	❑
9. Carries out Standard Steps X, Y, and Z.	❑	❑

Successfully completed   ❑

Needs practice and retesting ❑

Comments:

Instructor: _____

Skill 38-3 Applying a Wet-to-Damp or Wet-to-Dry Dressing

Student:_____

Date: _____

	S	U
1. Carries out Standard Steps A, B, C, D, and E as indicated.	❑	❑
2. Sets up equipment in logical order.	❑	❑
3. Using standard precautions, removes old dressing, inspects it, and discards appropriately.	❑	❑
4. Removes gloves; pours wetting solution into sterile basin.	❑	❑
5. Dons sterile gloves.	❑	❑
6. Wets dressings and wrings them out.	❑	❑
7. Fluffs gauze to be packed in wound.	❑	❑
8. Packs wound and covers with second moist dressing.	❑	❑
9. Places dry dressing over moist dressings.	❑	❑
10. Removes gloves and discards them; washes hands.	❑	❑
11. Secures dressings with tape or binder.	❑	❑
12. Carries out Standard Steps X, Y, and Z.	❑	❑

Successfully completed ❑

Needs practice and retesting ❑

Comments:

Instructor: _____

Skill 39-1   Cast Care

Student:_____

Date: _____

	S	U
1. Carries out Standard Steps A, B, C, D, and E as need indicates.	❑	❑
2. Examines cast for any dents.	❑	❑
3. Examines cast for areas where blood has seeped through, outlines them and notes date and time. Reports excessive increase in seepage.	❑	❑
4. Checks cast for sharp edges and tightness.	❑	❑
5. Pads or covers any rough edges.	❑	❑
6. Notifies MD or cast technician of any areas which are too tight or any skin damage from rough or tight areas.	❑	❑
7. Elevates extremity with cast so hand or foot is at the level of the heart.	❑	❑
8. Places the bed in slight Trendelenburg position during the first day or two for body casts, unless contraindicated by the patient's condition or physician orders.	❑	❑
9. Turns the patient at intervals so that all surfaces of the cast are exposed to air to facilitate even drying.	❑	❑
10. Instructs the patient in the dangers of using objects to scratch under the cast.	❑	❑
11. Smells the open edges of the cast to assess for odor which may indicate infection under the cast.	❑	❑
12. Carries out Standard Steps X, Y, and Z.	❑	❑

Successfully completed   ❑

Needs practice and retesting ❑

Comments:

Instructor: _____

Skill 39-2 Care of the Patient in Traction

Student:_____

Date: _____

	S	U
1. Carries out Standard Steps A, B, C, D, and E as need indicates.	❑	❑
2. Checks order for desired amount of weight for traction.	❑	❑
3. Assesses traction apparatus for correct function.	❑	❑
4. Assesses skin, distal circulation, and sensation.	❑	❑
5. Realigns patient in bed as needed.	❑	❑
6. Performs pin or tong care as ordered or according to agency protocol.	❑	❑
7. Carries out Standard Steps X, Y, and Z.	❑	❑

Successfully completed ❑

Needs practice and retesting ❑

Comments:

Instructor: _____

Skill 39-3   Transferring with a Mechanical Lift

Student:_____

Date: _____

	S	U
1. Carries out Standard Steps A, B, C, D, and E as need indicates.	❑	❑
2. Obtains another person to assist.	❑	❑
3. Positions chair, wheelchair, or stretcher as necessary and clears away any obstructions.	❑	❑
4. Elevates bed and locks wheels.	❑	❑
5. Correctly places the lift sling under the patient with the assistance of the other nurse.	❑	❑
6. Widens the stance of the lift base and locks into place.	❑	❑
7. Positions the lift correctly over the bed.	❑	❑
8. Lowers the sling hooks in a controlled manner and attaches to the sling.	❑	❑
9. Assures that all tubes are positioned so they will not be pulled or dislodged during transfer.	❑	❑
10. Asks or assists the patient to fold arms over chest.	❑	❑
11. Safely elevates the patient and moves to destination with assistance of other person.	❑	❑
12. Safely lowers patient into place.	❑	❑
13. Provides verbal reassurance to the patient throughout the procedure.	❑	❑
14. Positions patient in good alignment.	❑	❑
15. Covers patient, places security vest if needed, and places call light within reach.	❑	❑
16. Monitors the patient at least every 15 minutes for sitting tolerance.	❑	❑
17. Maintains visual contact with any patient unable to effectively use call light.	❑	❑
18. Returns patient to bed using lift as before, following all safety precautions.	❑	❑
19. Carries out Standard Steps X, Y, and Z.	❑	❑

Successfully completed ❑

Needs practice and retesting ❑

Comments:

Instructor: _____

Collaborative Success Plan for Retesting

Student: _____

Date: _____

Skill: _____

Problem areas: _____

_____

_____

_____

Plan for correction: _____

_____

_____

_____

_____

_____

Date of satisfactory performance: _____

Instructor: _____